Living Pharmaceutical Lives

Increasingly, pharmaceuticals are available as the solution to a wide range of human health problems and health risks, minor and major. This book portrays how pharmaceutical use is, at once, a solution to, and a difficulty for, everyday life.

Exploring lived experiences of people at different stages of the life course and from different countries around the world, this collection highlights the benefits as well as the challenges of using medicines on an everyday basis. It raises questions about the expectations associated with the use of medications, the uncertainty about a condition or about the duration of a medicine regimen for it, the need to negotiate the stigma associated with a condition or a type of medicine, the need to access and pay for medicines and the need to schedule medicine use appropriately and the need to manage medicines' effects and side effects. The chapters include original empirical research, literature review and theoretical analysis, and convey the sociological and phenomenological complexity of 'living pharmaceutical lives'.

This book is of interest to all those studying and researching social pharmacy and the sociology of health and illness.

Peri J. Ballantyne is Professor, Department of Sociology, Trent University, Peterborough, Ontario, and adjunct Assistant Professor, Leslie Dan Faculty of Pharmacy, University of Toronto, Toronto, Ontario, Canada. A health sociologist, Peri has focused her research on employment and work as social determinants of health, and on pharmaceutical use across the life course. In her research, Peri seeks to make explicit the ways in which pharmaceuticals are subject to social, political and economic forces that influence who accesses them and to what outcome.

Kath Ryan is Professor Emerita of the School of Pharmacy, University of Reading. She is an academic pharmacist and experienced qualitative researcher who has devoted her career, along with international colleagues, to the development of Social Pharmacy as a discipline for improved understanding of the use of medicines.

Routledge Studies in the Sociology of Health and Illness

For more information about this series, please visit: https://www.routledge.com/
Routledge-Studies-in-the-Sociology-of-Health-and-Illness/book-series/RSSHI

Living Pharmaceutical Lives

Edited by
Peri J. Ballantyne and Kath Ryan

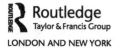

Routledge
Taylor & Francis Group

LONDON AND NEW YORK

First published 2021
by Routledge
2 Park Square, Milton Park, Abingdon, Oxon OX14 4RN

and by Routledge
605 Third Avenue, New York, NY 10158

Routledge is an imprint of the Taylor & Francis Group, an informa business

British Library Cataloguing-in-Publication Data
A catalogue record for this book is available from the British Library

Library of Congress Cataloging-in-Publication Data
Names: Ballantyne, Peri J., editor. | Ryan, Kath, editor.
Title: Living pharmaceutical lives / edited by Peri J. Ballantyne and Kath Ryan.
Description: Milton Park, Abingdon, Oxon ; New York, NJ : Routledge, 2021. | Series: Routledge studies in the sociology of health and illness | Includes bibliographical references and index.
| Identifiers: LCCN 2020052305 (print) | LCCN 2020052306 (ebook) | ISBN 9780367359553 (hardback) | ISBN 9780367772482 (paperback) | ISBN 9780429342868 (ebook)
Subjects: LCSH: Drugs–Research. | Drug development.
Classification: LCC RM301.25 .L5827 2021 (print) | LCC RM301.25 (ebook) | DDC 615.1/9–dc23
LC record available at https://lccn.loc.gov/2020052305
LC ebook record available at https://lccn.loc.gov/2020052306

ISBN: 978-0-367-35955-3 (hbk)
ISBN: 978-0-367-77248-2 (pbk)
ISBN: 978-0-429-34286-8 (ebk)

Typeset in Goudy
by SPi Global, India

Peri: I dedicate this collection to the many students of my Sociology of Pharmaceuticals and Sociology of Health Care courses who have provoked my continuing interest in the broad determinants and implications of 'pharmaceutical lives'. I am always encouraged to see students' initial grasp of the topic and its relevance in their own worlds, where pharmaceuticals are typically taken-for-granted – until issues and concerns such as are illustrated in this collection are encountered. I hope this collection will inspire social science and health studies scholars to teach social pharmacy and provoke continued critical studies of pharmaceuticals that will impact optimal outcomes for pharmaceutical users.

Kath: I dedicate this collection to my Pharmacy Practice and Sociology colleagues who teach the social determinants of health and illness and use narrative methods to create understandings of people's lived experiences of medicines. I hope it will further the development of Social Pharmacy as a discipline and enable teachers to inspire students and emerging health professionals to listen to people's stories when helping them to optimise their use of medicines. I also hope it might begin/add to a call for the invention and production of more essential and user-friendly medicines and regimens with users, their varied needs, lifestyles and autonomy in mind.

Contents

Figure

Tables

Contributors

Anna Birna Almarsdóttir is Professor of Social and Clinical Pharmacy at the University of Copenhagen, Denmark and Head of the WHO Collaborating Centre for research and training in the patient perspective on medicines use. Her research interests include the patient perspective on medicines use and pharmaceutical policy analysis.

Peri J. Ballantyne is Professor, Department of Sociology, Trent University, Peterborough, Ontario, and adjunct Assistant Professor, Leslie Dan Faculty of Pharmacy, University of Toronto, Toronto, Ontario, Canada. A health sociologist, Peri has focused her research on employment and work as social determinants of health, and on pharmaceutical use across the life course. In her research, Peri seeks to make explicit the ways in which pharmaceuticals are subject to social, political and economic forces that influence who accesses them and to what outcome.

Abisola Balogun-Katung is a qualitiative researcher and Research Associate with the Health Professions Education Unit, Hull York Medical School, University of York, United Kingdom. She has worked on various projects in health, social and medical education research. Her research interests include but are not limited to mental health, public health promotion/prevention, HIV, health behaviour, marginalised populations and qualitative research approaches.

Paul Bissell is Professor of Public Health and Dean of the School of Human and Health Sciences, University of Huddersfield, United Kingdom, with a background in the social sciences. Most of his academic career has been spent working in an inter-disciplinary capacity in the health sciences. While remaining an active researcher, Paul is equally passionate about learning and teaching and strongly committed to ensuring that students get the best possible experience and outcome from their studies.

Richard J. Cooper is a senior lecturer in public health at the School of Health and Related Research (ScHARR) at the University of Sheffield in the United Kingdom. His research and publications have explored different aspects of medical sociology, healthcare ethics, health service research and the supply and misuse of prescribed and over-the-counter medicines.

Sharon Davis is a Registered Pharmacist and Research Associate at the School of Pharmacy, Faculty of Medicine and Health, and the Woolcock Institute of Medical Research, University of Sydney, Sydney, Australia. Her research interests include the quality use of medicines, particularly in asthma and other respiratory diseases, and the training of healthcare providers in disability and chronic illness.

Jenny Epstein works in Toppenish, Washington, USA, as a pharmacist specializing in ambulatory care. She is also a medical anthropologist whose research focuses disease chronicity and pharmaceutical use. She is especially interested in how spatiotemporal forms shape subjectivity, self-care practices and everyday life.

Daniela Eassey is a practicing pharmacist and research associate at the University of Sydney School of Pharmacy, Sydney, Australia. Her research interests focus on patient experiences on living with and managing chronic conditions, particularly in respiratory diseases.

Flavia Ghouri is a Graduate Teaching Assistant in Pharmacy Practice at the University of Reading, and a practising community pharmacist in the United Kingdom. Her research focuses on qualitative exploration of the prescribing and use of antibiotics to provide behavioural insights into tackling antimicrobial resistance.

Amelia Hollywood is a Lecturer in Health Services Research within the School of Pharmacy at the University of Reading, United Kingdom. She is a Health Psychologist with extensive experience designing and evaluating behaviour change interventions within the National Health Service in the United Kingdom. Her research interests focus on supporting people to change their behaviour to improve health outcomes.

Karen C. Lloyd is a Senior Research Fellow in the Institute for Global Health at University College London, United Kingdom. She is a medical sociologist and qualitative researcher with interests in digital sexual health, personal engagements with digital technologies for HIV self-management, and constructions of identity through HIV bio- and digital technologies.

Michele J. McIntosh is Associate Professor of Nursing at the Trent-Fleming School of Nursing; Chair, Research Ethics Board, Trent University, Peterborough, Ontario, Canada; and Adjunct Professor in the School of Health Sciences, Queen's University, Kingston, Ontario. Current projects include the Breastfeeding Friendly Campus Initiative (@bfcampuses), a critical analysis of Canada's stance on breastfeeding in the context of HIV and the impact of COVID on infant feeding.

Bjarke Oxlund is a professor with special responsibilities and Head of Department of Anthropology at the University of Copenhagen, Denmark. His research and publications have been divided between aspects of youth, gender and HIV/AIDS in Africa and aging, biomedicine and the life course at large in Denmark. He has also worked as an advisor for the United Nations Population Fund (UNFPA), Save the Children Denmark, and The Danish Institute for Human Rights.

Adam Pattison Rathbone is an Advanced Clinical Pharmacist and Lecturer in Social and Clinical Pharmacy at the School of Pharmacy, Faculty of Medical Sciences, Newcastle University, United Kingdom. Dr Rathbone's academic research focuses on aspects of medication use; including individual and patient-specific factors, healthcare professional factors and health system and regulatory factors.

Sofie Rosenlund Lau is a trained pharmacist with a PhD degree in anthropology. She currently holds a postdoctoral position at the Department of Public Health, University of Copenhagen, Denmark. She works ethnographically at the cross section of social pharmacy, medical anthropology and science and technology studies.

Kath Ryan is Professor Emerita of the School of Pharmacy, University of Reading, United Kingdom. She is an academic pharmacist and experienced qualitative researcher who has devoted her career, along with international colleagues, to the development of Social Pharmacy as a discipline for improved understanding of the use of medicines.

Muhammad Saddiq is a senior university teacher in health systems management and leadership at the School of Health and Related Research (ScHARR) at the University of Sheffield in the United Kingdom. His teaching and research interests are in areas of cross-disciplinary health management and leadership capacity development for health organisations.

Lorraine Smith is a Research Psychologist and Professor of Patient Self-Management in the School of Pharmacy, Faculty of Medicine and Health, University of Sydney, Sydney, Australia. Her research interests focus on patient perspectives of self-management of long-term conditions.

Alison Thompson is Associate Professor at the University of Toronto's Leslie Dan Faculty of Pharmacy, Dalla Lana School of Public Health and a member of the University of Toronto Joint Centre for Bioethics, Toronto, Canada. Her interdisciplinary research is located at the intersection of philosophy and critical sociology, within the field of public health ethics.

1 Introduction

Living pharmaceutical lives

Peri J. Ballantyne and Kath Ryan

Introduction

Increasingly, pharmaceuticals are available as the solutions to human health problems, health risks, and to the challenges of everyday life. This is reflected in the growth in expenditures for pharmaceuticals in Organization for Economic Cooperation and Development (OECD) countries, as has been observed over several decades (Sarnak, Squires & Kuzmak, 2017). Country-specific data illustrate this trend. For example, in England, it is estimated that NHS spending on medicines grew from £13bn in 2010–2011 to £17.4bn in 2016–2017, a growth rate of about 5% per year (Ewbank, Omojomolo, Sullivan & McKenna, 2018). In Canada, in 2018, total drug spending was estimated to account for almost 16% of all health expenditures, at about $1,074 CDN per capita (Canadian Institute for Health Information, 2018). The Canadian Institute of Health Information reported that prescribed drug spending grew steadily, at an average rate of 10.6% per year from 1985 and 2005, and 7.6% between 2005 and 2010. Expenditures in 2017 were 5.5% higher than 2016 (Canadian Institute for Health Information, 2017, p. 7). In the United States – having the highest per capita spending on prescription drugs relative to other OECD countries (Sarnak, Squires & Kuzmak, 2017) – an IMS Health report that total spending on medicines in that country was $310bn USD in 2015, up 8.5% from the previous year (IMS Health, 2016), contextualises the current prominence of pharmaceuticals in health care and in people's lives.

Given figures like these, our attention has been turned to a consideration of how pharmaceuticals have modified the nature and expectations of 'health care' – of where it is provided, to whom, and to what effect; and to consider pharmaceutical use in non-health care contexts. While many (but not all) pharmaceuticals are prescribed by a health professional, most are consumed in the community, under the control of the user, and not the prescriber. Relative to other forms of health care, as small, portable technologies, pharmaceuticals occupy an unusual space in the lives of users. That is, once in hand – the user assumes the responsibility to use (or resist), and to observe a pharmaceutical's effects – to *negotiate* pharmaceutical use (Ballantyne, Mirza, Austin, Boon & Fisher, 2011; Dew, Chamberlain, Hodgetts, Norris & Radley, 2014). Pharmaceuticals are social objects then, with expectations of them and of the medicine user, for their use.

Obtaining them, however, is not unproblematic. Pharmaceuticals comprise a for-profit economy – and in many countries, or in subpopulations within them, the distinction between need for medicines and accessibility to them is problematic (Orbinski, 2004, 2018; Quick, Hogerzeil, Velásquez & Rägo 2002). This reflects the contradictory character of medicines as consumer goods – available to those who can purchase them (Law, Cheng, Kolhatkar, Goldsmith, Morgan, Holbrook & Dhalla, 2018; Lopert, Docteur & Morgan, 2018), and as necessary health care (Baker, 2006; Quick et al., 2002). An optimal scenario is one in which a needed medicine is available, and a medicine's use is limited to the need for it. However, many potential medicine users may be unable to access them when their costs are prohibitive, while others may be provided or may seek out and obtain unnecessary medicines because they are accessible and affordable, or because users (or prescribers) are persuaded by pharmaceutical advertisements that they are needed or desired (Every-Palmer, Duggal & Menkes, 2014; Mole, 2019).

In the context of the distinctive and bifurcated place of pharmaceuticals as essential health care and as consumer goods is the increasing demand for them. This is evident in the activist-driven building of mass markets for essential medicines for marginalised populations, for example, such as for persons living with HIV/AIDS (Lyttleton, Beesey, & Sitthikriengkrai, 2007; Nyugen, Ako, Niamba, Sylla & Tiendrébéogo, 2007). This activism was motivated by recognition of this group's shared 'therapeutic citizenship' (Nyugen et al., 2007) and claims for state-sponsored health protection through access to antiretrovirals. Other markets have emerged supporting the diversion of drugs intended for 'legitimate' medical treatments to an underground economy supported by those seeking to enhance their academic performance and future social positioning (Dubljević, Sattler & Racine, 2014; Ram, Hussainy, Henning, Jensen & Russell, 2015; Vrecko, 2013, 2015) or by the illegal opioid trade (Florence et al., 2013). Additional new and 'legitimate' applications of pharmaceuticals for prophylactic or enhancement purposes have been envisioned (Greely et al., 2008; Kamienski, 2012; Rose, 2003) and enacted (De Serres et al., 2017; Sugden, Housden, Aggarwal, Sahakian & Darzi, 2012; Trego & Jordan, 2010). The causes and consequences of people accessing medicines via all of these routes are sociologically important.

For health professionals like physicians, pharmacists and other prescribers – the gatekeepers of 'appropriate' consumption – pharmaceuticals are problematic because of the user's autonomy over their use – or perhaps to be clearer, pharmaceutical users are problematic because their negotiation of medicines may be 'unscientific' and based on influences deriving from the messy realities of peoples' social (and economic) worlds. These 'lay' worlds reflect and determine the public's understandings of both their health and social needs, and their views of the meaning and utility of 'health care'. While the massive research literature on medication non-adherence (see reviews by DiMatteo, 2004; Haynes et al., 2008) reflects the tension of lay-control over medicines from the gatekeeper perspective, a different one has emerged on users' negotiations of medicine use, for example, focusing on the management of the stigma attached both to chronic illness and medicine use (Hansen, Holstein & Hansen, 2009; Price, Cole & Goodwin, 2009; Ridge, Kokanovic, Broom, Kirkpatrick, Anderson & Tanner, 2015; Singh, 2005) or on making sense of the effects of chronic medicine use on identity and sense of self (Cheung & Free, 2005; Fullagar, 2009; Littlejohn, 2013; Malpass, Shaw, Sharp, Walter, Feder, Ridd & Kessler 2009; Pound, Britten, Morgan, Yardley, Pop, Daker-White & Campbell, 2005; Singh, 2011).

Pharmaceuticals have other properties that complicate users' experiences of them, and that have helped to construct a particular lay knowledge of pharmaceuticals as potentially 'remedy and poison' (Martin, 2006). While pharmaceuticals are consumed with the intention to benefit the user's physical or mental health status – they can and do produce both intended and unintended effects. That is, while drugs are marketed on the basis of evidence from clinical trials illustrating their primary benefit for some intended application, they may also produce unintended 'side' effects. Identification of these (intended and unintended) effects is part of the calculus of receiving a license to market a new pharmaceutical product. That is, a manufacturer is required to adhere to rules to document and report (intended and) unintended effects and to duly inform the future user of them (Abraham, 2008; Lexchin, 2013). Yet, a body of research on idiosyncratic drug reactions illustrates that pharmaceutical effects may be non-specific and unanticipated (i.e., see Kaplowitz, 2005; Uetrecht, 2008). Another issue – focused on the so-called 'off-label' uses of licensed pharmaceuticals – reveals and makes problematic the autonomy given health care professionals to experiment with pharmaceuticals for conditions that have not undergone trials for specific clinical applications (Stafford, 2008), and whose impacts have not been systematically evaluated. All of this is part of the context in which the public accesses and negotiates the use of medicines.

It is evident, then, that pharmaceuticals have transformed health care practice and the experiences of both the health professional, who might recommend them, and the person who will negotiate their uses; and that these transformations are driven by and/or effect a variety of interests – lay, professional, regulatory and commercial (Ballantyne, 2016). Moving forward in this collection, our interest is in depicting the lay-perspective and experience of the negotiation of medicines, and in illustrating and theorising the complexities and problematics of being a 'pharmaceutical person'. Ballantyne and colleagues initially depicted the older person as a pharmaceutical person – 'who draws on a lifetime of experience and knowledge – who takes responsibility for adherence (or non-adherence) to medicines and their associated effects on their own bodies' (Ballantyne et al., 2011, p. 69). More recently, Ballantyne et al., (2018) characterised the young and middle aging 'pharmaceutical person' as one who navigates their access to and use of a range of available medicine types having documented risk/benefit profiles. This analysis provides a picture of medication uptake across an important part of the life course, from young adulthood towards middle age, and shows the extent to which medicines are an integral part of young adult lives. These authors reason that, given the medicine use profiles shown, the cohort members who were the subject of their analysis would have both participated in defining their bodily experience as problematic, and seeing their body/mind as amenable to pharmaceutical management, 'the living of medicated lives, the becoming a "pharmaceutical person"' (Ballantyne et al., 2018, p. 42).

Everyday use of pharmaceuticals in social and interactional contexts

In the collection that follows, the contributions illustrate the opportunities and challenges of the everyday negotiation and use of medicines – showing that medicine use is broadly consequential – negotiated by users in their unique personal, social, cultural and political contexts. Authors address the problematics of medicine use – the opportunities, barriers, benefits and challenges they pose, as these relate to the expectations associated with their use; the uncertainty about a condition or about the duration of a medicine regimen for it; the need to negotiate the identity effects of being a medication user, and for some, the stigma associated with a condition or a type of medicine used to treat it; the need to access and pay for medicines; the need to schedule medicine use, and for many types of medicines, create routines for their long-term use; the need to notice and manage medicines' effects and side effects, etc.

While most of the chapters in this collection relate to the theme of living in tenuous circumstances – related to illness or the risk of future illness – we begin with one that illustrates how people sustain their physical and mental capacity for work through the use of pharmaceuticals. In *Drugs at work: implicated in the making of the neoliberal worker*, Peri J. Ballantyne examines the labour market as a particular context for pharmaceutical lives. Against a backdrop of neoliberal ideals of individual responsibility for health, the expansion of medicines on the market, and the growing availability of pharmaceutical 'enhancement' drugs, Ballantyne examines – through a review of the literature – how drugs are being envisioned, or used, to manage common chronic illnesses of working-age populations, to mitigate occupation-specific risks and treat occupational-related stressors, or to extend human limits and enhance productivity. Ballantyne's discussion focuses on the ethical challenges related to inequalities in access to medicines, informed consent, freedom from coercion to medicate and knowledge gaps related to the impacts of long term use of pharmaceuticals described in her review. She concludes that there are broad implications of 'drugs at work' – which pose both opportunities and risks for workers and for workplaces.

Four papers that follow examine users' perspectives of negotiating pharmaceuticals for commonly diagnosed conditions – and show the disruption of the conditions and challenges of using medications confronting persons in these circumstances. In *Medication-use narratives on the margins: managing type 2 diabetes without medical insurance*, Jenny Epstein addresses the medication practices of working-poor residents in Tacoma, Washington, United States, living with type 2 diabetes (T2DM). Epstein documents diabetes self-care histories to understand patterns of change in self-care practices over time. By reference to the notion of 'healthwork' and to the spatiotemporal forms in everyday practices of self-care, Epstein distinguishes three groups of T2DM actors: those individuals who had barely begun to manage diabetes; those who cycled through periods of management; and those who had achieved sustained control of blood sugars. Her results reveal the work necessary to integrate diabetes medications into daily life and the myriad ways people use medications to manage (or not) diabetes. Her narrative data show that for people struggling to make sense of diabetes, emphasis on medication adherence as a simple, rational decision, based on scientifically defined facts, can itself form a barrier to the creation of positive self-care practices by not addressing the complex social contexts surrounding medication use. Epstein concludes that for many of her participants, the promise of medications to restore order in daily life did not hold true. Instead, chronic use of diabetes medications meant a dependency on drugs and a loss of autonomy. For women in particular, she shows how an emphasis on learning medical facts and skills to measure, monitor and schedule diabetes management adversely affects diabetes control by alienating self-care practices from the lived experience. Epstein argues that to understand medication use in real-life, researchers must engage with how medication practices emerge as meaningful over time and within the particular contexts of a person's daily life.

In *Medicines use for severe asthma: people's perspectives*, Danielle Eassey, Lorraine Smith, Kath Ryan and Sharon Davis address the experience of long-term medicine-taking by persons diagnosed with severe asthma – whose lives are punctuated with the daily and nightly management of their condition. As a severe asthma diagnosis indicates that a person's asthma is not readily controlled, even when medicines are taken as directed, living with severe asthma involves an ongoing tension between the external pressures of taking medicines, obtaining and enacting action plans and attending health professional appointments so as to keep the condition under control, and one's internal wrestling with one's illness identity and the emotional labour needed to manage oneself on an on-going basis. In this chapter, the effects of long-term medicines use on illness identity and perceptions of control by 38 participants from diverse backgrounds and locations in Australia are explored to provide an understanding of what it is like to incorporate medicines and their attendant side effects into a life lived with severe asthma.

In *Pregnancy, urinary tract infections and antibiotics: prenatal attachment and competing health priorities*, Flavia Ghouri, Amelia Hollywood and Kath Ryan illustrate the complexities that arise due to conflicting priorities for women when managing infections in pregnancy against the backdrop of antimicrobial resistance as a prevalent health threat affecting society. Drawing on research conducted to explore women's perceptions of urinary tract infections during pregnancy and their beliefs about antimicrobial resistance, the authors found that women's illness perceptions and how they conceptualise antimicrobial resistance play a key role in their behaviour. Participants described a medical model of their illness where they view pregnancy as a deviation from the norm that leads them to rely solely on antibiotic treatment without adopting behavioural management of urinary tract infections, and antimicrobial resistance is relegated to be the responsibility of health professionals. Ultimately, prenatal attachment and prioritising the health of their unborn child shapes women's decision-making. These authors conclude that antibiotic use for urinary tract infection in pregnancy occurs in a setting where the solution is also the problem, but that prenatal attachment becomes the determining factor that shapes women's perceptions around the competing priorities affecting their health.

In '*What the medications do is that lovely four-lettered word – hope*': A phenomenological investigation of older people's lived experiences of medication use following cancer diagnosis, Adam Pattison Rathbone examines older people's experiences of taking medications for cancer. Reporting that older people with cancer have been found to have high rates of treatment discontinuation, Rathbone brackets his own expectation that those diagnosed with cancer 'ought' to be adherent, and seeks to understand what it is like to use medication following cancer diagnosis. Participants reported life-changing experiences of cancer diagnosis, as well as their responses to being supplied with a wide variety of pharmaceuticals they identified as 'cancer medications'. This included chemotherapy and adjuvant therapies as well as medications used to control the side effects of cancer-targeting treatments. While taking cancer medications presented many challenges that are discussed by Rathbone, for most of his study participants, cancer medications were given 'special status' compared to medications for other conditions, and this was attributable to cancer diagnosis being perceived as life-threatening, and cancer medications 'life-giving'. Recognising that his research did not help to account for the discontinuation of cancer medications reported in the literature, Rathbone's participants articulated the profound impact of a cancer diagnosis and their perceptions that cancer medications could be managed so as to give life and hope for the future.

The complex topic of pharmaceuticals-as-prevention of future disease is taken up in three chapters. In *The paradox of vaccine hesitancy and refusal: public health and the moral work of motherhood*, Alison Thompson observes that while routine childhood vaccination has been widely hailed as one of the most effective and important developments in public health, the phenomenon of vaccine hesitancy is growing in middle-class populations of high income countries. Biomedical discourses assume that the skewed risk perceptions of parents, misinformation about vaccines found on the internet, or the general lack of scientific literacy in parents account for this trend. Drawing on Crawford's concept of 'healthism' and Foucault's notions of governmentality and resistance, Thompson challenges these accounts. By reference to findings from a qualitative, narrative study of maternal experiences with childhood immunisation, she suggests that neoliberal public health has created the very maternal subjectivities that inevitably allowed the emergence of this form of resistance: mothers who are hypervigilant risk managers, and whose experiences with vaccination are embedded within their ideals of good public health citizenship.

In *The pharmaceutical imaginary of heart disease: pleasant futures and problematic present*, Sofie Rosenlund Lau, Oxlund Bjarke and Anna Birna Almarsdóttir observe that taking statins can be interpreted as a practice of anticipation, that is, a way to manage uncertain health futures and actively reorient possible future lives towards imagined safe and healthy trajectories. These authors explore what this kind of anticipation entails from the perspective of individual statin users. Framing statin use as *abductive work*, the findings show that taking statins as means of optimisation of the future demands of the individual a certain mode of *biopreparedness* in the present. They conclude that some statin users become trapped between the pharmaceutical imaginary of statins as the right way to keep future disease at bay and unpleasant experiences of side effects or moral failures in the present.

A third contribution focused on pharmaceutical-prevention addresses the intended and unintended outcomes of a state-sponsored human papilloma virus (HPV) vaccination program. In *Gardasil: a shot in the dark for adolescent girls*, Michele McIntosh describes the impacts of a publicly funded, school-based HPV vaccination program, initiated in Ontario, Canada in 2007. In Ontario, concomitant with the vaccine program where aged 12–13 year old girls were provided the Gardasil vaccine free of charge, was a change in girls' ability to access pap smears in the Ontario Health Insurance program. Prior to the change, girls were eligible to have a pap smear after first intercourse and typically annually afterwards. After the change in schedule, first pap-test coverage was only provided to women at 21 years of age and then every 3 years afterwards. Two particular concerns are taken up by McIntosh: a) the lack of informed decision-making about Gardasil, where through interviews, she determines that girls did not understand the risks, benefits or alternatives to the vaccine; and b) the increasing rates of sexually transmitted infections and pelvic inflammatory disease that are documented in Ontario. Her chapter presents an analysis of both the top-down institutional implementation of the HPV vaccination program, and the bottom-up experiences of it as conveyed by girls who represented its target population.

Two chapters approach the topic of stigma and marginalisation from different perspectives. In *Reflections on the use of antiretrovirals among HIV+ men who have sex with men (MSM) in Nigeria*, Abisola Balogun-Katung, Paul Bissell and Muhammad Saddiq argue that while the evidence is clear that optimal adherence to antiretroviral treatment (ART) is associated with virological suppression, reduction of ART resistance and a reduction of HIV transmission, in contemporary Nigeria, the criminalisation and marginalisation of men who have sex with men who are HIV positive means that adherence becomes a secondary concern. Based on narrative qualitative interviews with 21 HIV positive men who have sex with men who were receiving ART, Balogun-Katung and colleagues describe the barriers and facilitators to adherence encountered by study participants. ART use was facilitated by the men's perception that consistent use provided many important health benefits, however, the need to conceal their HIV status while often not having enough personal space in shared habitation to be able to do so, stigma and discrimination in a context of institutionalised homophobia, poverty, unemployment and food insecurity were barriers that impacted optimal use of ART. The authors conclude that in this and similar socio-political environments, men who have sex with men who are HIV positive encounter a hostile environment, making concealment of their status an everyday necessity, and call for greater openness and awareness of this and similar situations and action to reduce the broad, harmful consequences, including those related to suboptimal use of ART.

In *Opioid Analgesics, Stigma, Shame and Identity*, Richard Cooper explores how the lives of individuals affected by the consumption of opioid analgesics for pain relief are typically framed as clinical or public health concerns, to the neglect of additional psychosocial consequences such as stigma, shame and identity effects. The chapter provides an overview of the current issues relating to opioid analgesics, then considers the significance of different forms of stigma, shame and identity work more broadly in a health context, and provides examples of where research has sought to explore the connection between opioid analgesic use and stigma, shame and identity. It is argued that acknowledgement of these significant adverse manifestations of opioid analgesic use is imperative if clinicians and the public are to recognise and respond to minimise them.

While medicine use can reinforce stigma and discrimination associated with a condition, or can be stigmatising and delegitimising itself, one chapter shows that medicines can serve as tools for making illness experiences meaningful, and potentially legitimise illness in the face of medically unexplained symptoms. In *The drama of medicines: narratives in stories of living with postural tachycardia syndrome*, Karen Lloyd, Paul Bissell, Kath Ryan and Peri J. Ballantyne argue that telling stories about living with illness and taking medicines to manage illness is a critical form of embodied meaning making. Their chapter presents an analysis of 'medication narratives', or stories told about medicines, by persons living with postural tachycardia syndrome, a rare dysfunction of the autonomic nervous system. Drawing on Arthur Frank's work on the dramas of illness narratives, stories told about medicines are presented as dramas that illustrate the 'work' that medicines do or have done with and to them. Three kinds of dramas are revealed in stories accessed from online/digital support group 'communities of practice' involving persons living with postural tachycardia syndrome: (1) dramas of medicines in the body, (2) dramas of signification and the self, and (3) dramas of experimentation. The authors argue that conceiving of medication narratives as dramas and illuminating how people living with illness use medicines to make sense of and negotiate their lives, is particularly effective in the context of medical uncertainty for conditions such as postural tachycardia syndrome.

Finally, given that this collection was being organised at the same time that COVID-19 emerged as a global pandemic, in the final chapter, we examine COVID-19 from the perspective of the anticipated pharmaceutical therapies and vaccines that are hoped to quell it. In *(Developing) pharmaceutical solutions to COVID-19: navigating global tensions around the distribution of therapeutics and vaccines*, Peri J. Ballantyne, Kath Ryan and Paul Bissell outline the emergence of coronavirus-19 disease, and problematise the observed social gradient in the distribution of illness and death attributed to it. Describing the development of therapeutic medicines and vaccines for COVID-19, they examine the competing public health and political and commercial interests in the 'race' to approve and access them. The authors draws on the concepts of biological citizenship – the shared biological identity of persons at risk of COVID-19; and therapeutic citizenship – relating to claims to biomedical resources including pharmaceuticals – to suggest that we are at an historic juncture where global political leadership is called on to prioritise the needs of citizens – especially the most vulnerable – over commercial opportunities emanating from the COVID-19 pandemic.

We encourage readers to take in the contributions that follow, that include original empirical research, literature review and theoretical analysis of pharmaceuticals as, at once, the solution to, and a problem for, everyday life. Each of the submissions included in the collection demonstrate the myriad ways in which taking pharmaceuticals is consequential in ways that are both anticipated and unanticipated; emerging from the social, cultural, political and interpersonal contexts in which their uses are negotiated by users. Here then, by reference to select social settings, life stages and interactional contexts, contributions to this collection convey the complexity of 'living pharmaceutical lives'.

References

Abraham, J. (2008). Sociology of pharmaceuticals development and regulation: A realist empirical research programme. *Sociology is that Health and Illness, 30*(6), 869–885.

Baker, B.A. (2006). Placing access to essential medicines on the human rights agenda. Chapter 22 in Cohen, J.C.C., Illingworth, P. and Schuklenk, U. (Eds.), *The Power of Pills. Social, Ethical and Legal Issues in Drug Development, Marketing and Pricing*. London: Pluto Press.

Ballantyne, P.J., Norris, P., Parachuru, V.P., & Thomson, M. (2018). Becoming a 'Pharmaceutical Person': Medicine use trajectories from age 26 to 38 in a representative birth cohort from Dunedin, New Zealand. *SSM: Population Health, 4*, 37–44. doi:10.1016/j.ssmph.2017.11.002.

Ballantyne, P.J. (2016). Understanding users in the field of medications. *Pharmacy, 4*(2), 19. doi: 10.3390/pharmacy4020019.

Ballantyne, P., Mirza, R.M., Austin, Z., Boon, H.S., & Fisher, J.A. (2011). Becoming old as a "pharmaceutical person": Negotiation of health and medicines by Canadian immigrant and non-immigrant older adults. *Canadian Journal of Aging, 30*(2), 169–184.

Canadian Institute for Health Information. (2018). *National Health Expenditure Trends, 1975 to 2018*. Ottawa, ON: CIHI.

Canadian Institute for Health Information. (2017). *Prescribed Drug Spending in Canada, 2017: A Focus on Public Drug Programs*. Ottawa, ON: CIHI.

Cheung, E., & Free, C. (2005). Factors influencing young women's decision-making regarding hormonal contraceptives: A qualitative study. *Contraception, 71*, 426–431.

Dew, K., Chamberlain, K., Hodgetts, D., Norris, P., Radley, A., & Gabe, J. (2014). Home as hybrid centre of medication practice. *Sociology of Health and Illness, 36*, 1, 28–43.

De Serres, G., Skowronski, D.M., Ward, B.J., Gardam, M., Lemieux, C., Yassi, A., … Carrat, F. (2017). Influenza vaccination of healthcare workers: Critical analysis of the evidence for patient benefit underpinning policies of enforcement. *PLoS ONE, 12*(1), e0163586.

DiMatteo, M.R. (2004). Variations in patients' adherence to medical recommendations: A quantitative review of 50 years of research. *Medical Care, 42*(3), 200–209.

Dubljević, V., Sattler, S., & Racine, E. (2014). Cognitive enhancement and academic misconduct: A study exploring their frequency and relationship. *Ethics and Behaviour, 24*(5), 408–420.

Every-Palmer, S., Duggal, R., & Menkes, D.B. (2014). Direct-to-consumer advertising of prescription medication in New Zealand. *The New Zealand Medical Journal, 127*(1401), 102–110.

Ewbank, L., Omojomolo, D., Sullivan, K., & McKenna H. (2018). *The rising cost of medicines to the NHS. What's the Story?*. The King's Fund. Retrieved from https://www.kingsfund.org.uk/sites/default/files/2018-04/Rising-cost-of-medicines.pdf.

Florence, C.S., Zhou, C., Luo, F., & Xu, L. (2013). The economic burden of prescription opioid overdose, abuse and dependence in the United States. *Medical Care*, *54*(10), 901–906. doi:10.1097/MLR.0000000000000625.

Fullagar, S. (2009). Negotiating the neurochemical self: Anti-depressant consumption in women's recovery from depression. *Health: An Interdisciplinary Journal for the Social Study of Health, Illness and Medicine*, *13*(4), 389–406.

Greely, H., Sahakian, J., Harris, J., Kessler, R.C., Gazzaniga, M., Campbell, P., … Farah, M. (2008). Towards responsible use of cognitive enhancing drugs by the healthy. *Nature*, *456*, 702–705.

Hansen, D.L., Holstein, B.E., & Hansen, E.H. (2009). "I'd rather not take it, but…": Young women's perceptions of medicines. *Qualitative Health Research*, *19*(6), 829–839.

Haynes, R.B., Ackloo, E., Sahota, N., McDonald, H.P., & Yao, X. (2008). Interventions for enhancing medication adherence (Review). *The Cochrane Library*, *4*, 1–159.

IMS Health. (2016). IMS health study: U.S. drug spending growth reaches 8.5 percent in 2015. Retrieved from https://www.businesswire.com/news/home/20160414005904/en/IMS-Health-Study-U.S.-Drug-Spending-Growth

Kamienski, L. (2012). Helping the postmodern Ajax: Is managing combat trauma through pharmacology a Faustian bargain? *Armed Forces & Society*, *39*(3), 395–414.

Kaplowitz, N. (2005). Idiosyncratic drug hepatotoxicity. *Nature Reviews Drug Discovery*, *4*, 489–499.

Law, M.R., Cheng, L., Kolhatkar, A., Goldsmith, L.J., Morgan, S.G., Holbrook, A.M., & Dhalla, I.A. (2018). The consequences of patient charges for prescription drugs in Canada: A cross-sectional survey. *CMAJ Open*, *6*(1), E63–E70. doi:10.9778/cmajo.20180008.

Lexchin, J. (2013). Health Canada and the pharmaceutical industry: A preliminary analysis of the historical relationship. *Healthcare Policy*, *9*(2), 22–29.

Littlejohn, K.E. (2013). Gender and the social meanings of hormonal contraceptive side effects. *Gender and Society*, *27*(6), 843–863.

Lopert, R., Docteur, E., & Morgan, S. (2018). Body count [PDF]. The human cost of financial barriers to prescription drugs. *Canadian Federation of Nurses Unions*. Retrieved from https://nursesunions.ca/wp-content/uploads/2018/05/2018.04-Body-Count-Final-web.pdf.

Lyttleton, C., Beesey, A., & Sitthikriengkrai, M. (2007). Expanding community through ARV provision in Thailand. *AIDS Care*, *19*(1), S44–S53.

Malpass, A., Shaw, A., Sharp, D., Walter, F., Feder, G., Ridd, M., & Kessler, D. (2009). "Medication career" or "moral career"? Two sides of managing antidepressants: A meta-ethnography of patients' experience of antidepressants. *Social Science & Medicine*, *68*(1), 154–168.

Martin, E. (2006). The pharmaceutical person. *Biosocieties*, *1*, 273–287.

Mole B. (2019). Prescripton for bank – Big Pharma shells out $20B each year to schmooze docs, $6B on drug ads. Persuading Doctors and Direct-to-Consumer ads Land 1-2 Punch for Knockout sales. *ARS Technica*. Retrieved from https://arstechnica.com/science/2019/01/healthcare-industry-spends-30b-on-marketing-most-of-it-goes-to-doctors/.

Nyugen, V.K., Ako, C.Y., Niamba, P., Sylla, A., & Tiendrébéogo, I. (2007). Adherence as therapeutic citizenship: Impact of the history of access to antiretroviral drugs on adherence to treatment. *AIDS*, *21*(5), S31–S35. doi:10.1097/01.aids.0000298100.48990.58.

Orbinski, J. (2018). AIDS, Médecins Sans Frontières, and access to essential medicines. Chapter 8 in P.I. Hajhal (ed.) *Civil Society in the Information Age*. 1st electronic edition. London, Routledge. doi:10.4324/9781315186924.

Orbinski, J. (2004). Access to medicines and global health: Will Canada lead or flounder? *CMAJ, 170*(2), 224–226.

Pound, P., Britten, N., Morgan, N., Yardley, L., Pope, C., Daker-White, G., & Campbell, R. (2005). Resisting medicines: A synthesis of qualitative studies of medicine taking. *Social Science & Medicine, 61*, 133–155.

Price, J., Cole, V., & Goodwin, G.M. (2009). Emotional side-effects of selective serotonin reuptake inhibitors: A qualitative study. *British Journal of Psychiatry, 195*, 211–217.

Quick, J.D., Hogerzeil, H.V., Velásquez, G., & Rägo, L. (2002). Twenty-five years of essential medicines. *Bulletin of the World Health Organization, 80*(1), 913–914.

Ram S., Hussainy, S., Henning, M., Jensen, M., & Russell, B. (2015). Prevalence of cognitive enhancer use among New Zealand tertiary students. *Drug and Alcohol Review, 35*(3), 345–351. doi:10.1111/dar.12294.

Ridge, D., Kokanovic, R., Broom, A., Kirkpatrick, S., Anderson, C., & Tanner, C. (2015). "My dirty little Habit": Patient constructions of antidepressant use and the `crisis` of legitimacy. *Social Science & Medical, 146*, 53–61.

Rose, N. (2003). The neurochemical self and its anomalies. In R. Ericson (Ed). *Risk and Morality* (pp. 407–437). Toronto: University of Toronto Press.

Sarnak, D.O., Squires, D. & Kuzmak, G. (2017). Paying for prescription drugs around the world: Why Is the U.S. an outlier?. *The Commonwealth Fund*. Retrieved from https://www.commonwealthfund.org/publications/issue-briefs/2017/oct/paying-prescription-drugs-around-world-why-us-outlier.

Singh, I. (2011). A disorder of anger and aggression: Children's perspectives on attention deficit/hyperactivity disorder in the UK. *Social Science & Medicine, 73*, 889–896.

Singh, I. (2005). Will the 'real boy' please behave: Dosing dilemmas for parents of boys with ADHD. *American Journal of Bioethics, 5*(3), 34.

Stafford, R.S. (2008). Regulating off-label drug use: Re-thinking the role of the FDA. *NEJM, 358*, 1427–1429. doi:10.1056/NEJMp0802107.

Sugden, C., Housden, C.R., Aggarwal, R., Sahakian, B.J., & Darzi, A. (2012). Effect of pharmacological enhancement on the cognitive and clinical psychomotor performance of sleep-deprived doctors: A randomized controlled trial. *Annals of Surgery, 255*(2), 222–227.

Trego, L.L., & Jordan, P.J. (2010). Military women's attitudes toward menstruation and menstrual suppression in relation to the deployed environment: Development and testing of the MWATMS-9. *Women's Health Issues, 20*(4), 287–293.

Uetrecht, J. (2008). Idiosyncratic drug reactions: Past, present, and future. *Chemical Research in Toxicology, 21*(1), 84–92.

Vrecko, S. (2015). Everyday drug diversions: A qualitative study of the illicit exchange and non medical use of prescription stimulants on a university campus. *Social Science & Medicine, 131*, 297–304.

Vrecko, S. (2013). Just how cognitive is "Cognitive Enhancement"? On the significance of emotions in university students' experiences with study drugs. *AJOB Neuroscience, 4*(1), 4–12.

2 Drugs at work

Implicated in the making of the neoliberal worker[1]

Peri J. Ballantyne

Introduction

As outlined in the introduction to this collection, pharmaceutical use has become a normal aspect of peoples' lives: a central technology of health care, and increasingly, of non-health-care human enhancement. There has been little systematic analysis of the place of pharmaceuticals in the lives of workers, but as shown in this chapter, it is a phenomenon that has emerged as a sort of transformation by stealth, supporting the labour market need for 'healthy' and functional workers, and workers' need for employment. As I argue below, a medicated workforce can be examined as a feature of the neoliberal turn, reflecting both the ways workers are subjected to disciplinary power of the market, and their subjectification and self-discipline as neoliberal citizens (Davies, 2017; McGuigan, 2014).

The socio-political context of neoliberalism

Emerging in response to perceived market restrictions of post-WWII 'Keynesian' welfare capitalism, neoliberal capitalism is a political–economic ideology that organises the social world and individuals' roles within it in particular ways. Its major feature is a commitment to an unrestricted, free market, and its policies emphasise economic growth and consumerism, de-regulation of markets and a minimal role for government social programs (Davies, 2017; McGuigan, 2014). Neoliberalisation is a social process involving the transformation of the state to meet, maintain and cater to capitalist markets (Jensen & Prieur, 2016, p. 98). This is accomplished through state support in creating and maintaining markets; in supporting the creation of a specific form of subjectivity – the individual as rational agent – and in 'interfering in the lives of human beings in order to make them valuable by the standards of the market' (Jensen & Prieur, 2016, p. 98). Neoliberalisation transforms a welfare state to a competition state, with specific implications for individuals as workers and as citizens.

The neoliberal worker

Bal & Dóci (2018) address three interrelated ways neoliberalism affects workplaces and individual experiences in them. *Instrumentality*, closely aligned with the principle of commodification, refers to how people and resources are valued: 'in neoliberalism, everything becomes instrumental to generate profit, including labour and people in organizations' (Bal & Dóci, 2018, p. 539). In the neoliberal workplace, *individualism* conveys the expectation that each individual act in a self-interested way and assume responsibility for their actions. Finally, aligned with a commitment to privatisation, in neoliberalism, organisations are expected to be *competitive*, and 'organizational practices… support a system of competition among employees for the best careers, jobs and positions' (Bal & Dóci, 2018, p. 539). The fate of the neoliberal worker depends on the ability to compete based on the market value of one's skills, traits and characteristics (Jensen & Prieur, 2016, p. 99).

These features of neoliberalism have shaped the way individual health is defined and they operate to facilitate the making of the 'good' and 'healthy' citizen required for the labour market (Ayo, 2012). This includes the expectation and/or obligation of individuals to pursue health to meet the needs of the capitalist economy for a productive workforce and for a population that consumes its goods. Ayo (2012) draws on the Foucauldian concept of governmentality to describe how individuals are made into particular types of subjects. For Foucault, governmentality described the political power that operates, via the state and other institutions, to bring about 'desirable behaviours' (Ryan, Bissell, & Morgall Traulsen, 2004, p. 46), not through force or coercion but through the willing actions of autonomous individuals who regulate themselves (Ayo, 2012, p. 100). To achieve or maintain health, the neoliberal citizen is expected to seek the support of experts who offer their goods and services through the market (Ayo, 2012). In this way, 'individuals are seen as being both the cause and the solution to potential and actual health problems and are… accountable for their own health….' (Ayo, 2012, p. 104).

Medical neoliberalism

The transformation of a regulated, welfare state economy to a neoliberal political economy and the parallel transformation in citizen subjectivity requires that 'attention is paid to those social institutions and practices avowedly charged with the management of subjective life' (Davies, 2017, p. 193). One such institution is the health care system. Fisher (2007) outlines three features of medical neoliberalism. First is a focus on *privatised health care*, linked to ideals about the free market and consumer choice, and epitomised in the US managed care system whose services and remuneration are set by private insurance providers (Fisher, 2007, p. 5). Second, the *commodification of health care* transforms patients into consumers who are obligated to utilise products and services to ensure health and manage illness, and who bear the responsibility for the choices they make – or fail to make – regarding their health (Fisher, 2007, p. 4). Third, medical neoliberalism also *commodifies the body* – fragmenting it so that body parts and discrete bodily problems are commodified along with the products designed to maintain, cure or enhance them (Fisher, 2007, p. 4).

Neoliberal health care supports and reinforces a particular kind of subject/patient who views illness in reductionist terms and consumes services and goods while pursuing the duty to be well. This is reinforced through pharmaceutical-isation – 'the translation or transformation of human conditions, capabilities and capacities into opportunities for pharmaceutical intervention' (Williams, Martin, & Gabe, 2011, p. 711). Pharmaceuticalisation 'ties together the com-modification of health care with the fragmentation of the body where illness is treated in terms of discrete systems for which there are tailored products' (Fisher, 2007, p. 5), while turning 'public issues into personal problems' that are med-ically defined and pharmaceutically managed (Davies, 2017, p. 204). Pharma-ceutical solutions to worker health and productivity reflect what Dew (2019) describes as 'pharmaceuticalised governance' – 'the routines of pharmaceutical consumption that are embedded in relations of power and domination' (p. 6). Dew draws on Foucault's governmentality, asserting that 'domination can come from many sources, such as the state, corporations, households, workplaces', but that 'we are ourselves always implicated in processes of domination' (2019, p. 7). Pharmaceuticalised governance captures the government of the self by the neo-liberal worker who has internalised the logics of instrumentality, individualism and competition in the neoliberal workplace.

In sum, contemporary health systems assist individuals to 'work for' the neo-liberal economy as producers and consumers. Through commodification of bod-ies, health services and products, the achievement of health is individualised as a private trouble, and the neoliberal worker manages health and health risks through the consumption of health services and products, including pharmaceu-ticals. In the remainder of this paper, I examine pharmaceutical use in the labour market, showing the settings, rationale and consequences of pharmaceutical use by the contemporary neoliberal worker. The review here shows the diverse ways pharmaceuticals have become integral to workers' bodies/minds: to manage the common chronic illnesses of working-aged populations; to treat occupational-related stressors and workloads and to mitigate occupation-specific risks; and to extend human limits and enhance productivity.

Pharmaceuticals for common chronic illnesses and conditions in working-aged populations

Scholars examining chronic illnesses of the working-aged often concern them-selves with the economic burden of different conditions, related to absenteeism and 'presenteeism' (reduced performance) of workers (see, for example, Zhang, McLeod, & Koehoorn, 2016). In the section that follows, we consider the poten-tial implications of pharmaceutical use for three chronic health problems com-monly reported in working-aged populations: pain, mental illness and diabetes.

Pain is a common chronic condition – its management an economy unto itself (Smith & Hillner, 2019). While estimates of the prevalence of chronic pain in adult populations vary widely, the risks of pharmaceutical treatment of pain – especially when used chronically – are well documented. These include gastrointestinal, renal, hepatic, cardiovascular, cardiac and respiratory effects, intoxication, interactions and adverse reactions, dependence and abuse poten-tial, non-fatal self-poisoning, overdose and suicide (see Ballantyne, Norris,

Parachuru, & Thomson, 2018. p. 41). Serious adverse effects may be experienced with the use of analgesics even with recommended doses over short periods of time (Paulose-Ram et al., 2003).

Not unsurprisingly, particular kinds of work appear to produce a heightened risk of pain and chronic pain. In a recent US national survey of opioid prescribing, workers in particular occupations – construction, extraction, farming, service and production, transportation and material moving occupations – were more likely than those in other occupations to obtain opioid prescriptions (Asfaw, Alterman, & Quay, 2020). In another study, Badzi & Ackumey (2017) reported that among 206 construction workers randomly sampled from seven construction sites around an urban municipality in Ghana, more than 95% reported using analgesics – mostly to relieve aches and pain or to induce sleep. Respondents reported being frequent users of analgesics, often using multiple types simultaneously; about a third had no knowledge of possible side effects of continuous use of analgesics (Badzi & Ackumey, 2017). These findings suggest that users may be unaware of the negative consequences of chronic use of pain medications, and that those negative consequences for workers may never be documented or remediated. For example, Cooper's analysis of shame and stigma associated with pain management using opioid-type analgesics (this volume), suggests that users may not seek support for the safe use of such medicines, and that their iatrogenic effects may extend beyond their physiological consequences.

The treatment of mental illness in the working-aged population is also of major concern. For example, the Canadian Mental Health Association reports that by age 40, 50% of Canadians will have or have had a mental illness (CMHA, n.d.); in England, it is estimated that 15% of the workforce had symptoms of a mental health problem in 2016 (Stevenson & Farmer, 2017). Stanfeld, Rasul, Head, & Singleton (2011) documented varied prevalence of common mental disorders across different occupational groups in the United Kingdom, concluding that occupations with higher risk of common mental disorders are those with high levels of job demands, especially emotional demands, and lack of job security.

While mental illnesses include many different conditions that vary in degree of severity, and mental health conditions may remain undiagnosed, profiles of psychotropic drug prescribing suggest the high prevalence of experienced mental distress in working-aged populations. This is illustrated in a recent systematic review of psychoactive drug consumption among truck-drivers (Dini, Bragazzi, Montecucco, Rahmani, & Durando, 2019), where 27.6% of truck drivers reported any psychotropic drug use – an alarming level when compared to the general population (i.e., looking at detailed data, these authors reported 31.3% vs. 0.7% use of amphetamines for truck drivers and general population, respectively). Dini et al. interpreted the data as indicating that truck drivers are using stimulants as performance enhancing drugs to maintain or increase their productivity on the job – of course suggesting fatigue and other emotional and mental consequences of the occupation, and perhaps also, the imperative to be competitive. Other studies also document the relationship between stressful conditions of work and psychotropic drug use (Kowalski-McGraw, Green-McKenzie, Pandalai, & Schulte, 2017; Milner, Scovelle, King, & Madsen, 2019).

The known risks of psychotropic medicines vary by type (i.e., antidepressants, antipsychotics, benzodiazepines, stimulants), but present particular concerns for their use in the workplace. For example, these types of medicines are reported to 'reduce users' sensitivity to their surroundings, especially to subtle environmental cues, such as the behaviour of other people; they diminish users' ability to react creatively, to take initiative, and to think laterally' (Moncrieff, 2017, p. 76). Some psychotropic medicines produce euphoria and are thus subject to overuse, and for some, dependence and addiction is of concern (Moncrieff, 2017). The positive effects of one major class of psychotropics – antidepressants – need to be weighed against the documented negative physical effects such as stomach complaints, insomnia, fatigue, headaches and emotional effects such as detachment and personality changes (see Ballantyne et al., 2018, p. 42). A study of working people with depression found that those taking antidepressants had more time off work than non-users, and the authors here could not report any evidence that antidepressant treatment improved work performance (Dewa, Hoch, Lin, Paterson, & Goering, 2003).

Turning to another prevalent chronic condition, it is estimated that about 9–10% of the adult population across the globe has diabetes (Saeedi et al., 2019); the American Diabetes Association (2018) estimated that in 2017, diabetes cost the nation $237 billion in direct medical cost and $90 billion in lost productivity. Poorly managed diabetes is associated with serious health risks such as stroke and heart attack, kidney failure, lower limb amputation, blindness and depression (Diabetes Canada, 2019). The fact that labour market participation is more tenuous for those newly diagnosed with diabetes (Pedron, Emmert-Fees, Laxy, & Schwettmann, 2019) suggests that its management in the workplace may be difficult.

Several occupational factors associated with the development of diabetes – sedentary work, schedules that limit a person's time to rest, or to participate in physical activities, schedule medications, access healthy food and eat regularly (Canadian Centre for Occupational Health and Safety, n.d.) – suggest the kind of workplace support needed by workers with diabetes. Yet, the topic of diabetes management in the workplace appears to be under-researched (de Wit, Trief, Huber, & Willaing, 2020). Findings of two empirical studies raise concern: in one, workers with diabetes reported poor support from managers, felt obligated to prioritise work requirements, and adapted their disease management to fit the job, that is, keeping blood glucose levels higher than optimal to avoid hypoglycaemia (Ruston, Smith, & Fernando, 2013). Authors in another empirical study similarly documented the priority given work demands over diabetes management and raised concern about the likely consequences: seriously worsening diabetes, a move to insulin for treatment, and the eventual inability to retain employment at all (Bissell, May, & Noyce, 2004). In her empirical study problematising the expectation of adherence to medication regimens for diabetes, Epstein (this volume) illustrates how the experience of diabetes and its medical management is influenced by social-structural forces that may be outside the control of the individual, asserting that 'learning what pharmaceuticals could and could not do was a process that included how factors such as employment, housing and personal relationships affected the effectiveness of medications'.

This brief overview suggests that many workers are living with chronic conditions and that the demands of work may either create such conditions or exacerbate them. In neoliberalism, pain, mental illness, and diabetes are individual problems whose solutions are pharmaceuticalised. Using pharmaceuticals in the workplace complicates the worker's life – to obtain optimal outcomes, pharmaceuticals have to be appropriately managed and manageable at work; they may produce side effects that impact a worker's ability to perform their work; and chronic pharmaceutical use may, therefore, threaten a worker's employability.

Pharmaceuticals to treat occupational-related stressors and workloads, and to mitigate occupation-specific risks

In this section, the ways in which pharmaceuticals have been used to manage occupation-specific stressors, workloads and work schedules, and occupational risks are illustrated by reference to military and health care workers.

Pharmaceuticals have become modern solutions to occupational stressors or high-risk situations faced by military enlistees in several ways. For example, menstrual suppression using combined oral contraceptives has been promoted for enlisted women – who in 2019 made up 14.6% of total military personnel in the United States (US Medicine, 2019). In a study designed to describe and assess enlisted women's views of menstrual suppression, most participants expressed a guarded interest along with concern about the short- and long-term safety profile and side effects of combined oral contraceptives (Trego, 2007). Their risks mimic those of traditional oral contraceptives – stroke or blood clots, with increased risk with age, smoker status or hypertension (National Women's Health Network, 2015). Possible long-term outcomes of menstrual suppression are unknown, and the potential benefit of menstruation to women's health (see Howes, 2010) could render its suppression disadvantageous.

With regard to the global movement of enlisted troops to tropical regions, the use and harms of the anti-malarial drug mefloquine from the mid-1980s and well into the early 2000s by thousands of Canadian, American, British, EU and other military personnel illustrate how pharmaceuticals may be both rational and perilous. While initially downplayed or unknown, over time many acute and long-term or permanent side effects of mefloquine have been identified including physical symptoms such as dizziness, tinnitus, insomnia, seizures and psychiatric outcomes – paranoia, anxiety and depression, suicidal and homicidal thoughts, among others (Nevin, 2017; Ringqvist, Bech, Glenthøj, & Petersen, 2015). Enlistees and their advocates have organised class action lawsuits in response to coercion to use mefloquine, the lack of informed consent for its use, the harm, suffering and lack of support to veterans experiencing long-term consequences of its use (Burton, 2004; Davis, 2020; Haines, 2019).

Other studies have examined the high levels of psychiatric drug-use by enlisted personnel. For example, O'Meara reported that in the US military between 2005 and 2011, prescriptions for psychoactive drugs increased almost 700%; that one in six American service members were taking at least one psychiatric medication in 2010, and that more than 110,000 Army active duty personnel were given antidepressants, narcotics, sedatives, antipsychotics and anti-anxiety drugs in 2011 (O'Meara, 2014). Concerns were raised over a 2013–2014 report on the quality of care delivered by the US military health system that failed to address the serious side effects of psychiatric drugs prescribed to service members diagnosed with post-traumatic stress disorder or depression (Billings, 2017).

Similar concerns have been expressed over another treatment used to manage mental health vulnerability among enlistees (Donovan, 2010; Kamienski, 2012). The drug *propranolol*, used in the military to prevent or treat post-traumatic stress disorder, influences the bodily system responsible for response and memory formation and the emotional response associated with a memory, and 'may both dampen memory formation and dissociate the memory from the emotional response' (Donovan, 2010, p. 64). Medical ethicists present two irreconcilable positions on its use in the military. On the one hand, in disrupting memory formation, propranolol causes a disruption of self/identity, reducing the opportunity for moral or social learning of the consequences of war; it enables sociopathic behaviour, enhancing the risk of physical harm of combat while attempting to lower its psychological harms. On the other hand, considering the poor prospects of veterans diagnosed with post-traumatic stress disorder, an economic and humanitarian argument favours the use of propranolol as a low cost and effective intervention (Kamienski, 2012, p. 403).

In health care occupations, pharmaceutical solutions to work- and workload-related demands associated with fatigue, stress, burnout, and psychological symptoms have also come under the research spotlight. For example, in a study to assess the level of use of illicit and prescription drugs for cognitive or mood enhancement by German surgeons, Franke et al. (2013) documented 9–20% utilisation rates (based on different survey techniques). Respondents indicated their use to be in response to intense workloads and perceived workload and private stress. Franke et al. expressed concerns about the addictive potential of the drugs used, and the riskiness of surgeons overestimating their capabilities while under the medications' influence (p. 8). In another study, Sugden, Housden, Aggarwal, Sahakian, & Darzi (2012) conducted a randomised controlled trial to assess the effects of modafinil – a drug used to treat sleep disorders – on healthy resident doctors, concluding that 'fatigued doctors might benefit from pharmacological enhancement in situations that require efficient information processing, flexible thinking, and decision making under time pressure' (p. 222). It is notable that these researchers viewed sleep deprivation in doctors as an individual problem rather than one caused by the organisation of medical work:

> sleep-deprived and fatigued doctors pose a safety risk to themselves and their patients. Yet, because of the around-the-clock nature of medical practice, doctors frequently care for patients after periods of extended wakefulness or during circadian troughs.
>
> (p. 222)

That the use of pharmaceutical drugs by stressed and fatigued medical professionals may be interpreted to reflect not only rational but also responsible behaviour was taken up by Goold & Maslen (2014). These authors examined arguments regarding whether surgeons and other medical professionals should be morally obliged to take cognitive enhancing drugs, and whether surgeons who make fatigue-related errors during patient care should be legally obliged to use drugs for physical endurance and held accountable for their failure to medicate.

Another example of pharmaceutical management of risk in health care settings is the 'vaccine or mask' policy for health professionals at the front lines of patient care. In Canada, the vaccine or mask policy started in British Columbia hospitals in 2012 was later adopted by health-care facilities in two other provinces. This policy forced nurses and other hospital workers who do not get the influenza vaccine to wear an unfitted surgical mask for the entire flu season (Leslie, 2015). Two legal rulings – in 2015 and 2018 – struck down the policy in Ontario (Canadian Federation of Nurses' Unions, 2018; Leslie, 2015), supported by the lack of evidence that the practice impacts patient outcomes (DeSerres et al., 2017).

The examples above illustrate the ways in which the bodily and mental experiences of workers in two occupational groups are pharmaceuticalised – fitted to working environments that – in the case of military deployment – are frequently and predictably hostile to 'natural' human bodies/minds, or are otherwise organised around institutional efficiencies and economic imperatives. The potential short- and long-term iatrogenic effects of the drugs profiled here, coercion to use them, and failures around informed consent for their use render the pharmaceutical management of medical and military work problematic.

Extending human limits and enhancing productivity

While some of the examples above illustrate pharmaceutical enhancement to prevent or pre-empt anticipated health risks or harms to workers (i.e., think of the sleep-deprived surgeon, or the influenza risk for nurses), in this section, I examine the use of pharmaceuticals by healthy individuals seeking to extend their natural capacities and enhance their productivity in the workplace and elsewhere.

Non-medical cognitive enhancement involves the use of pharmaceuticals such as pain relievers, stimulants, or anti-anxiety medications by healthy people. Few general population studies of non-medical cognitive enhancement have been conducted, but a large number have targeted post-secondary students (i.e., Brandt, Taverna, & Hallock, 2014; Dubljević, Sattler, & Racine, 2014; Micouland-Franchi, MacGregor, & Fond, 2014; Petersen, Nørgaard, & Traulsen 2015; Ram, Hussainy, Henning, Jensen, & Russell, 2016). A smaller body of empirical literature is focused on non-medical cognitive enhancement in occupations like law (Krill, Johnson, & Albert, 2016), medicine (Franke et al., 2013) and academia (Maher, 2008; Wiegel, Sattler, Goritzs, & Diewald, 2016). As with studies involving post-secondary populations, these document varying prevalence rates – that is, ranging from 5% to 20% in the examples here. Common reference is made to Maher's (2008) findings from a survey of academics who subscribed to the journal *Nature* that one in five reported taking drugs like Ritalin (methylphenidate), Provigil (modafinil) and beta blockers – drugs prescribed for cardiac arrhythmia but that also provide an anti-anxiety effect – to stimulate focus, concentration or memory. That among those attorneys who reported using stimulants, 74% indicated using these weekly (Krill et al., 2016, p. 49) indicates the potential scale of non-medical cognitive enhancement in the 'knowledge' economy should its uptake continue to grow.

The use of pharmaceuticals for non-medical cognitive enhancement provokes strong responses from both opponents and proponents. For example, cognitive enhancement in the post-secondary population has been framed as an 'epidemic of abuse' (Brandt, Taverna, & Hallock 2014), a form of cheating (Dubljević et al., 2014), or an illegal practice involving the 'diversion' of drugs prescribed for legitimate medical reasons (Vrecko, 2015). Additional concerns include safety and uncertainty about long-term side effects, the potential for coercion to use them, fairness and ethics – that non-medical cognitive enhancement undermines human agency and effort and exacerbates existing social inequalities (Brühl, d'Angelo, & Sahakian 2019; Cederström, 2016; Mohamed & Sahakian, 2012; Maher, 2008). Proponents observe that many drugs used for performance enhancement have already been approved for the treatment of psychiatric conditions and have proven safety profiles. For example, Greely et al. (2008) noted that stimulants used to treat attention deficit hyperactivity disorder also affect healthy people's attention levels, working memory and response rates; and that modafinil – prescribed for sleep disorders like narcolepsy – is effective for others experiencing fatigue-related problems (p. 702). Arguments in favour of non-medical cognitive enhancement include the potential to 'level the playing field' in educational competition and effect 'substantive improvements in the world' (Greely et al., 2008, p. 704). Brühl et al. (2019) offer the argument that, from a public health or preventive medicine perspective, cognitive enhancers could empower people to perform well, particularly in stressful environments, and therefore protect them from the negative effects of stress (p. 5). Greely et al. (2008), make the case for the *inevitability* of increasing uptake of non-medical cognitive enhancers:

> The new methods of cognitive enhancement are 'disruptive technologies' that could have a profound effect on human life in the twenty-first century. A laissez-faire approach to these methods will leave us at the mercy of powerful market forces that are bound to be unleashed by the promise of increased productivity and competitive advantage.
>
> (p. 704)

Non-medical cognitive enhancement – used to become 'better than well' (Caplan & Elliott, 2004) could be viewed as a rational strategy for workers vying for advantage in the neoliberal labour market. Indeed, Sales, Murphy, Murphy, & Lau (2019) found in their recent qualitative study that users of pharmaceuticals for non-medical cognitive enhancement viewed their use as normal, safe and destigmatised because their use was for increased productivity and not for intoxication. As Bloomfield & Dale (2015) explain, workers benefit when their use of pharmaceuticals for non-medical cognitive enhancement reinforces and benefits existing employment relations and structures:

> The development of human enhancement technologies like pharmaceutical drugs has helped to foster the normalisation of working extremely – enabling longer working hours, greater effort or increased concentration – and yet at the same time promote the conditions of possibility under which workers are able to work on themselves so as to go beyond the norm, becoming extreme workers.
>
> (p. 552)

The discussion above illustrates the contexts and rationales for the use of cognitive enhancing drugs for non-medical purposes but is not a comprehensive review. Indeed, the related matter of performance enhancement in athletics is not taken up in this chapter. The complexity of this issue is captured in the assertion by Greely et al. (2008) that '*in the context of sports, pharmacological performance enhancement is indeed cheating. But of course, it is cheating because it is against the rules*' (p. 703)! Without attempting to tackle the ethical implications of their statement, I offer the discussion above as indicating a blurring of the line between the use of pharmaceuticals for the treatment of illnesses and health risks and the 'treatment' of healthy individuals to have enhanced capacity to meet the demands of the neoliberal workplace. The implications of this trend for workers are far reaching, as I address below.

Discussion

In this paper, I have outlined the principles of neoliberal political economy: individualism, instrumentality and commodification, and competition in the privatised market; and the role of contemporary health care systems and products in supporting individuals to 'work for' the neoliberal economy as producers and consumers. Through the commodification of bodies, health services and products, the task of achieving and maintaining health is individualised as a private trouble that is increasingly tackled through the consumption of pharmaceuticals. I have illustrated the prominent role of pharmaceuticals in contemporary working-aged populations, used to manage common chronic illnesses or conditions, to mitigate or prevent specific occupational-related stressors, workloads and risks, and to extend human limits and capacities. The use of pharmaceuticals for these purposes supports the needs and aims of neoliberalism for productive workers who compete for work in competitive labour markets. But what are the implications of the pharmaceuticalisation of the working body/mind for the individual pharmaceutical user? Four points are addressed.

First, Davies' (2017) assertion that pharmaceutical solutions transform public issues into private troubles can be examined by reference to military and medical examples discussed above. The examples of malaria prophylaxis using mefloquine or 'therapeutic forgetting' using propranolol illustrate how military workers' private troubles related to their 'fitness' for work are prioritised over problematising the high risk social and physical settings of military work. The individual 'solution' to risky environments may even appear to be 'progressive', that is, when enlisted women are enabled to suppress menstruation. Similarly, in medical work, Sugden et al. (2012) normalise both the 'around-the-clock nature of medical practice' and the use of modafinil as a solution to the burden this poses for medical workers. In these and other examples, attention to the public issue of the organisation of work and to the imperative of safe work – in which every worker has a stake – is deflected when the limitations of the worker are instead the focus.

Second, the 'relations of power and domination' that support pharmaceuticalised governance (Dew, 2019) in the workplace are evident where coercion to use pharmaceuticals has been documented. Examples include the 'vaccinate or mask' policies imposed on front line health care workers (and successfully challenged in some settings), and where accepting mefloquine was a requirement for enlistees' deployment to tropical settings (Davis, 2020). More subtly, competitive forces in law, academia or in business, when perceived as natural, are likely to inhibit the possibility that workers' view non-medical cognitive enhancement as coercive or potentially harmful. Pharmaceuticalised governance reinforces the neoliberal status quo – whose logics may dictate that pharmaceutical solutions are not only rational but also responsible or legally imperative (Goold & Maslen, 2014).

A third concern is that the organisation and structure of work may produce suboptimal outcomes for pharmaceuticalised workers. Examples above suggest that the nature and settings of work may cause or exacerbate common health problems such as chronic pain, diabetes or mental illness; or that the organisation of work – that is, scheduling that suits the organisation rather than workers' physical or mental health needs – may mean that pharmaceutical benefits are not realised or their unintended effects create new, sometimes unrealised health risks. In these cases, new kinds of problems arise – the need for and costs of new health care, the prescribing of new pharmaceuticals to manage the iatrogenic effects of older ones, workers' diminished capacity to sustain employment.

Finally, while the examples here suggest that taking pharmaceuticals can enable a worker's economic participation, and may enhance it, taking pharmaceuticals is risky. Their risks may be heightened when their use occurs 'at work' and becomes an ongoing feature of working life. Examples above suggest that workers' may be unaware of risks and side effects associated with pharmaceuticals (i.e., Badzi & Ackumey, 2017). Frequently, the effects of the long-term use of pharmaceuticals such as non-medical cognitive enhancers or combined oral contraceptives have never been established. For others, long-term effects of short-term use of a drug like mefloquine emerged too late to avert its harm to users. On the other hand, pharmaceuticals may avert risk to both users and their clients (or patients) (Franke, 2013; Sugden et al., 2012). Then the concern is when their use is based on an imbalanced cost/benefit analysis, where benefits are assumed, and risks are minimised 'in the fine print' or are unknown. As the recipients of the benefits and harms of medicines, users should expect to be fully informed of the known benefit/risk profiles of any recommended drug, and as with other medical procedures, to provide fully informed consent prior to use. If adequate information about their long-term effects is unavailable, that should be part of the informed decision-making afforded the prospective user.

Conclusion

Pharmaceuticals are quintessentially a commodity targeted for individual consumption, affecting individual health, illness and risk. In the review above, pharmaceuticals are shown to be used instrumentally, to support the worker at work, and to enable the worker to better 'work for' the neoliberal economy – to govern oneself to become and remain competitive in the labour market. To obtain optimal outcomes, however, pharmaceuticals must be appropriately managed and manageable at work; they may produce side effects that impact workers' ability to perform their work; and chronic pharmaceutical use may, therefore, threaten a worker's employability. These 'entanglements' of pharmaceutical use based on the 'the interconnections between institutions, people and processes' (Dew, 2019, p. 7) in the workplace are suggested here to influence pharmaceutical consumption by workers, and to have broad reaching implications for workers' lives. Kevin Dew's assessment is appropriate as a conclusion: 'the desire to find a pill for every ill is a strong one, perhaps more so in societies where the productive worker is viewed as the central character in economic life, and economic life takes precedence over other issues' (Dew, 2019, p. 25).

Note

1 A version of this paper was presented at the International Social Pharmacy Workshop symposium "Living Pharmaceutical Lives" Leuven, Belgium, July 23–26, 2018.

References

American Diabetes Association. (2018). Economic costs of diabetes in the U.S. in 2017. *Diabetes Care, 41*, 917–928.

Asfaw, A., Alterman, T., & Quay, B. (2020). Prevalence and expenses of outpatient opioid prescriptions, with associated sociodemographic, economic and work characteristics. *International Journal of Health Services, 50*(1), 82–94.

Ayo, N. (2012). Understanding health promotion in a neoliberal climate and the making of health conscious citizens. *Critical Public Health, 22*(1), 99–105.

Badzi, C.D., & Ackumey, M.M., (2017). Factors influencing use of analgesics among construction workers in the Ga-East municipality of the Greater Accra region, Ghana. *Ghana Medical Journal, 51*(4), 156–163.

Bal, P.M., & Dóci, E. (2018). Neoliberal ideology in work and organizational psychology. *European Journal of Work and Organizational Psychology, 27*(5), 536–548.

Ballantyne, P.J., Norris, P., Parachuru, V.P., & Thomson, M. (2018). Medicine use trajectories from age 26 to 38 in a representative birth cohort from Dunedin, New Zealand. *SSM: Population Health, 4*, 37–44.

Billings, B. (2017). New report shows high percentage of active duty soldiers prescribed psychiatric drugs. *Citizens Commission on Human Rights International.* Retrieved August 5, 2020, from http://news.cchrint.org/2017/08/17/high-percentage-active-duty-soldiers-receiving-psychiatric-drugs/.

Bissell, P., May, C., & Noyce, P. (2004). From compliance to concordance: Barriers to accomplishing a reframed model of health care interactions. *Social Science & Medicine*, 58(4), 851–862.

Bloomfield, B., & Dale, K. (2015). Fit for work? Redefining 'normal' and 'extreme' through human enhancement technologies. *Organization*, 22(4), 552–569.

Brandt, S.A., Taverna, E.C., & Hallock, R.M. (2014). A survey of nonmedical use of tranquilizers, stimulants, and pain relievers among college students: Patterns of use among users and factors related to abstinence in non-users. *Drug & Alcohol Dependence*, 143, 272–276.

Brühl, A.B., d'Angelo, C., & Sahakian, B.J. (2019). Neuroethical issues in cognitive enhancement: Modafinil as the example of a workplace drug? *Brain and Neuroscience Advances*, 3, 1–8.

Burton, B. (2004). Australian army faces legal action over mefloquine. *British Medicine Journal*, 329(7474), 1062.

Canadian Centre for Occupational Health and Safety (n.d.). *OSH answers facts sheets. Diabetes in the workplace.* Retrieved August 5, 2020 from https://www.ccohs.ca/oshanswers/diseases/diabetes.html#:~:text=Employers%20and%20employees%20should%20work,to%20maintain%20a%20prescribed%20diet.

Canadian Federation of Nurses' Unions. (2018). *ONA Wins Second Decision on 'Unreasonable and Illogical' Vaccine or Mask Influenza Policies.* Retrieved August 5, 2020 https://nursesunions.ca/vaccinate-or-mask-influenza-policy-struck-down/

Canadian Mental Health Association (n.d.). *Fast Facts About Mental Illness.* CMHA National. Retrieved July 27, 2020 from https://cmha.ca/about-cmha/fast-facts-about-mental-illness.

Caplan, A., & Elliott, C. (2004). Is it ethical to use enhancement technologies to make us better than well? *PLoS Medicine*, 1(3), e52.

Cederström, C. (2016). Like it or not, "Smart Drugs" are coming to the office. *Harvard Business Review.* Retrieved from https://hbr.org/2016/05/like-it-or-not-smart-drugs-are-coming-to-the-office

Davies, J. (2017). Political pills: Psychopharmaceuticals and neoliberalism as mutually supporting. In J. Davies (Ed.), *The Sedated Society* (pp. 189–225). Cham, Switzerland, Palgrave Macmillan.

Davis, C. (April 9, 2020). Canadian Armed Forces Veterans Set to File Lawsuits against Mefloquine. *TopClass Actions.* Retrieved August 10, 2020 https://ca.topclassactions.com/uncategorized/canadian-armed-forces-veterans-to-file-lawsuits-against-mefloquine/.

De Serres, G., Skowronski, D.M., Ward, B.J., Gardam, M., Lemieux, C., Yassi, A., Patrick, D.M., Krajden, M., Loeb, M., Collignon, P., & Carrat, F. (2017). Influenza vaccination of healthcare workers: Critical analysis of the evidence for patient benefit underpinning policies of enforcement. *PLoS ONE*, 12(1), e0163586. doi:10.1371/journal.

Dew, K. (2019). *Public Health, Personal Health and Pills. Drug Entanglements and Pharmaceuticalised Governance.* Abington, Oxon: Routledge.

Dewa, C.S., Hoch, J.S., Lin, E., Paterson, M., & Goering, P. (2003). Pattern of antidepressant use and duration of depression-related absence from work. *British Journal of Psychiatry*, 183, 507–513.

de Wit, M., Trief, P.M., Huber, J.W., & Willaing, I. (2020). State of the art: Understanding and integration of the social context of diabetes care. *Diabetic Medicine*, 37, 473–482.

Diabetes Canada (2019). *Diabetes in Canada*. Retrieved July 28, 2020 https://www.dia-betes.ca/DiabetesCanadaWebsite/media/About-Diabetes/Diabetes%20Charter/2019-Backgrounder-Canada.pdf.

Dini, G., Bragazzi, N.L., Montecucco, A., Rahmani, A., & Durando, P. (2019). Psychoactivie drug consumption among truck-drivers: A systematic review of the literature with meta-analysis and meta-regression. *Journal of Preventive Medicine and Hygiene*, 60(2), E124 – E139.

Donovan, E. (2010). Propranolol use in the prevention and treatment of posttraumatic stress disorder in military veterans: Forgetting therapy revisited. *Perspect in Biology and Medicine*, 53(1), 61–74.

Dubljević, V. Sattler, S., & Racine, E. (2014). Cognitive enhancement and academic misconduct: A study exploring their frequency and relationship. *Ethics and Behaviour*, 24(5), 408–420.

Fisher, J. (2007). Coming soon to a physician near you: Medical neoliberalism and pharmaceutical clinical trials. *Harvard Health Policy Review*, 8(1), 61–70.

Franke, A., Bagusat, C., Dietz, P., Hoffmann, I., Simon, P., Ulrich, R., & Lieb, K. (2013). Use of illicit and prescription drugs for cognitive or mood enhancement among surgeons. BMC *Medicine*, 11(102), 1–9.

Goold, I., & Maslen, H. (2014). Must the surgeon take the pill? Negligence duty in the context of cognitive enhancement. *The Modern Law Review*, 77(1), 60–86.

Greely, H., Campbell, P., Sahakian, B., Harris, J., Kessler, R., Gazzaniga, M., & Farah, M.J. (2008). Towards responsible use of cognitive enhancing drugs by the healthy. *Nature*, 456, 702–705.

Haines, A. (April 30, 2019). *Canadian veterans suing government over anti-malarial drug's adverse effects*. CTV News, Toronto, Canada. Retrieved August 5, 2020 from https://www.ctvnews.ca/w5/canadian-veterans-suing-government-over-anti-malarial-drug-s-adverse-effects.

Howes, M. (2010). Menstrual function, menstrual suppression and the immunology of the human female reproductive tract. *Perspectives in Biology and Medicine*, 53(1), 16–30.

Jensen, S.Q., & Prieur, A. (2016). The commodification of the personal: Labour market demands in the era of neoliberal post industrialization. *Distinktion: Journal of Social Theory*, 17(1), 94–108.

Kamienski, L. (2012). Helping the postmodern Ajax: Is managing combat trauma through pharmacology a Faustian bargain? *Armed Forces & Society*, 39(3), 395–414.

Kowalski-McGraw, M., Green-McKenzie, J., Pandalai, S.P., & Schulte, P.A., (2017). Characterizing the interrelationships of prescription opioid and benzodiazepine drugs with worker health and workplace hazards. *Journal of Occupational and Environmental Medicine*, 59(11), 1114–1126.

Krill, P.R., Johnson, R., & Albert, L. (2016). The prevalence of substance use and other health concerns among American attorneys. *Journal of Addiction Medicine*, 10, 46–52.

Leslie, K. (September 10, 2015). Vaccinate or mask' policy struck down by Ont. *Nurses' union*. *The Canadian Press*. Retrieved August 10, 2020. https://www.ctvnews.ca/health/vaccinate-or-mask-policy-struck-down-by-ont-nurses-union-1.2556697.

Maher, B. (2008). Poll results: Look who's doping. *Nature*, 452, 674–675.

McGuigan, J. (2014). The neoliberal self. *Culture Unbound*, 6, 223–240.

Micouland-Franchi, J.A., MacGregor, A., & Fond, G. (2014). A preliminary study on cognitive enhancer consumption behaviors and motives of French medicine and pharmacology students. *European Review for Medical and Pharmacological Science*, 18(13), 1875–1878.

Milner, A., Scovelle, A.J., King, T.L., & Madsen, I. (2019). Exposure to work stress and use of psychotropic medications: A systematic review and meta-analysis. *Journal Epidemiology and Community Health*, 73(6), 569–576.

Mohamed, A.D., & Sahakian, B.J. (2012). The ethics of elective psychopharmacology. *The International Journal of Neuropsychopharmacology*, 15, 559–571.

Moncrief, J. (2017). Opium and the people: The prescription psychopharmaceutical epidemic in historical context. Chapter 4 in Davies J. (Ed). *The Sedated Society. The Causes and Harms of our Psychiatric Drug Epidemic* (pp. 73 – 99). Cham, Switzerland, Palgrave Macmillan.

National Women's Health Network. (2015). *Menstrual Suppression*. Retrieved August 11, 2020 from https://www.nwhn.org/menstrualsuppression/.

Nevin, R.L. (2017). A serious nightmare: Psychiatric and neurologic adverse reactions to mefloquine are serious adverse reactions. *Pharmacology Research & Perspectives*, 5(4), e00328.

O'Meara, K.P. (December 2, 2014). Drugging our military to death. *Citizens Commission on Human Rights (CCHR) International*. Retrieved August 10, 2020. https://www.cchrint.org/2014/12/02/drugging-our-military-to-death/.

Paulose-Ram, R., Hirsch, R., Dillon, C., Losonczy, K., Cooper, M., & Ostchega, Y. (2003) Prescription and non-prescription analgesic use among the US adult population: Results from the third National Health and Nutrition Examination Survey (NHANES III). *Pharmacoepidemiology Drug and Safety*, 12(4),315–326.

Pedron, S., Emmert-Fees, K., Laxy, M., & Schwettmann, L. (2019). The impact of diabetes on labour market participation: A systematic review of results and methods. *BMC Public Health*, 19(25), 1–13.

Petersen, M.A., Nørgaard, L.S., & Traulsen, J.M. (2015). Going to the doctor with enhancement in mind – an ethnographic study of University Students' use of prescription stimulants and their moral ambivalence. *Drugs: Education, Prevention and Policy*, 22(3), 201–207.

Ram, S.S., Hussainy, S., Henning, M., Jensen, M., & Russell B. (2016). Prevalence of cognitive enhancer use among New Zealand tertiary students. *Drug Alcohol Review*, 35(3), 345–351.

Ringqvist, Å., Bech, P., Glenthøj, B., & Petersen, E. (2015). Acute and long-term psychiatric side effects of mefloquine: A follow-up on Danish adverse event reports. *Travel Medicine and Infectious Disease*, 12(1), 80–88.

Ruston, A., Smith, A., & Fernando, B. (2013). Diabetes in the workplace – diabetic's perceptions and experiences of managing their disease at work: A qualitative study. *BMC Public Health*, 13(386), 1–10.

Ryan K., Bissell P., & Morgall Traulsen, J. (2004). The work of Michel Foucault: Relevance to pharmacy practice. *International Journal of Pharmacy Practice*, 12, 43–53.

Saeedi, P., Petersohn, I., Salpea, P., Malanda, B., Karuranga, S., Unwin, N., Colagiuri, S., Guariguata, L., Motala, A.A., Ogurtsova, K., Swah, J.E., Bright, D., Williams, R., & IDF Diabetes Atlas Committee. (2019). Global and regional diabetes prevalence estimates for 2019 and projections for 2030 and 2045: Results from the International Diabetes Federation Diabetes Atlas, 9th edition. *Diabetes Research and Clinical Practice*, 157, 1–9.

Sales, P., Murphy, F., Murphy, S., & Lau, N. (2019). Burning the candle at both ends: Motivations for non medical prescription stimulant use in the American workplace. *Drugs: Education, Prevention and Policy*, 26(4), 301–308.

Smith, T.J., & Hillner, B.E. (2019). The cost of pain. *JAMA Network Open*, 2(4), e191532.

Stanfeld, S.A., Rasul, F.R., Head, J., & Singleton, N. (2011). Occupation and mental health in a national UK survey. *Social Psychiatry and Psychiatric Epidemiology*, 46, 101–110.

Stevenson, D., & Farmer, P. (2017). *Thriving at work: The Stevenson Farmer review of mental health and employers*. Retrieved July 30, 2020 from https://www.gov.uk/government/publications/thriving-at-work-a-review-of-mental-health-and-employers

Sugden, C., Housden, C.R., Aggarwal, R., Sahakian, B.J., & Darzi, A. (2012) Effect of pharmacological enhancement on the cognitive and clinical psychomotor performance of sleep-deprived doctors: A randomized controlled trial. *Annals of Surgery*, 255(2), 222–227.

Trego, L.L. (2007). Military women's menstrual experiences and interest in menstrual suppression during deployment. *Journal of Obstetrical Gynaecological and Neonatal Nursing*, 36, 342–347.

US Medicine (October 20, 2019). *Menstrual suppression could help deployed women avoid discomfort, inconvenience*. Retrieved August 7, 2020 from https://www.usmedicine.com/agencies/department-of-defense-dod/menstrual-suppression-could-help-deployed-women-avoid-discomfort-inconvenience/

Vrecko, S. (2015). Everyday drug diversions: A qualitative study of the illicit exchange and non medical use of prescription stimulants on a university campus. *Social Science & Medicine*, 131, 297–304.

Wiegel, C., Sattler, S., Goritz, A.S., & Diewald, M. (2016). Work-related stress and cognitive enhancement among university teachers. *Anxiety, Stress & Coping: An International Journal*, 29, 100–117.

Williams, S.J., Martin, P., & Gabe, J. (2011). The pharmaceuticalisation of society? A framework for analysis. *Sociology of Health & Illness*, 33(5), 710–725.

Zhang, W., McLeod, C.B., & Koehoorn, M. (2016). The relationship between chronic conditions and absenteeism and associated costs in Canada. *Scandinavian Journal of Work Environment & Health*, 42(5), 413–422.

3 Medication-use narratives on the margins

Managing type 2 diabetes without medical insurance[1]

Jenny Epstein

Introduction

The increasing use of pharmaceuticals to manage all aspects of everyday life has prompted scholars to examine how this use shapes relationships between body and self. The myriad ways people use medications, particularly for type 2 diabetes mellitus (T2DM)[2], and how medication use can change over time is a process I have observed over decades as a clinical pharmacist. In this chapter, I use this experience and expand on previous work to examine how pharmaceutical use mediates particular spatial and temporal forms, which in turn shapes relationships between body and self. This spatiotemporal lens allows new avenues to examine how the social spaces humans design and live within (including bodies) shape the ways we conceive and take care of ourselves.

As a mass-produced technology, pharmaceuticals are designed (ideally) to deliver uniform and mechanically predictable effects with every dose taken. In turn, the bodies they work on become (again ideally) equally uniform and predictable, inseparable from routinised medication schedules and greater regimentation of the user's daily life. In contrast, I show how successful diabetes control comes from creating social space that is local, unique and rooted in embodied experience. Focusing on the spatial and temporal forms provides a unique insight into the ways alienation between body and self is both produced and resisted through pharmaceutical use. It moves the focus away from individual psychology or labels of 'non-adherence' and studies how people creatively construct (or struggle to construct) medication self-care practices within the macro forces of modern capitalism.

I use Henri Lefebvre's (1991, 1979) conception of social space as a way to more fully grasp how a global, mass-produced technology like pharmaceuticals shapes everyday life. Composed of heterogeneous forms of space and inseparable from time, social space is not simply a detached backdrop or passive frame for human practice, but plays an active role in all aspects of cultural production. Lefebvre used spatial and temporal forms as a way to understand how power is produced and resisted in modern capitalism, with a particular focus on the production of and resistance to alienation in everyday life. In what Lefebvre defines as the 'abstract' social space of modern capitalism, relationships between things are made measureable, uniform and interchangeable; time becomes predicable and routinised. Here, I apply this theoretical frame to ethnographic research that took place in Tacoma, WA, USA. I use life-story narratives of working-poor residents living with T2DM as a way to illustrate how less obvious, but powerful social forces shape the ways people construct medication practices over time.

Lefebvre (1991) defines the ways the body is quantified through self-measurement and the ways time is routinised as 'abstract space', a social space that increasingly dominates everyday life, mediated through the global flow of commodities, such as pharmaceuticals. Through this mediation, relationships between body and self are made interchangeable, impersonal and measurable – mirroring the qualities of social relations (and social space) that dominate our larger social world. This process orders self-care practices so that the necessity for meaning-creation and self-contemplation become hidden. Instead, technical skill, self-measurement and routinisation are deemed essential qualities of self-care.

Mastering T2DM self-care is the transcendence of routine through meaning-creation. Methodologically, diabetes life histories uncover how this process unfolds over time. Analysis of these life histories showed that the ability to create new meanings was an essential piece of the struggle to make life-saving change worth the effort. The data I collected shows people slowly coming to terms with using (or not) medications, so managing their symptoms meant profoundly rearranging existing ways of understanding embodied experience. Most importantly, the struggles people experienced centred on what I argue is an underlying contradiction of long-term medication use: namely, the self-measurement, routine-creation and technical monitoring skills, which form the foundation of T2DM self-care protocols, exacerbate an already existing sense of disconnection many people feel towards their own bodies and health.

In this chapter, I explore how these principles apply to pharmaceutical use and how, as a mass-produced technology, pharmaceuticals shape the ways people must rethink their bodies and everyday schedules. With this framework in mind, I focused on the following questions: What patterns can be identified surrounding diabetes medication use over time? How do these patterns correlate to practices of self-care and ultimately relationships between body and self? Who had to make the greatest changes and why? What were the motivators and barriers to self-transformation?

Routinisation and meaning-creation

I also build on the concept of 'healthwork', which defines chronic medication use as the 'everyday/everynight activities through which people look after health (Mykhalovskiy et al., 2004, p. 323)'. The authors analyse the ways people use medications to understand how forms of power are expressed through daily self-care practices. Medication use is therefore much more complex than cognitive remembering or simple acts of swallowing or injecting. Instead, the effort needed to create and sustain chronic medication practices is defined as *work*. Past research on healthwork by McCoy (2009) and Huyard et al. (2019) have emphasised the temporal qualities of pharmaceutical self-care practices. Both papers argue that using pharmaceuticals chronically requires the creation of scheduled habits that are repetitive from day to day and year to year; they view the creation of medication routines as stabilising practices. Although their work shows how routinised medication habits are dynamic and context-driven processes, they leave out why and how this particular temporal form (routinisation) is often a barrier and thus resisted by many people, or the interconnections of temporal and spatial forms so that the qualities of routinised time and scientifically uniform bodies are tightly intertwined.

By narrowing in on routinisation to frame medication use, Huyard et al. (2019) and McCoy (2009) leave out the body. The routinisation pharmaceutical use requires is inseparable from other technical skills, such as self-measurement and monitoring, which quantify one's body. Left out of the relationship between body and self are the ways cultural forms, particularly abstracted social space, is integral to the production of power. Indeed, routinisation reflects the domination of 'abstract space' in everyday life (Lefebvre 1991): mass production, commodification and instrumental reason. Instead, quantification and routinisation are barriers for many people, particularly affecting those who already have a tenuous relationship between body and self. The collected narratives show how long-term 'healthwork' requires creatively transforming universal bodies and mechanistic routines into uniquely meaningful self-care practices. Following Lefebvre's lead, I connect routinisation with the production of alienation in everyday life. I identify the decades of work required to create sustainable self-care practices as processes of dealienation.

For many of the people I interviewed, T2DM brought not only the symptoms of high glucose levels, but also the necessity to create time for self-contemplation of one's health as a positive concern. As I discuss later in three cases, this often was a new and difficult life-skill on top of the necessity for skills such as self-measurement and scheduling taught through biomedical patient education programs to manage blood sugars. The spatiotemporal forms of these new demands contrasted sharply. On the one hand, people learned biomedical constructions of T2DM as an impersonal progression of cellular dysfunction and on the other, they understood T2DM in terms of their own history and embodied knowledge. As I discuss next, life history methodology provides a way to understand how people meld these different ways of understanding over time. However, the intent here is *not* to create a dichotomy between different spatiotemporal forms. Instead, Lefebvre's conception of social space as a dialectical whole provides a framework to examine healthwork as a process of integration that sometimes lasts over decades.

Methodology: Medication use narratives

In Tacoma, WA, as everywhere, T2DM arises from conditions of everyday life. For the residents I interviewed, these conditions were marked by long hours of work, cheap and/or high caloric food, stress, and little inclination and/or time for self-reflection and self-care. As a methodology, life histories of T2DM demonstrate how lived experience is held in tension with scientific abstraction as people learn to manage their bodies (or not) over time. Sociologist Steph Lawler (2002) uses the work of Paul Ricoeur to explain these differences of temporal form. Lawler thinks of narrative as a process of self-reflection, which requires reinterpreting the past from the present: a kind of looping back and forth through time. She contrasts this with Ricoeur's description of conventional time as being linear and 'conceived as a series of instants succeeding one another along an abstract line oriented in one direction' (Ricoeur 1980:174). Lawler argues that life history methodologies allow for both backward and forward perspectives of time, in which experiential knowledge dominates. For this project, I was interested in the interplay of linear and 'looping' temporal forms as people learned to manage T2DM. Life history interviews made visible the different forms of social space and rhythms centred on the body, particularly the 'work' of objectifying one's own body through self-monitoring and measurement.

The interview tool I designed combined two life history methodologies (Davis, 2006; Griffiths et al., 2007) to reflect the different spatiotemporal perspectives I was trying to collect. The first part of the interview consisted of three interconnected timelines of living with diabetes: medical events, social history and what people learned and felt about these events.[3] The three timelines worked out chronological details of an individual's medical history as understood by the individual, since I did not access the participant's medical chart. The timelines uncovered forgotten events and revealed a great amount of contextual and historical data. During the interview, the timelines quickly became intertwined. A frequent question was, 'Is this *really* what you want to hear about?' After being encouraged to keep talking, people then understood the interview was not about creating a medical evaluation, but about their own thinking and process of self-care. Interviewees knew I did not have access to their medical charts, nor did I ask them to provide blood glucose logs. Many times, numbers were volunteered, or I asked if people remembered a reading at a particular event. In this way, the 'tangential' information formed the crux and unique perspective of each interview.

The second part of the interview consisted of a 'care diagram' where people explained the degree of importance of six quality-of-life domains, in relation to the timelines they just narrated. These domains were: Social, Spiritual, Environmental, Psychological, Economic and Physical. After narrating a chronological history, the circular domain diagram gave participants space to reassemble and explain this history further, providing opportunity for the looping back and forth needed for contemplation Lawler (2002) discusses. Without the discussion of domains, many crucial insights that contextualised how people felt and what they had learned would have been lost.

I conducted 58 interviews in 2013–2014, each taking 1–3 hours. To qualify, participants had to have lived with T2DM for at least 5 years, giving them time to develop (or not) self-care practices. Of the 58 people interviewed, 37 were women and 21 were men. Ages of interviewees ranged from 34 to 72 years, with half between 50 and 60 years old. The youngest age at diagnosis was 27. The average age of diagnosis was 49 years, and the average time living with diabetes was almost 9 years. Of the 58 interviewees, 42 were Anglo-American, 10 were African-American, four were Latino, one was Samoan-American and one was Micronesian. This population breakdown reflected the population of the clinics I recruited from, and not the population of Tacoma.

Participants were recruited from two ambulatory-care clinics. One was a volunteer clinic (Volunteer Care) and the other a federally funded Community Health Clinic (CHC). Both served lower-income residents, a demographic reflecting the city residents most affected by T2DM. A similar system to recruit interviewees was used in each setting: a nurse or medical assistant identified people diagnosed with T2DM as they checked in and I discussed participating in my project as they waited for their appointments. In total, I interviewed 34 from Volunteer Care and 26 from CHC. Because of its smaller size and patient population, I talked to every person diagnosed with T2DM at Volunteer Care. The CHC clinic was busy, with medical staffing in flux, which made negotiating interviews more difficult. The larger size and greater impersonality of the clinic made people less willing to be interviewed and made selection at CHC more biased due to convenience sampling; however, the retrospective nature of the interviews served (at least partially) as an internal control for this bias. Except for a few, most people experienced periods of 'noncompliance' with medical treatment, sometimes for decades. How people integrated (or not) the tension between the need for greater routinisation and quantification on the one hand and the need for self-contemplation and transformation on the other, formed the crux of the analysis.

Findings and analysis

Analysis of the narratives revealed three distinct patterns of controlling diabetes, which I labelled: 'Just Beginning', 'Cycling' and 'Care of the Self'. The groups do not represent a linear procession, but where people were when I interviewed them, although many had experienced better or worse control over time. Rather, these categories correlate to how Lawler (2002) discusses differences in narrative types between the linear progression of medical discourse and the reflexive back-and-forth of narratives of medication use. Using this distinction, I defined control as the ability to examine one's past behaviours and to put learned experience into practice. In the Just Beginning group, people were still struggling to integrate abstract and embodied knowledge. In the Just Beginning group, routinisation and quantification were not integrated or were actively resisted. In this group, narratives revealed how clinicians presented routinisation and quantification as useful tools for orderliness often at odds with the marginal social control many people actually experienced. Instead of being a useful tool, routinisation and quantification were resisted as another added burden. In the Cycling group, people cycled between Just Beginning and Care of the Self. Rational decision-making and medical facts could be incorporated into self-care practices, but this did not motivate sustained transformation. Control was therefore not defined in terms of medication compliance, technical skills or creating routines, but rather in terms of the meanings underlying practices of self-care. This triangulation of meaning/practice/self was never divorced from social context as analysis showed how gender, disability or homelessness were overly represented in the Just Beginning group. And yet, in spite of social instability, limited economic means and/or lack of health insurance, individuals in the Care of the Self group were able to create or maintain meanings and practices that sustainably controlled diabetes symptoms.

The interviews also showed how medication use formed a continuum that mirrored the groups of control. In the Just Beginning and Cycling groups, judgment arose from self-measurement of blood glucose, weight and calories and the inability to meet numerical goals of 'good diabetes control'. Medications in these groups were often blamed for not working or were a reminder of having T2DM and therefore avoided altogether. In contrast, among the Care of the Self group, there was an acceptance of what medications could and could not do. This acceptance was more than a learned skill, as it also correlated with greater social stability and/or a sense of place in the world. Using medications to control T2DM turned ordinary daily routines into sites for reflexive reasoning, but this process also held the possibility of further alienation. As I discuss in the next section, changes in social stability had important effects on people's ability to maintain disciplined habits and judgment.

Judgment: Linearity and stasis

I can't get my ducks in a row. The world is too chaotic.

Just Beginning. Lisa, 57

Trying to get back to [my] life. I can't cope with work, can't cope with nothing anymore. I blame my body for what it's doing to me and that's not a good feeling.

Just Beginning. Janice, 69

In the Just Beginning group, simply taking medications did not restore order in daily life. Instead, medication use was dominated by a sense of judgment and two contrasting practices that enabled little change in daily routines. At one extreme, medications were avoided entirely; as one man told me, medications reminded him of diabetes, so he didn't take them. At the other extreme, medications were overly relied on to 'fix diabetes' with all responsibility for self-care placed on prescribed medications. Both patterns allowed people to maintain familiar practices and to side-step responsibility for creating new practices of self-care.

When she could afford diabetic medications, Laura (Just Beginning) was compliant, but she used them with little trust and made few changes to her life. For Laura, medications provided a way to maintain her ability to work two jobs and little else. As another woman, Jane (Care of the Self), told me, 'I thought the medications didn't work for me and I blamed them for not working'. For Jane, medications only began to 'work' after 12 years of living with diabetes when she was no longer able to do her job due to complications of diabetes. Jane found herself with time to experiment with healthier foods, exercise and change her life. Her willingness developed from a more reciprocal treatment relationship at Volunteer Clinic and her new work as a translator at a hospital. All of these changes in Jane's life helped to shape self-care practices. Underlying this new control was new insight in her abilities to figure out what self-care practices worked for her, particularly the extent and limitations of medications. In contrast, Laura couldn't make any other changes and was dependent on medications to control blood sugars, even after living with T2DM for 25 years.

Both overdependence and underuse strongly correlated to contextual factors such as the demands of low-paying work and working two jobs or unemployment, family health issues, lack of health insurance and overwhelming stress. In this group, medication routines were a reminder that one's life had irrevocably changed, and was now tied to external, numerical scales and self-measurement. In the next three cases, one story from the Just Beginning group and two from the Cycling group are used to illustrate the interconnections between social stability, self-care and medication use.

Learning the value of health (Just Beginning)

Taking care of one's body for good health, or even the idea of valuing one's health were not priorities for many of those interviewed. 'Working just to live' and maintaining an often-times precarious social stability through low-paying jobs took priority. Valuing one's health, or even that the concept existed was a slowly learned process. Financially stable at the time of the interview, Marie was one of the few people who was able to articulate how growing up poor connected with a disregard for one's health. She described how daily care for one's health was a luxury, not a necessity:

> I grew up in a poorer area and people just lived that way [with poor health]. Now I see 103-year-old women at my condominium making turkey dinners for Thanksgiving. Or, there's this 89-year-old lady complaining about her knee and I'm thinking 'Well, you're 89 years old', but she has such expectations for herself. I never saw that as a kid.

Later, Marie went on to say, 'When I was younger, it was taking care of the kids [her siblings] and stuff and then I started working and working overtime. I've never had time to just think about the way I feel'. In addition to working long hours, Marie also worked evenings and graveyard shifts, so her work schedule never matched a 'normal' day. She 'couldn't be bothered' to figure out when to check glucose levels and used food, especially junk food, to stay awake. She had gained about 100 pounds before her diagnosis. Marie's primary concern was working:

> To me, just keeping working was the deal. All I wanted was to sleep and feel halfway decent to get up and keep working. Just keeping my sanity was my concern. I couldn't be bothered with diabetes. I was just like a little savage girl before running through life.

Shortly after her diagnosis approximately 20 years earlier, she had done her own research and requested to be prescribed metformin, a new approach at the time to reduce insulin resistance. Despite this promising start, taking medication was the extent of Marie's efforts to manage diabetes; 'I think my MD realized I was a lost cause'. Now Marie finds herself with a new willingness to value her health and life:

> I never wanted to do that [take care of herself]. Now I'm stuck with living and the realities of all this stuff. So, now, okay. I don't know. I'm here and I have to play. I'm an unwilling participant. [pause] And I have it good, I'm very thankful for what I have. I mean, it doesn't seem like it, but I am... You've got me crying.

Loss of stability (Cycling)

Rick's story describes how routinisation is dependent on larger structural forces that provide social stability and a positive sense of one's place in the world. Losing a sense of place and connection to a larger purpose can be devastating to maintaining the routinisation pharmaceutical use requires.

In his late 50s, Rick was diagnosed with T2DM 15 years prior to our meeting, at a time when his job and place in the world were unquestioned. Rick's world turned upside down over the course of a few years. After his long-time employer declared bankruptcy, Rick lost his job and future retirement pension. After 30 years, he had been the most senior and second highest paid employee on 'the floor'. His job had provided a structure of progression to his life, from 'pushing a broom to management, the whole bit'. Although he quickly found another job, 2 years later, he was injured badly at his new job and was no longer working when we talked. When I asked Rick how he felt about using insulin he told me:

> Well, that's one thing that bothers me is I'm OK being on insulin. 'Well, why don't you want to get to a point where you can take less or quit altogether?' Answering his own question, he said, 'I've lost this mental push'. 'I need to be part of something greater than myself. My job was part of that. Working in the sawmill [his first job], I was good at what I did. Before I got hurt [at his second job], I was just starting to get to be the guy that was needed again. Now that's been taken away from me'.

Without work to organise his day, measuring, monitoring and scheduling to control T2DM had no purpose. Since losing his job, Rick was casting about, trying to get back the motivation, to get out of:

> 'the state I call "Poor me" (whiny voice). The more work I do, the more active I am, the less insulin I use. I know this. I know this'. Babysitting his grandkids gave Rick enjoyment and some structure, but he was looking for 'this calm feeling you get from having a purpose'. 'I think this disease [T2DM] is as much physical as mental. And it's really hard for me, just dealing with that part. I know how to take care of myself, but it's not enough to get me

out there. There's something to be said for being scheduled. Everything was set up, everything fell into order. Now it doesn't feel that way. Now it's just 'Oh, I'll get to it'.

The power of food (Cycling)

Cedric was 42 year old and diagnosed with T2DM 14 years prior to his interview. For a few months after his diagnosis, Cedric took medications and made a few changes to his diet. Within a month or so he felt much better; the fatigue, thirst, and just 'feeling really bad' disappeared. After he was first diagnosed, his attitude towards diabetes was:

> I ignored it. I thought I was invincible; it [complications] won't happen to me. I can handle it. I can just stop it at any time. Just put down sodas, do a few push-ups, it won't bother me. When I'm ready [to deal with diabetes], I'll be fine.

After taking medications for about 2 years, Cedric moved to a new city and 'lived life as though I was no longer a diabetic. I mean, I just stopped all my medications. I stopped everything. I didn't take care of myself at all'. Cedric did not have medical insurance after his move, which helped him ignore diabetes. 'Since I felt fine I didn't see the sense in me trying to monitor anything. I just wanted to be normal, whatever that is, no hang-ups, no diseases'. However, Cedric's life changed abruptly when he was incarcerated and placed in a prison 'boot camp' program for 5 months. Unlike many people I interviewed, Cedric had no choice about diet and exercise. His blood sugars dropped within a non-diabetic range and he lost 50 pounds from enforced daily exercising and a 2,000 calorie per day diet.

No junk food was allowed in prison. But Cedric described the enticement of junk food after he was released:

> Your body feels the difference immediately [junk food after the boot camp diet]. Automatically. I mean it was just so powerful. When I got out, all I could think of is 'I want Burger King. I. Want. Burger King'. I went to Burger King, I took one bite and I got so sick. Like, 'This is not real food'. Oh my goodness, it was terrible. But [pause] I just kept on doing it until I got back to that old way of feeling. Looking to food for comfort, that habit of thinking, everything starts from there. When you're in a negative place you want something to comfort you and I took comfort in food [pause] and that was the enemy. I mean especially bad foods.

It didn't help at all that Cedric was assigned to a job at McDonalds on work release.

Marie's, Rick's and Cedric's stories illustrate the complex interplay of social structure, routinisation and quantification. Throughout all the interviews, willingness or unwillingness to create and perform medication routines was indicative of the larger context of one's life and opportunities. Marie's story shows how simply taking medications does little to change existing disconnections between body and self. Rick's story shows how loss of connection and purpose can result in resistance to routinisation. Cedric's story illustrates how people resist self-measurement and scheduling that disrupt existing practices of self-care that can be self-destructive. For Marie, Cedric and many others, poor-nutritional food played an important role in alleviating stress, feelings of boredom and loneliness, while facilitating work schedules that allowed little means or time for buying and experimenting with healthy foods. Throughout all the stories in the Just Beginning and Cycling groups, a similar theme played out: routinisation and quantification were impossible or could not be sustained without the time and space for critical self-reflection. To create practices of self-care that really addressed the condition of diabetes meant confronting not just the increased alienation brought into one's life through self-measurement and scheduling; it also would have required dismantling unhealthy practices that provided comfort and coping. Routinisation was not a neutral tool and did not provide sustaining structure in and of itself.

Acceptance: Embodied learning and contemplation

In contrast to judgment in Just Beginning and Cycling, medication use in the Care of the Self group was incorporated into a whole regimen of purposeful self-care practices. Although medical facts and self-measurement were necessary parts of self-care, especially at beginning stages, they were not the drivers for creating control of T2DM. Instead, control came from transforming what was uniform and impersonal into practices that were unique expressions of self-worth and purpose. Within the process of Care of the Self, medications became *one piece* of multiple parts of control. Acceptance was a process that included making new sense of one's body, and figuring in the extent to which medications could and should play in controlling T2DM. The expression of learning to 'take diabetes seriously' was used often to describe a process that unfolded over time. However, Rick's story illustrates how structural forces that upend social stability can overwhelm individual self-care practices. Medication use therefore always fits within abilities and opportunities to connect one's own history and purpose with self-care. Rather than simply creating habitual medication practices, the diabetes life histories revealed the interplay between reimagining one's relationship between body and self and the structural forces shaping this relationship. As I describe in the next story, what may appear as a process of learning to be a 'compliant patient' was actually a complicated process of figuring out what T2DM was, how medications acted within one's own body and fitting that within one's own history.

Finding pieces to a puzzle (Care of the Self)

Maggie was 60 years old and a patient at CHC clinic at the time of our interview. A cashier at Walmart, she told me she was enjoying the healthiest and happiest period of her life. Maggie's story began 6 months before losing her previous cashier job after calling in sick too many times. She had been feeling constantly fatigued and not herself:

> It just got to the point where I couldn't do anything anymore. I couldn't figure out what was going on with my body. I had so many unanswered questions it was unreal. I had just unbelievable fatigue and that didn't make any sense. I've always been a go-getter and healthy person, OK? So, when all of a sudden this started happening it confused me and then I lost my job, the depression…

Months after losing her job, she and her high school-aged son lost their apartment and then lost the belongings they had in storage. From the details of this period Maggie related to me, she was unable to separate the extreme financial stress she was under after losing her job from the fatigue and 'fog' of high blood sugars. The fatigue, irritability and not 'being able to cope' seemed a part of who she was, and Maggie kept waiting for 'something to give me the why's and why not's, something to grasp onto to' while her life spun out of control.

Things began to change after a chance meeting at a bus stop with an outreach worker from a local non-profit. When he asked Maggie if she was doing okay:

> 'I just broke down. Normally I don't do that but I was just in so much turmoil'. Maggie had no knowledge of the social safety net that existed in Tacoma to help people get back on their feet. 'Oh, you go here, you go there, yeah, I actually had someone positive in my life who was helping me. Once he gave me the clues and the numbers and whoever I could get a hold of, everything went into place. I could look to the positive instead of that dreary negative'.

Maggie was able to get diagnosed with diabetes, receive disability allowance, find an apartment and get a new job at Walmart. At the time of our conversation, Maggie was still in disbelief at the kind interest an unknown person took in her. 'Why? Why did he stop and talk to me when no one else was taking any interest in me? Then I stop and think 'Well, the Lord works in mysterious ways'. But as Maggie talked about herself, I became aware that making sense of the world through her own ability to analyse situations was an inherent part of who she was.

For Maggie, T2DM was a process of becoming aware of possibilities:

> It [diabetes] made me more aware of the things I could control… The physical part of diabetes has opened up new doors for me… when I figured out what my body's doing, you know exactly that, and he [her physician] was telling me the diagnosis of a diabetic and, yeah, it all made sense, it all came together into a little puzzle and I was like 'Wow, I know now'. It's made me stronger.

Similar to Marie and Cedric, Maggie had little concern for her health before being diagnosed with T2DM. A self-described 'junk food addict', adamant that she could not use needles and inject insulin, diabetes was a process of fitting together pieces of a puzzle. She took pride in her ability to put the right pieces into place.

Maggie is constantly aware of her body. She explained to me details of what her physician has told her, but in her own terms:

> Putting in insulin in my body, [at first] it didn't know why it's in there... It took it [her body] a little bit for it to figure out 'I got to have it', you know what I'm saying? So now, with what I'm doing, cause it knows and it will tell me. And it's really weird. I don't know if you can understand that. Sometimes in the morning it [her body] will automatically get me up and tell me that 'This is time for you to do insulin'. Anymore, I don't have to set the clock or nothing. I just get up, get into the refrigerator and get my insulin because it knows. It's hard to explain. But it's amazing to me how your body learns, yeah, like it really knows.

On the surface, Maggie appears to be compliant with medication use, but her 'compliance' was a hard-won victory over an extremely dark period of her life. Instead of further alienating body and self as discussed in the previous cases, Maggie more firmly unites them to create an understanding of T2DM that is unique to her. Maggie told me she had dealt with overwhelming odds from a young age:

> 'My whole life. Ever since I was little, let's see since I was 5 years old. Not fun. But there's always a new, there's always something to look forward to'. When I asked Maggie who helped her learn this, she said, 'By me, by me, because there was nobody there. When you don't have nothing, you have to piece it together. I was always finding things on my own. I always thought there was a different road, there's a different road I can take. So that gives me hope to find out who I am. ... Now, I don't have to go back to who I was [before diabetes], to not controlling who I am. ... Life keeps going on no matter what. Because of all the bad things that have happened to me, it [T2DM] was going to take over me. I was never going to let it, that was instilled in me at an early age'.

Gender

Maggie's story is remarkable, not just because of her hard-won ability to make sense of and overcome difficult odds; she was also an exception in a gender pattern between men and women across the self-care groups. After categorising the collected narratives, I found that women made up the majority of the 'Just Beginning' group, even though many had had diabetes for decades. As Table 3.1 shows, men are overly represented in the 'Care of the Self' group, particularly married men and women, mostly unmarried, are overly represented in the 'Just Beginning' category.

Women related abusive relationships, jobs that were low-paying and/or required less-skilled labour and a sense of being buffeted by life that men in the Care of the Self group did not report. The overall dynamics that distinguished men and women were the more financially dependent roles women played as

Table 3.1 Self-care groups by gender

	Men	Women
Just Beginning	6 (1 married man)	14 (1 married women)
Cycling	13 (3 married men)	11 (4 married women)
Care of the Self	18 (6 married men)	6 (3 married women)
Total	37	21

wives, past histories of abuse and the greater responsibilities of day-to-day caregiving to others. This pattern reinforces what the narratives also reveal; controlling T2DM is not simply a process of understanding facts and creating habits but a complicated interplay of how structural forces shape relationships between body and self and how this relationship plays out in self-care practices.

Medication mistrust

> I hate taking pills. I have to do this [take T2DM medications]. That's the worst thing about diabetes. I hate the idea that I need to take medication. You know, it seems to me like there is a dependency there.
>
> Cycling. Brad, 48

> Everything in the [diabetes] class was built around medications and I didn't want to be dependent like that. We were told, 'If you have cake, use a little more insulin'. It wasn't making a whole lot of sense to me. Why eat it in the first place if you shouldn't be eating it? It felt like you were giving up.
>
> Care of the Self. Lillian, 59

> Now I know through experience that without medication you can't feel healthy and then you can't be fit for living. I know that to keep moving [controlling T2DM] I have to take the meds. It's kind of like a new page in my life. I have to keep track of how I feel, the meds I take, and how I am mentally.
>
> Care of the Self. James, 64

Looking back on his life with T2DM and thinking about his future, Cedric (Cycling) saw using medications as a temporary necessity:

> Right now, medications are a stepping-stone, which will get my blood sugars under control, which will free me up. As long as I have a clear mind, my body will react in the way I want it to. The foods I was eating that got me to this point, they just have to go.

For Cedric, self-care is about giving up self-destructive comforts; medications are a temporary fix until he can change those practices.

Across all the groups, medication use did not impart a sense of control; instead, people expressed the opposite view: that medications were a sign of dependence or of losing control of one's body. However, in the Care of the Self group, this distrust of medications was minimised by having learned the limits of what pharmaceuticals could or could not do to control T2DM within the constraints and opportunities of their own lives. As Marie's (Just Beginning) story shows, simply taking medications was not enough over the long-term to prevent the symptoms of high blood sugars. For all the interviewees, learning what pharmaceuticals could and could not do was a process that included how factors such as employment, housing and personal relationships affected the effectiveness of medications. A further step was the ability to make changes in one's life to meet these gaps of pharmaceutical effectiveness. This process of overcoming medication distrust and gaining a sense of internal control was therefore a process of positive meaning-creation: of integrating self-measurement and routinisation of pharmaceutical schedules with knowledge gained through embodied experience. However, as Rick's and Cedric's stories relate, or the greater number of single women in the Just Beginning group shows, this process of meaning creation is always shaped by structural forces beyond individual control.

Meaning-creation, denial and psychology

As mass-produced commodities, pharmaceuticals demand users create new biographies of self that incorporate a universal biological body and mechanised rhythms of daily life. Yet, the narratives presented here show how medication use is also a process of meaning-creation, tightly welded to an individual's life 'plot' and the ways people learned to care for themselves over time. They explain the struggles people experienced as they came to terms (or not) with the depersonalisation of their bodies and daily events that self-measurement and medication schedules can bring to everyday life. Thus, instead of viewing medication use as a straightforward rational habit, these narratives reveal the importance of meaning-creation as a skill to control diabetes, and how this skill must always be examined within the context of larger structural forces.

As the narratives show, alienation can be produced through what are intended to be life-saving self-care practices. Too often, self-care is conflated under effectiveness of pharmaceutical and medical treatment, with emphasis placed on learning to convert the complexity of everyday life into numbers and schedules. Individual psychology or denial is then often used to explain why people resist or cannot adopt 'the facts' of medical care. With the growing prevalence of treatment chronicity, understanding meaning-creation as an important aspect of healthwork, provides professionals, clients and other stakeholders a way to reorient care. Instead, overcoming self-disregard, learning to value positive self-care and concretely addressing the structural forces that make self-transformation impossible are the real components of care of the self. Finally, the heterogeneity of the stories told here does not provide a uniform pattern of practices to be widely applied. Instead, the narratives can be used to remember that healthwork is a critically reflexive individual *process*. Following Lefebvre's emphasis on the role of social space in cultural production, clinicians should remember that scientific abstraction is not a neutral tool, but an active player in these processes and often times a barrier to self-care transformations.

Notes

1 A version of this paper was presented at the International Social Pharmacy Workshop symposium "Living Pharmaceutical Lives" Leuven, Belgium, July 23–26, 2018.
2 Throughout the chapter, I use the terms diabetes and T2DM interchangeably.
3 The research was approved through Washington University IRB.

References

Davis, P. (2006). Poverty in time: Exploring poverty dynamics from life history interviews in Bangladesh. CPRC Working Paper 69. www.chronicpoverty.org/uploads/publication_files/WP69_Davis.pdf.

Griffiths, T., Giarchi, G., Carr, A., & Horsham, S. (2007). Life mapping: A therapeutic document approach to needs assessment. *Quality of Life Research, 16*(3), 467–481.

Huyard, C., Haak, H., Derijks, L., & Lieverse, L. (2019). "When patients' invisible work becomes visible: Non-adherence and the routine task of pill-taking" *Sociology and Health, 41*(1), 5–19.

Lawler, S. (2002). "Narrative in social research" In T. May (ed.), *Qualitative Research in Action* (pp. 242–258). Sage: London.

Lefebvre, H. (1979). "Space: Social product and use value" In J.W. Freiberg (ed.), *Critical Sociology* (pp. 285–296). John Wiley & Sons: London.

Lefebvre, H. (1991). *The Production of Space: Translated by Donald Nicholson-Smith.* Cambridge: Blackwell.

McCoy, L. (2009). Time, Self and the Medication Day: A closer look at the everyday work of 'adherence'. *Sociology of Health, 31*(1), 128–146.

Mykhalovskiy, E., McCoy, L., & Breslier, M. (2004). Compliance/adherence, HIV, and the critique of medical power. *Social Theory and Health, 2,* 315–340.

Ricoeur, P. (1980) Narrative time. *Critical Inquiry, 7*(1), 269–290.

4 Medicines use for severe asthma

People's perspectives

Daniela Eassey, Lorraine Smith, Kath Ryan and Sharon Davis

Introduction

Living with severe asthma is, for many people, an all-consuming experience. Some days, simply being able to breathe is a struggle. Relying on medicines that do not always have the desired effect even when taken according to instructions, undertaking treatments, interacting with healthcare professionals and making emergency visits to hospital regularly punctuate the lives of those with severe asthma. Many people with severe asthma cannot work or study full time, or care for their loved ones. They experience stigma from others because their condition is often invisible and misunderstood.

Making a clinical diagnosis of severe asthma requires specialist assessment and will exclude modifiable problems such as misdiagnosis, incorrect inhaler technique and poor adherence (Chung et al., 2014). A diagnosis of severe asthma indicates that a person's asthma cannot be medically controlled, despite high doses of medicines that are taken as directed. Thus, severe asthma is indeed a 'pharmaceutical life', and there is often a tension between the external pressures of taking medicines and meeting action plans and health professional appointments, and one's internal struggle with perceptions of illness identity, emotions, and keeping an often uncontrollable disease under control.

In this chapter, we explore the effects of long-term medicine use on illness identity and perceptions of control, in the context of severe asthma, to provide an understanding of what it is like to incorporate medicines and their attendant side effects into a life lived with severe asthma. We use the Common-Sense Model of Self-Regulation (CSM) (Leventhal, Phillips, & Burns, 2016) as our theoretical lens to guide our interpretations of the narratives shared with us by 38 people from diverse backgrounds and locations in Australia who have severe asthma.

Background

Respiratory conditions impose an immense global heath burden and are leading causes of mortality and morbidity (Forum of International Respiratory Societies, 2017). Of all chronic respiratory conditions, asthma and chronic obstructive pulmonary disease (COPD) are the most common. Asthma is a condition of the lungs, affecting people of all ages (Masoli, Fabian, Holt, & Beasley, 2004; Papi, Brightling, Pedersen, & Reddel, 2018) and can range from mild to severe, based on the level of treatment required to control symptoms and prevent asthma attacks. Mild, moderate and severe asthma affects approximately 330 million people worldwide with approximately 250,000 annual deaths (Lenzen, Daniëls, van Bokhoven, van der Weijden, & Beurskens, 2017; Pinnock, 2015; Williams, Steven, & Sullivan, 2011). Severe asthma is a complex and heterogeneous disease that affects 3-10% of individuals with an asthma diagnosis. It accounts for high morbidity and is estimated to contribute to half the healthcare costs associated with asthma (McDonald et al., 2017; Sadatsafavi et al., 2010).

Achieving control over a long-term condition is often, at least in part, influenced by how effective treatments are, and the extent to which prescribed medicines are taken as directed. It is widely recognised that for people with mild to moderate asthma, taking medicines as directed tends to be suboptimal (Chung et al., 2014; Pike, Levy, Moreiras, & Fleming, 2018; Sabate, 2003) with primary non-adherence rates ranging from 6% to 44% of asthma patients worldwide (Sabate, 2003). The reasons why people with asthma may not take their medicines as directed are multifactorial, including erroneous understanding of or use of treatment, simple forgetfulness, side effects or a misalignment between an individual's goals and those of their healthcare practitioner (Foster, McDonald, Guo, & Reddel, 2017).

In contrast, for people with severe asthma, taking medicines as directed is often a priority because they depend on the actions of the medicine to breathe sufficiently well to carry out even the most basic of daily activities, and to avoid regular flare-ups and hospitalisations. People living with severe asthma will use many of the same medicines used by people with mild to moderate asthma – often at higher doses – but without improvement, and often require additional treatments. The risk of developing serious side effects is higher for people with severe asthma who need to take high-dose inhaled corticosteroids, often with additional courses of oral corticosteroids (Shaw et al., 2015). These can have varying negative impacts on quality of life and health status (Lefebvre et al., 2015).

Living with a long-term condition by definition means that the individual with the condition is intimately involved in how a disease plays out. A sense of autonomy and personal control are key factors. Choices and decision-making are ultimately the privilege of the person with the condition, with many a decision or action taken contrary to what a health professional or treatment guideline would recommend. Unless a person is hospitalised, the management of a condition such as severe asthma is at least a shared process between patient and healthcare professional. From the healthcare delivery perspective, an underpinning principle of chronic condition self-management is that people with long-term conditions are encouraged to be involved in their health management. This principle is supported by the adoption of a biopsychosocial approach to health and illness, with the aim of reducing power hierarchies between patients and health professionals and incorporating the priorities, preferences and goals of those living with and managing their condition (Coleman & Newton, 2005; Jones, MacGillivray,

Kroll, Zohoor, & Connaghan, 2011). Recent theoretical work into self-management support emphasises the importance of taking into account the wider psychological, social and environmental contexts within which people seek to 'live well' with their conditions (Morgan et al., 2017). In healthcare policies, support for self-management is also depicted as part of an expanded role for health professionals providing care, shifting from solely delivering information to including roles that focus on empowering and engaging their patients with their health care (Coleman & Newton, 2005; Jones et al., 2011).

A variety of internal and external factors can influence the experience of having to take long-term medicines. The intersection of these external and internal pressures of navigating life for those with severe asthma presents numerous challenges. The CSM (Leventhal et al., 2016) is a widely used model to understand the environmental, cognitive and emotional factors that operate dynamically and transactionally to impact individual responses and behaviours (Chan & Mak, 2016; Huston & Houk, 2011; Leventhal et al., 2016; Mann, Lefort, & Vandenkerkhof, 2013). The model proposes that individuals create mental representations of their illness based on external stimuli (e.g., family, friends, medical providers and social environments) and internal stimuli (e.g., emotions, beliefs and perceptions of illness identity) (Leventhal et al., 2016). According to this model, people develop implicit beliefs and emotions about their illness and treatment within five domains: (1) identity: perception of their illness label and symptoms, (2) control/cure: perceptions of cure and ability to control their illness, (3) consequences: treatment side effects, social and financial costs, (4) timeline: beliefs about how long an illness may last and disease trajectory, and (5) perceptions of the cause of illness (Leventhal et al., 2016). We use the first three domains of this model to cast an investigative and interpretative lens over the 'pharmaceutical lives' of people with severe asthma.

Methods

This study was part of a larger project funded by the Australian National Health and Medical Research Council (NHMRC) Centre of Research Excellence (CRE) in Severe Asthma. One of the aims of the project was to develop an online, publicly available information and support resource for people with severe asthma, their families, friends and carers, and for health professionals. The resource is available through the Healthtalk Australia website (https:// healthtalkaustralia.org) of peoples' stories of living with various health conditions. The severe asthma web pages provide a range of interview clips and narratives to help patients and health professionals understand the variety of experiences (Ziebland S, Lavie-Ajayi M, & Lucius-Hoene G, 2015; Ziebland et al., 2016). The data collection method was developed by the Health Experiences Research Group (HERG) at the University of Oxford (Herxheimer et al., 2000). The authors were involved in the collection and analysis of data for this study. In addition to publishing findings in the peer-reviewed literature and on the Healthtalk website, the interview transcripts are stored in a data repository and are available for secondary analysis.

Recruitment to the study was via general practitioners and respiratory physicians from across Australia, who handed out 'Information Packs' detailing the study and inviting potential participants to contact the study investigators if they would like to take part. We aimed to include participants from as wide a range of ethnicities, geographical locations and sociodemographic backgrounds as possible. Participants had to be aged 18 years and above and have received a diagnosis of severe asthma from their physician. The interviewer was a trained qualitative researcher (DE). The study received Human Research Ethics Committee approval from the University of Sydney (Australia); approval number 2015/934.

Thirty-eight face-to-face interviews were conducted around Australia from October 2016 to October 2018. In-depth interviews were conducted in the participant's place of choice, including their home, community centre or library. Interviews explored participants' experiences and perspectives of living with severe asthma. Participants were asked to tell their own story from the point when they first noticed they had breathing problems. They were encouraged to talk about their experiences of living with this condition, with as little interruption as possible from the interviewer. The interviews, which ranged from one-and-a-half to four hours, were video and/or audio recorded and transcribed verbatim. Interviews were thematically analysed, summarised as individual topics, and published on the Healthtalk Australia website. To protect their anonymity participants were offered the opportunity to adopt a pseudonym.

A supra-analysis (secondary analysis of existing data from a new theoretical perspective) (Ziebland et al., 2016) was conducted using a framework analysis approach (Gale, Heath, Cameron, Rashid, & Redwood, 2013). We used this analytical process to explore peoples' experiences of using medicines for the management of their severe asthma. The analysis involved researchers (DE, SD) recoding and becoming familiar with the content from the narratives available and identifying key issues. The dimensions of the CSM informed analytical categories. These were then thematically analysed to identify patterns within and between categories. The process of coding, analysing and interpreting the data involved all authors, who are experienced qualitative researchers. To assist the reader, when presenting interview excerpts, we provide an identifier indicating a participant's gender, age and years of living with asthma.

Results

The 38 participants ranged in age from 19 to 74 years, and 21 were female (55%). The majority identified as Caucasian; approximately 60% resided in urban areas and the remainder were from regional areas of Australia. All participants spoke English fluently. There was an even split between those working, retired and unemployed.

Our analysis revealed that participants' perceptions of their illness were influenced by their experiences and reflections, emotional responses to challenges they faced, and their impressions of social and environmental support. Three of the five domains of the CSM – identity, consequences, and control/cure – resonated in participants' narratives about living with severe asthma, and in each, the relevance of pharmaceuticals was evident. We present our findings organised around these themes: (1) severe asthma as an illness identity, (2) living with severe asthma and its consequences and (3) the need for asthma control.

Theme 1: 'Severe asthma means to me that you can't function' – illness identities

The clinical management of 'severe asthma' emphasises promoting self-management and improving asthma control through supporting self-care practices such as taking medication regularly, awareness of symptoms and, in some cases, avoidance of triggers. In contrast, participants' narratives brought the experience of severe asthma to life, conveying the myriad ways it impacted their daily lives and showing the cognitive and emotional labour of its management. The narratives revealed an illness identity reflecting a personal interpretation of asthma symptoms and their impact on the lived experience. Individuals described their perceptions of 'severe' asthma as relating to symptom severity and/or requiring additional treatment to control their condition. Some individuals reported fearing the uncertainty that comes from a rapid transition from feeling 'stable' to becoming 'uncontrolled' in a matter of a few minutes. The CSM captures the dynamic nature of living with an unpredictable condition like severe asthma and the emotional and cognitive work that goes into managing it. For example, Marion described how unpredictable her condition is and how this made her feel uncertain about her ability to maintain a sense of productivity in society and preserve her social ties:

> I thought I was travelling along with [my asthma] reasonably well managed and, you know, at a point where I could live with it sort of thing. But now we know that's not the case, and that I don't know if it's just going to continue going up and down like this every couple of months or whether it will get to a point where it can get stable and reasonably well managed and go back to just, you know, being a catastrophe every couple of years or something. You know like I'm yet to find that out, really.
>
> Female, aged 60, 30 years living with asthma

Shannon reported that:

> Severe asthma means to me that you can't function. Yeah. You're always preparing. You're always – you're trying to do your best. You always prepare for that day. I don't know how people could do it during work because you just don't know when your triggers are going to happen. And with mine, with the amount of medications and all that I'm on, I just – yeah. It's really hard. Really hard to function, really hard.
>
> Female, aged 39, 23 years living with asthma

For others, the label of 'severe' in their illness was based on the level or amount of treatment required to manage their condition. This could mean going from using 'puffs of relievers' to 'need[ing] the machine'. Marg, for example, reported that the severity of her illness depended on the treatment she requires:

> I sat down and thought what does it mean to me? And to me it means I have treatment for asthma that I am dependent upon, so that to me is severe. I don't want any severer [sic] than that, then it'd be critical.
>
> Female, aged 74, 66 years living with asthma

Individuals' illness identities were also shaped by everyday interactions with the external environment. Of note were participants who reported experiencing negative interactions with healthcare professionals and the general population. Participants felt that, generally, others misunderstood their condition, particularly around the idea that all asthma is similar, and can be easily treated just by using relievers. Comments from other people were at times hurtful and stigmatising. Leanne felt frustrated that others didn't understand how debilitating her severe asthma can get compared to mild/moderate asthma:

> Everyone says the same thing, 'Well what's the difference?' There's a big difference, you know. And then you try and sit there and explain it to them, they just don't get it. You can sit there until you're blue in the face and unless you actually smack them with it, they don't get it. At all. They just think oh you get a bit puffy you take some puffers, you'll be fine.
>
> Female, aged 41, 25 years living with asthma

Participants dealt with the perceived stigma of taking medicines in front of others in different ways but in essence all wanted to be seen as normal and not different from everyone else. Denise took a fatalistic view:

> It's a necessity. If you want to stay alive you know you've got to use them, and that's it. You know you can't say, oh I'm too embarrassed to use that. Hey, do you want to live, or do you want to die? Take a choice. So, it's something that's got to be done. You've just got to go with it.
>
> Female, aged 69, 62 years living with asthma

In contrast, Joel talked about using inhalers in public:

> I'll turn away. People think you're [um] diseased and they take a couple of steps back and seeing them yeah, yeah and I don't like that.
>
> Male, aged 35, 22 years living with asthma

Justin summed it up in saying:

> Now that I'm older, it's no big deal. I've got asthma, deal with it. Um, but when I was 19, 20, 21, I was embarrassed. I was embarrassed because I didn't want to be different.
>
> Male, aged 54, 53 years living with asthma

A second aspect of illness identity that emerged from our participant interviews was a perception of the illness as severe, acute and/or chronic. For some individuals the term 'chronic' signified that the condition required long-term treatment for 'daily maintenance' to be able to breathe, whereas, terms such as severe or acute were, at times, used to describe their asthma as uncontrolled. John, for example, explained that his condition is chronic due to his reliance on daily medications:

> Because it's a chronic disease it impacts me all the time… see the label severe asthma is that your asthma is such that, if you weren't treated, you would be in and out of hospital continuously. In other words, severe asthma should be treated all the time. It's not something you can treat a little bit at a time… somebody with severe asthma always has lots of other drugs they take… [severe would be] an acute exacerbation of my asthma.
>
> Male, aged 67, 5 years living with asthma

In some cases, uncertainty expressed by individual participants' doctors about their diagnosis brought on emotions such as fear and frustration. For example, Wayne reported that his healthcare providers did not seem to agree on his diagnosis, and living with this uncertainty left him feeling frustrated and confused:

> So, the specialist at [the hospital], they say I've got chronic bronchiolitis and [another] specialist said it's asthma. So, I don't know what I've got to be honest. I'm just confused. I was admitted to hospital round about four weeks ago and the respiratory nurse there said that he'd never seen anybody with the amount of medications that I was on for, for asthma. He goes, 'what you've got isn't asthma', so I don't know what I've got to be honest, it's just under that label.
>
> Male, aged 58, 4 years living with asthma

This theme has illuminated the challenges to illness identity as perceived by our study participants. Pharmaceutical treatments and healthcare professionals' clinical decision-making were revealed as central to achieving (or not) asthma control. In turn, personal interpretations of the illness and its identification were underpinned by uncertainty, confusion, fear and frustration. Participants were heavily reliant on their asthma medicines simply to be able to function on a daily basis.

Theme 2: The consuming effects of severe asthma – illness consequences

As proposed by the CSM, treatment side effects, including social and financial costs are some of the consequences of long-term illness and contribute to individuals' emotional, cognitive and behavioural experiences. In this study, many participants related feeling that severe asthma stripped their sense of independence and ability to undertake day-to-day activities, for example, social engagements and in some cases tasks such as housework. Karen reported:

> I haven't worked at all for two and a half years, and so this has been the biggest adjustment ever. I mean my son was in the States, he came home… so

he's taken on so much housework and helping out with his brother, and my husband had to take, you know, on a lot of the things I used to do.

Female, aged 55, 30 years living with asthma

In response to the challenges faced when living with severe asthma, individuals described various coping strategies to deal with the consequences of their condition. These strategies included planning ahead and finding different ways to do things at their own pace. Additionally, participants reported the importance of having their reliever medicine with them at all times. Their narratives highlighted previous experiences where they were admitted to hospital due to not being prepared. Monique explained that she felt panic if she didn't have her reliever inhaler with her:

You always have to remember your Ventolin. If you forget your Ventolin, the panic, the panic that you feel, even if you're not having an asthma attack. You happen to look in your handbag for something and you realise that you don't have your Ventolin and you're just like, what am I going to do? So, we started carrying ones in the car so there was a spare there.

Female, aged 39, 36 years living with asthma

People described the importance of taking their regular medicine and establishing and maintaining a routine facilitated this. Although it was seen as vital to keep on top of their asthma, organising and taking medicines took quite a bit of time out of the day. Moreover, side effects of medicines were an important consideration affecting the health of people with severe asthma. So, although oral corticosteroids were reported by most participants as essential for getting their illness under control, the cure was sometimes viewed as worse than the disease itself. This was illustrated in Karen's description of the side effects of taking oral corticosteroids:

[It] makes your skin thin, it makes you bruise, it gives you a wonderful shaped face, it gives you, as a woman, hair growth where you don't want it. It can interfere with your bone density, when you were younger it interfered with your hormones, it can interfere with everything. I'm getting cataracts, terrible reflux, interferes with your sleep pattern. It made me a steroid induced diabetic. I was actually on insulin for 12 months.

Female, aged 55, 30 years living with asthma

For others, having to follow the same medicine routine for the rest of their lives impacted their mental health and physical energy levels. For example, Marg described understanding the consequences of not taking her medicine but reported feeling tired of having to do the same time-consuming routine daily:

I think oh I'm too bloody tired to do all this you know, I don't want to get up and go and do all the treatment, the coughing. And if I lie there a little bit longer then eventually my head says 'Well, stay in, that's going to be much worse. Get out of bed, sit at the end of your table, it's the same up there as it is here'. I sit down at the table and I go through the process. I get my blood pressure monitor out for a start. I check all that out... grab the nebuliser when I need Ventolin.

> Female, aged 74, 66 years living with asthma

Some treatments and their associated costs could have unwelcome consequences. For some participants, the side effects from medicines used to control their asthma led to surgical operations and unexpected expenses. For example, Tony described that:

> My whole life has been controlled by the asthma there. It really has in a lot of ways. A lot of money [has] been spent on operation procedures there too, because of the asthma, because of the prednisone, you know. Because of the side effects. It's controlled my life, it really has. You've got no idea. Plenty of operations there for the eyes. I was paying about $14,000 for this detached retina there. It only covered about $8,000 with the health fund. Out of pocket about $6,000 there, you know.
>
> Male, aged 66, 60 years living with asthma

In summary, in this theme, we have shown that taking medicines to achieve a measure of control often resulted in negative consequences for users. Drug side effects, financial pressures and psychological burdens were common. These 'pharmaceutical lives' were cognitively, emotionally and physically draining.

Theme 3: 'Asthma control means saving your life. It's as simple as that' – The need for asthma control

In line with the CSM domain 'cure/control', our analysis revealed participants' beliefs regarding the critical importance of asthma control, and the accompanying cognitive and emotional work involved. Both internal and external forces were at play, as shown through the personal efforts of those living with the condition as well as the impact of support received from others, including family, friends and health professionals. Achieving asthma control was of prime importance to participants, mainly because this goal focused on the most basic of physiological tasks – breathing. Such is the severity of severe asthma that simply breathing well enough to perform taken-for-granted daily tasks was often a challenge. In contrast to the experiences of many people with mild to moderate asthma, respondents maintained that making sure they took their medicines was important for them to achieve asthma control. Pharmaceutical therapy thus was an integral part of respondents' lives.

Participants described what asthma control meant to them, how they controlled their condition and the emotional consequences of being unable to control their asthma. Having 'asthma control' often meant being able to do the things they wanted to do and not be limited by their symptoms, and for many, this was possible because of medication. For example, for John B, control was expressed in terms of his medicine:

> well controlled meant... not needing to take any prednisone or anything [and] I can do everything I want.
>
> Male, aged 72, 70 years living with asthma

Making sure they took their medicines as directed, making sure they had an up-to-date asthma action plan and avoiding potential triggers were identified by participants as ways of maintaining a sense of control over their severe asthma. They described not having a choice about taking medicine if they wanted to keep their symptoms at bay. For Justin, taking his medicine has become an automatic routine:

> You just take it in the morning automatically. You've got to have a routine.
>
> Male, aged 54, 53 years living with asthma

Individuals reflected that over the course of their lives living with severe asthma, they were prescribed different medicines to control their condition, as not all medicines were effective for every person and often it was a case of trial and error. Clive, for example, described that a new injectable biological medicine helps 'a bit'. He stated, however, that it may not be appropriate for everybody as you need to:

> meet all the parameters for it and [access is] quite stringent, get on the list (of people eligible for biological medicine) type of thing.
>
> Male, aged 56, 26 years living with asthma

An Asthma Action Plan was considered by participants as an empowering tool to help them achieve control over their asthma. The plans are individualised and provide instructions on how to adjust medications in response to asthma symptoms. They are designed to help a person with asthma take early action to prevent or reduce the severity of an asthma flare up. While this is a positive strategy for those living with severe asthma, access to these plans is restricted; only a medical practitioner can write an asthma action plan. Other healthcare professionals such as pharmacists or respiratory care nurses cannot provide these plans. Apart from the problem of obtaining an action plan, participants reported that having an Asthma Action Plan helped develop a sense of control over their condition, as illustrated by Margie:

> I've got an asthma plan. Yeah. So, I mean you just take your medication as prescribed, and then if you're still sick you take... you can up the dose. If you're still sick, and you've got a cold or something, or its [unfavourable] weather, you just take a few prednisone for a week or ten days, and that usually makes you better, so start again. And you just go back on whatever dose you were on before, you know, twice daily, whatever you take.
>
> Female, aged 67, 58 years living with asthma

Making sure medications are taken as directed and having an Asthma Action Plan was not always an effective strategy for keeping asthma under control. Kim, for example, described that attacks came on with no warning, sometimes leading to being intubated, and she felt that she was being controlled by this condition:

I don't know what it's going to do to me. I don't know when it's going to do it. I'm good now. You could leave in an hour and [my carer] could be sitting here talking to me and then I'll go and say 'OK I'll go in there'; I need a rest and then I'd be gone (needing medical intervention).

Female, aged 51, years with asthma unknown

Similarly, Shannon described constantly feeling fearful and anxious:

It's got control over me. I don't have control over it whatsoever. I think that I do, and I do everything right, I do all the medications that they want me to do that they just… it's scaring me now at least this time because it's coming to winter, and as soon as it comes to winter, I'm scared and you know it seems to flare up more when it comes to winter time.

Female, aged 39, 23 years living with asthma

External influences such as the quality of support received from friends, family and health care professionals acted to both disable and enable participants' sense of control over their severe asthma. Support from these external sources made a difference to the emotional and physical capabilities needed for making decisions and choosing courses of action. Participants valued feeling empowered and heard by these external influencers. Some felt supported by their siblings and parents, while others felt they were a 'burden' to their friends and family. Jemma's partner had accepted her condition; however, she reported feeling guilty as her partner had to support her. She reported how her condition had affected her family life:

My partner looks after me and knows exactly what's going on, knows when I'm having asthma, knows… just about knows when to call the ambulance and she goes by me a bit, she's getting more confident in making the decision without me… it affects my relationship because my partner is my carer and she does everything for me.

Female, aged 59, 7 years living with asthma

Participants reported varied interactions with their healthcare providers. Some were happy with interactions with their doctors and felt able to voice their opinion when they felt their asthma was not well controlled, and others reported that they were blamed for their illness; or simply not heard. For example, Lauren was frustrated that she didn't feel heard and believed by her healthcare provider when discussing her asthma control:

I feel like at the moment maybe it's frustrating and maybe this is literally just me as a person, but I feel like you could tell someone about an experience and all they'll do is just nod. And I'm like I just need a bit of context. Like, was that bad? Should that not be happening? Like, all this sort of stuff or like is it normal and that, 'Yeah, that can happen when like blah, blah, blah'. Like I don't know, I just need some context. Whereas at the moment I guess it's, like, very one-way. Like, I'll just tell you what happens and it's like they'll nod and all that sort of stuff.

> Female, aged 27, living with asthma since childhood

Monique felt that her doctors blamed her for the uncontrolled nature of her condition:

> I'm like taking everything people tell me to take... it's not that I'm not doing something and, I felt that the doctors were putting it on me, that it was somehow my fault that my asthma wasn't well controlled, and I'm like no, you're the people who medicate me, you have to work out what controls me. I don't know what drugs do what. So that was confounding, that it seemed that I was to blame a bit.
>
> Female, aged 39, 18 years living with asthma

Taken together, findings from this theme show that good asthma control was considered by our participants to be essential to their quality of life so they could carry out even simple everyday tasks and express their autonomy and independence. Our participants had a range of strategies to achieve this – strict adherence to medicine use, obtaining and using an Asthma Action Plan, and enlisting support from family, friends, and healthcare professionals. Asthma control, however, was not always easy or attainable, despite the careful attention paid to making sure medicines were taken as directed. Lack of control resulted in a sense of powerlessness that can accompany living with severe asthma.

Discussion

In this chapter, we drew on the CSM (Leventhal et al., 2016) to illustrate the complexities of everyday life with severe asthma and to illustrate the role that medicines play in the lives of those with severe asthma. Living with this condition is indeed a 'pharmaceutical life'. Severe asthma is not curable: people living with it are aware that they will need to depend on medicines to accomplish the basic physiological task of breathing

Our findings show that people with severe asthma have a complex relationship with the medicines needed both for life, and for a life well-lived. While most asthma research points to poor adherence to medicines use and ways to improve it (McDonald & Yorke, 2017; Rau, 2005), our previously published work and other studies have shown that people with severe asthma prioritised taking their medicines as directed (Armour et al., 2007; Blake, 2017; Eakin & Rand, 2012; Eassey, Reddel, Ryan, & Smith, 2019). For many participants, medicines enabled them to accomplish their broader life goals and for some, taking a higher-than-recommended dose was required, despite serious side effects (Eassey et al., 2019).

Our analysis was organised around three domains of the Leventhal et al., (2016) CSM, and enabled us to show the emotional, cognitive and environmental factors regarding participants' illness identities related to living with severe asthma, its consequences, and the contexts associated with gaining (or feeling loss of) control over this serious illness. Organising our data in this way furthered our understanding of the complex and nuanced experiences of living long-term with asthma and severe asthma. As we illustrated, for people living with severe asthma living a pharmaceutical life is cognitively, emotionally and physically draining. At different times, participants conveyed a lack of personal control over the disease, uncertainty as to when a flare-up might occur, resentment and reluctance about having to rely on medicines; and gratitude for the benefits of medicines when control was achieved. In other words, participants both resented and depended on pharmaceuticals to live their lives. Navigating the at-times choppy waters of healthcare professionals' capacity for understanding of and respect for their experiences also presented challenges for participants living with this debilitating condition.

An examination of the narratives of people's experiences of living with severe asthma undermines many of the existing assumptions about managing this condition: (1) taking medications as directed is not common among people with asthma; (2) a biomedical focus on managing the clinical aspects of the condition will automatically convey better quality of life and (3) health professionals are expert in the field of severe asthma and united in their treatment approaches. On the contrary, our findings have shown that taking medicines as directed is seen as a task vital to daily life, 'control' over severe asthma is by definition very difficult to achieve, and communication with healthcare professionals might not be forthcoming, and might not be consistent or trustworthy. We suggest that health carers reflect on the tensions between the external pressures of taking medicines, establishing and enacting action plans, obtaining health professional appointments and the internal pressures of wrestling with perceptions of illness identity and strong emotions that are a common feature in the daily lives of people living with severe asthma.

References

Armour, C., Bosnic-Anticevich, S., Brillant, M., Burton, D., Emmerton, L., Krass, I., ...Stewart, K. (2007). Pharmacy Asthma Care Program (PACP) improves outcomes for patients in the community. *Thorax, 62*(6), 496–502. doi:10.1136/thx.2006.064709

Blake, K. V. (2017). Improving adherence to asthma medications: current knowledge and future perspectives. *Curr Opin Pulm Med, 23*(1), 62–70. doi:10.1097/mcp.0000000000000334.

Chan, R. C. H., & Mak, W. W. S. (2016). Common sense model of mental illness: Understanding the impact of cognitive and emotional representations of mental illness on recovery through the mediation of self-stigma. *Psychiatry Res, 246*, 16–24. doi:10.1016/j.psychres.2016.09.013.

Chung, K. F., Wenzel, S. E., Brozek, J. L., Bush, A., Castro, M., Sterk, P. J., . . . Teague, W. G. (2014). International ERS/ATS guidelines on definition, evaluation and treatment of severe asthma. *Europ Resp J, 43*(2), 343–373. doi:10.1183/09031936.00202013.

Coleman, M. T., & Newton, K. S. (2005). Supporting self-management in patients with chronic illness. *Am Fam Physician, 72*(8), 1503–1510.

Eakin, M. N., & Rand, C. S. (2012). Improving patient adherence with asthma self-management practices: What works? *Ann Allerg, Asthma Immunol: OfficPublic Am Coll Allerg, Asthma, Immunol, 109*(2), 90–92. doi:10.1016/j.anai.2012.06.009.

Eassey, D., Reddel, H. K., Ryan, K., & Smith, L. (2019). Living with severe asthma: the role of perceived competence and goal achievement. *Chronic Illn,* 1742395319884104. doi:10.1177/1742395319884104.

Forum of International Respiratory Societies. (2017). *The Global Impact of Respiratory Disease* 2nd ed. Sheffield, European Respiratory Society.

Foster, J. M., McDonald, V. M., Guo, M., & Reddel, Helen K. (2017). "I have lost in every facet of my life": The hidden burden of severe asthma. *Europ Resp J, 50*(3). doi:10.1183/13993003.00765-2017.

Gale, N. K., Heath, G., Cameron, E., Rashid, S., & Redwood, S. (2013). Using the framework method for the analysis of qualitative data in multi-disciplinary health research. *BMC Med Res Methodol, 13*(1), 117. doi:10.1186/1471-2288-13-117.

Herxheimer, A., McPherson, A., Miller, R., Shepperd, S., Yaphe, J., & Ziebland, S. (2000). Database of patients' experiences (DIPEx): A multi-media approach to sharing experiences and information. *The Lancet, 355*(9214), 1540–1543. doi:doi:10.1016/S0140-6736(00)02174-7

Huston, S. A., & Houk, C. P. (2011). Common sense model of illness in youth with type 1 diabetes or sickle cell disease. *J Pediatr Pharmacol Ther, 16*(4), 270–280. doi:10.5863/1551-6776-16.4.270.

Jones, M. C., MacGillivray, S., Kroll, T., Zohoor, A. R., & Connaghan, J. (2011). A thematic analysis of the conceptualisation of self-care, self-management and self-management support in the long-term conditions management literature. *J Nurs Healthc Chronic Illn, 3*(3), 174–185. doi:10.1111/j.1752-9824.2011.01096.x.

Lefebvre, P., Duh, M. S., Lafeuille, M. H., Gozalo, L., Desai, U., Robitaille, M. N.,…Dalal, A. A. (2015). Acute and chronic systemic corticosteroid-related complications in patients with severe asthma. *J Allergy Clin Immunol, 136*(6), 1488–1495. doi:10.1016/j.jaci.2015.07.046.

Lenzen, S. A., Daniëls, R., van Bokhoven, M. A., van der Weijden, T., & Beurskens, A. (2017). Disentangling self-management goal setting and action planning: A scoping review. *PloS One, 12*(11), e0188822. doi:10.1371/journal.pone.0188822.

Leventhal, H., Phillips, L. A., & Burns, E. (2016). The Common-Sense Model of Self-Regulation (CSM): a dynamic framework for understanding illness self-management. *J Behav Med, 39*(6), 935–946. doi:10.1007/s10865-016-9782-2.

Mann, E. G., Lefort, S., & Vandenkerkhof, E. G. (2013). Self-management interventions for chronic pain. *Pain Manag, 3*(3), 211–222. doi:10.2217/pmt.13.9.

Masoli, M., Fabian, D., Holt, S., & Beasley, R. (2004). The global burden of asthma: executive summary of the GINA Dissemination Committee report. *Allergy, 59*(5), 469–478. doi:10.1111/j.1398-9995.2004.00526.x.

McDonald V. M., & Yorke J. (2017). Adherence in severe asthma: time to get it right. *Europ Resp J, 50*(6), 1702191. doi:10.1183/13993003.02191-2017.

McDonald, V. M., Maltby, S., Reddel, H. K., King, G. G., Wark, P. A., Smith, L., …Gibson, P. G. (2017). Severe asthma: Current management, targeted therapies and future directions-A roundtable report. *Respirology, 22*(1), 53–60. doi:10.1111/resp.12957.

Morgan, H. M., Entwistle, V. A., Cribb, A., Christmas, S., Owens, J., Skea, Z. C., & Watt, I. S. (2017). We need to talk about purpose: a critical interpretive synthesis of health and social care professionals' approaches to self-management support for people with long-term conditions. *Health Exp, 20*(2), 243–259. doi:10.1111/hex.12453.

Papi, A., Brightling, C., Pedersen, S. E., & Reddel, H. K. (2018). Asthma. *Lancet, 391*(10122), 783–800. doi:10.1016/s0140-6736(17)33311-1.

Pike, K. C., Levy, M. L., Moreiras, J., & Fleming, L. (2018). Managing problematic severe asthma: beyond the guidelines. *Arch Dis Child, 103*(4), 392–397. doi:10.1136/archdischild-2016-311368.

Pinnock, H. (2015). Supported self-management for asthma. *Breathe (Sheff), 11*(2), 98–109. doi:10.1183/20734735.015614.

Rau, J. L. (2005). Determinants of patient adherence to an aerosol regimen. *Resp Care, 50*(10), 1346–1359.

Sabate, E. (2003). Adherence to long-term therapies: evidence for action. Retrieved from World Health Organization.

Sadatsafavi, M., Lynd, L., Marra, C., Carleton, B., Tan, W. C., Sullivan, S., & FitzGerald, J. M. (2010). Direct health care costs associated with asthma in British Columbia. *Can Resp J: J Can Thorac Soc, 17*(2), 74–80.

Shaw, D. E., Sousa, A. R., Fowler, S. J., Fleming, L. J., Roberts, G., Corfield, J., . . . Chung, K. F. (2015). Clinical and inflammatory characteristics of the European U-BIOPRED adult severe asthma cohort. *Eur Respir J, 46*(5), 1308–1321. doi:10.1183/13993003.00779-2015.

Williams, B., Steven, K., & Sullivan, F. M. (2011). Tacit and transitionary: an exploration of patients' and primary care health professionals' goals in relation to asthma. *Soc Sci Med, 72*(8), 1359–1366. doi:10.1016/j.socscimed.2011.02.038.

Ziebland, S., Lavie-Ajayi, M., & Lucius-Hoene, G. (2015). The role of the Internet for people with chronic pain: Examples from the DIPEx International Project. *Brit J Pain, 9*(1), 62–64. doi:10.1177/2049463714555438.

Ziebland, S., Powell, J., Briggs, P., Jenkinson, C., Wyke, S., Sillence, E., ...Farmer, A. (2016). Programme grants for applied research. In *Examining the Role of Patients' Experiences as a Resource for Choice and Decision-Making in Health Care: A Creative, Interdisciplinary Mixed-Method Study in Digital Health*. Southampton (UK): NIHR Journals Library.

5 Pregnancy, urinary tract infections and antibiotics

Prenatal attachment and competing health priorities

Flavia Ghouri, Amelia Hollywood and Kath Ryan

Introduction and background

Pregnancy is the period in which a foetus grows and develops inside a woman's body. The normal duration of a pregnancy is nine months or about 40 weeks. It is a physiological state in which women go through a number of physical and emotional changes. The physical changes can be accompanied by uncomfortable symptoms such as nausea or vomiting and cause women to seek medical support and advice. Among the many different types of health problems experienced during pregnancy, one common condition that can affect women is an infection of the urinary tract. A urinary tract infection (UTI) is normally caused by transfer of bacteria from the gut into the genitourinary tract where they can multiply and cause an infection (Flores-Mireles, Walker, Caparon, & Hultgren, 2015). Behaviours such as not drinking adequate water or wiping the genitals from back to front after urination are associated with developing urinary infections (Ghouri, Hollywood, & Ryan, 2018). UTIs are among the most frequently occurring infections in pregnancy and cause symptoms such as increased frequency of urination and burning pain when passing urine (Delzell & Lefevre, 2000). Infections can also be asymptomatic, however, meaning that bacteria can infect the urinary tract without any outward signs or symptoms.

Asymptomatic infections are estimated to affect 2–12% of pregnant women (UK National Screening Committee, 2017) and are normally diagnosed through routine screening in the first trimester of pregnancy. Previous studies have shown that UTIs, both symptomatic and asymptomatic, are associated with a number of negative outcomes in pregnancy. For example, there are studies which associate UTIs with preterm birth, restricted foetal growth and even miscarriage (Matuszkiewicz-Rowińska, Małyszko, & Wieliczko, 2015). Due to these risks, routine screening for UTIs in pregnant women is a standard practice in many countries. Treatment is essential upon a positive diagnosis and a short course of a suitable antibiotic is prescribed to clear the infection. Although women and health professionals can sometimes be concerned about using medicines in pregnancy, due to a risk of teratogenicity (i.e., harm to the developing foetus), most antibiotics used to treat UTIs are effective and have a good safety profile (Crider et al., 2009).

Despite their value in avoiding complications arising from UTIs, antibiotic use is not without risks. One major issue with antibiotics, regardless of the state of pregnancy, is the problem of antimicrobial resistance. Antimicrobial resistance (AMR) is a naturally occurring phenomenon by which microorganisms such as bacteria undergo spontaneous changes in their genetic make-up to develop resilience against antibiotic medicines. The genetic changes allow bacteria to resist antibiotic treatment and cause infections that can eventually progress to life-threatening conditions if no effective antibiotic is available. AMR is fuelled by antibiotic use therefore a conservative approach to using antibiotics is vital and discouraging excessive use has been the focus of attention in multiple health campaigns (McNulty & Johnson, 2008; McNulty, Nichols, Boyle, Woodhead, & Davey, 2010). Considered within the context of pregnancy, it is also evident that AMR infections can be a particular challenge for women. This is because suitable antibiotics to treat infections in pregnancy are those that are not only effective at treating the infection but also do not cause any negative impact on foetal development. The requirement to ensure foetal safety can thus limit antibiotic treatment options which might otherwise be available to non-pregnant women (Rizvi, Khan, Shukla, Malik, & Shaheen, 2011).

Methods

We conducted two qualitative research studies with pregnant women to explore their experience of developing a UTI in pregnancy (Study One), and their perceptions of AMR (Study Two). The first study analysed the views of women as expressed through their posts on an online pregnancy forum (Ghouri, Hollywood, & Ryan, 2019). The online forum serves as a digital space, predominantly for women, where people can share their experiences on different topics or 'conversational threads'. Topics discussed on the forum vary and can range from health issues to political and social agendas. The conversation threads were searched using the search function on the website under the topic of UTIs in pregnancy. The search results were then downloaded and analysed using inductive thematic analysis. Although the exact demographics are difficult to ascertain, a census described subscribers to this website as predominantly White, British, women in their 30s or 40s with a degree qualification (Mumsnet Census, 2009). The second study was conducted by interviewing 15 women about their views on AMR. The demographic details of the women in the interview study were similar to the women in the first study. Women were invited to participate in this research study through online advertisements on social media. A single telephone interview was then conducted with women who lived in the United Kingdom and had experienced a UTI during pregnancy. The interviews were recorded for the purpose of transcription and then analysed using inductive thematic analysis. Both studies revealed multiple concerns within the context of UTIs in pregnancy. The benefits and risks to the women, the foetus, and society are weighed and assigned priority. This chapter collates and presents the research using excerpts from participants in the two research studies with a focus on women's perspectives of experiencing a UTI during pregnancy, in an era where AMR is a growing and pressing health threat.

This research was reviewed and granted ethical approval by the University of Reading's Research and Ethics Committee (Ref: 17/30).

Findings

Illness perceptions

The term 'illness perception' describes people's knowledge and beliefs about their illness (Boltz et al., 2013). It can be defined as 'a patient's common-sense beliefs about their illness' (Leventhal, Meyer, & Nerenz, 1980) which determines how they behave in response to becoming ill. UTIs are the most frequent type of infection affecting women during their pregnancy and this was a common perception held by the majority of women in both studies. As well as viewing UTIs as being common in pregnancy, however, women also attributed the pregnancy as the cause of the UTI. Many women had the perception that they had a lowered state of immunity while they were pregnant which when combined with hormonal changes in the body, puts them at a greater risk of developing a UTI compared to when not pregnant:

> You're so susceptible when you're pregnant because your immune system seems to be so uhm… compromised when you're pregnant.
>
> Study Two, Participant 1, 31 years

Most women thought that the physiological changes due to pregnancy meant that diagnosis through a dipstick test was trickier compared to when not pregnant. A dipstick test refers to a diagnostic test in which a chemically treated strip of material is dipped into a urine sample to indicate the presence of an infection. Similarity between the symptoms of a UTI, and the uncomfortable symptoms that women might experience in the normal course of pregnancy, such as increased frequency of urination and back or abdominal pain, were also thought to contribute to this diagnostic difficulty. The problem with differentiating the symptoms also led to women's feelings of uncertainty about the need for antibiotics:

> I also had trouble getting diagnosed when pregnant and was told by the midwife that it's because there are so many things present in your pee and altering what's in your pee when pregnant that it can be hard to get a dip result indicating a UTI.
>
> Study One, Bella

Women who had a history of UTIs, however, felt more confident that they had an infection when they experienced UTI-like symptoms. Knowing their own bodies, and having experienced UTI symptoms in the past, meant that they felt certain about when they had a UTI as opposed to a symptom of their pregnancy.

In such cases, women felt that they were right in seeking medical assistance and demanding the care that they needed:

> I suffer cystitis awfully regularly and really painfully when I'm not pregnant and knew exactly what was wrong with me but for whatever reason, there was not enough bacteria to show in my pee. I had to fight for antibiotics to put it right and it was only due to my medical history that I was prescribed anything!
>
> Study One, Brenda

There was also a perception that the development of a UTI during pregnancy was a greater cause for concern than when not pregnant. The reason behind this perception was the association of UTIs with negative pregnancy outcomes such as preterm birth or miscarriage. Most women's views are reflected in the following two quotes that demonstrate the fear and anxiety felt due to a UTI in pregnancy:

> I'm really worried as I'm aware UTIs, if left untreated, can cause miscarriage. I feel like a sitting duck! I'm obviously glugging away at the water and cranberry juice, but the pains are worrying me.
>
> Study One, Rachel

> I decided that I would take the antibiotics because normally when I had UTIs outside of pregnancy I would just take lots of water and let it ride it out but because I was pregnant I knew there was a risk of early birth so I was happy to take the antibiotics at that point.
>
> Study Two, Participant 3, 31 years

In contrast, there were a small number of women who did not think that UTIs were anything to be overly concerned about as they are fairly common and easily treatable with antibiotics:

> I had the same around 20 weeks pregnant and I've had 4 more since (I'm now 36 weeks) the antibiotics should clear it up pretty quick and they are forever testing your urine... I wouldn't worry.
>
> Study One, Nicole

The majority of women expressed concern and a keenness to obtain prompt antibiotic treatment to clear the infection. The uncertainty about the cause of the symptoms, either pregnancy or an infection, combined with an awareness that UTIs can negatively affect pregnancy caused increased expectation to use antibiotics as an insurance option 'to be on the safe side' and 'just in case' of an infection. Most women did not consider preventative behaviours, such as maintaining adequate fluid intake, to be effective at avoiding UTIs and indicated an automatic reliance on antibiotics if symptoms of a UTI were experienced.

Furthermore, combined with the previously mentioned risks that UTIs pose to pregnancy, most women felt obliged to use antibiotics even when some might have preferred alternative management options:

> Um well, you know, normal hygiene that everyone knows. Sort of wiping from front to back and general cleanliness – although I mean I suppose that doesn't make much difference.
>
> Study Two, Participant 12, 43 years

> If you weren't pregnant you could maybe take your friend's advice to drink water and cranberry juice and wait it out but given that you are pregnant it's irresponsible advice to be honest.
>
> Study One, Nikita

The preference to use antibiotics was demonstrably clear in the descriptions surrounding antibiotic use. Understandably, however, a few women were concerned about using antibiotics while they were pregnant because of uncertainty and a fear relating to how the medication might affect their baby as seen in the following quote:

> They gave me antibiotics for what they suspect is a UTI... just worried now after seeing the heartbeat that taking the antibiotics will do something to baba
>
> Study One, Sally

Despite the concerns, most women felt that antibiotics were safe in comparison to the risks of a UTI. They used their doctor's prescription as evidence of the safety of the antibiotics because they trusted their doctor not to prescribe something that might cause harm to their baby:

> Doc wouldn't prescribe if dangerous. It's more dangerous to leave a UTI, as at its worst it can cause kidney issues and miscarriage.
>
> Study One, Carey

The illness perceptions of women experiencing a UTI indicate that they thought they had reduced 'self-efficacy' for maintaining their own health in pregnancy. Self-efficacy is a theoretical construct developed by Bandura in his Social Cognition Theory (Bandura, 1986). It refers to the belief a person has in their own ability to perform an action to bring about a desired change. Self-efficacy is linked with personal agency, which is the sense of control and power a person feels, about performing a task or behaviour. A review by Luszczynska & Schwarzer (2015) described how an individual's expectancy about a behaviour and their self-efficacy determines their performance of that behaviour. Women's illness perceptions showed that, on the whole, they expected UTIs to have highly negative outcomes and therefore relied on pharmaceuticals, that is, antibiotics in this case. Similarly, they expected prevention measures to be ineffective and therefore did not consider them to be an important part of their personal health routine thus demonstrating low self-efficacy in managing their health in pregnancy.

Ogden et al. have described health models where the cause of an illness and its resolution could be attributed to internal individual or external uncontrollable factors (Ogden et al., 1999, 2001). Women's illness perceptions, described above, are reflected in a 'biomedical model'. The biomedical model, as defined by Ogden (2012) refers to associating the cause of an illness as external and beyond the control of the self. In the biomedical model, an ill person assigns the cause of an illness to involuntary factors beyond their direct influence, for example, germs or their genetic make-up. The biomedical model encourages medical solutions to problems and unsurprisingly pharmaceuticals, in these cases antibiotics, were seen as the main solution for UTIs according to women and their accounts of the healthcare professionals they consulted.

As previously mentioned, a number of women attributed lowered immunity due to pregnancy as the cause of the infection. As a result, the solution to disease and illness was also viewed to be external from the self, provided by healthcare professionals through interventions such as antibiotics. Since the biomedical model focused on external factors as the cause and solution to an illness, it overlooks internal factors, such as one's own health behaviours, which can play a key part in causing and solving health issues. Most women in the two studies attributed the cause of their UTI to lowered immunity in pregnancy that resulted in increased pharmaceuticalisation in their lives. This led them to rely on antibiotics for a quick, albeit efficient, cure. The reliance on antibiotics was strongly indicated by the following quote, 'How will I ever get rid of this without antibiotics [is the] question that really dragged me down' (Study One, Lynn).

Conceptualisation of antimicrobial resistance

Women's conceptualisation of AMR in the two studies was not considerably different from what has previously been described in the literature on public perceptions of AMR (Brookes-Howell et al., 2012; Brooks, Shaw, Sharp, & Hay, 2008; Norris et al., 2013). The majority of women had heard about AMR and described it as a health threat due to antibiotics losing their effectiveness. Despite this awareness, however, uncertainty about the problem still existed. The main area where women expressed uncertainty was with regards to how AMR affects society versus an individual who is prescribed and uses antibiotics. Most women were unclear about how resistant bacteria transfer among people in close contact and spread across the social community to cause a rise in AMR infections:

> Well I assumed that it was an individual that built up resistance because they were given a lot of antibiotics and that eventually it stops working on that person. I'm not sure how it works if you've never taken antibiotics and then you need them.
>
> Study Two, Participant 1, 31 years

AMR was often referred to as a hypothetical problem that had the potential to be a significant health issue in the future if antibiotics were to 'eventually stop working'. It was not described as a current health threat that affects people in the present:

> I think I've heard in the media that they've [antibiotics] been overprescribed in the past and – and, we might end up at a point where some of us are resistant to uh, like, they won't help us.
>
> Study Two, Participant 11, 29 years

Despite viewing it as a future problem, AMR was acknowledged as a health risk that needed to be tackled. A few women suggested focusing on improving diagnostic support and increasing efforts to educate the public, however, most women were unsure about how they should respond to this issue. In this vein, they considered AMR as a problem affecting the healthcare sector that could therefore be best addressed through the increased awareness and efforts of healthcare professionals rather than members of the public:

> I would say there is a bit of an issue with GPs over prescribing antibiotics and there needs to be more awareness at the healthcare professional level.
>
> Study Two, Participant 7, 32 years

The uncertainty surrounding antibiotic use and how individuals could respond to AMR was often referred to in relation to the beneficial effects of antibiotics. As these medicines are valuable in treating infections, AMR posed a dilemma around how they could be used appropriately. As one interview participant (Study Two, Participant 8, 38 years) mentioned, antibiotics caused problems but they 'also save lives'.

Uncertainty surrounding AMR was also particularly apparent when women expressed confusion due to 'conflicting messages' about the consumption of antibiotics. Treatment with antibiotics normally occurs over a defined period of days, which is termed as the 'antibiotic course'. Traditional health advice encourages people to finish the treatment course, even if they feel they have recovered, to prevent reinfections with resistant bacteria. A small number of women, however, reported feeling a conflict with regards to whether they should finish the antibiotic course after being exposed to a different message in the news. For example,

> You get the odd media report saying that, you know, you shouldn't finish the course and your doctor's telling you to finish the course, so I think there is a lot of misinformation about resistance.
>
> Study Two, Participant 3, 31 years

The way women conceptualised AMR demonstrated a picture of uncertainty about their own role in tackling this health issue. They recognised AMR as a threat but one that affected the health of the individual taking antibiotics rather than society as a whole. It was seen as a risk that might become problematic in the future, in contrast to a current and pressing issue. This way of conceptualising AMR reduces 'self-efficacy', that is their belief that they can do anything to reduce the rise of AMR, a construct that was introduced earlier. The uncertainty surrounding AMR coupled with anxiety over the risk of a UTI in pregnancy meant that most women delegated responsibility to health care professionals. They felt disempowered about the decision-making affecting their health, even though they recognised AMR as a health threat. In a small number of cases, because the short-term worry about UTIs upstaged the longer-term concerns about using antibiotics, women felt like they had to argue their case to ensure they were treated:

> The walk-in centre doctor tried to turn me away too with a negative dip result but I argued the toss with her because I'd had so many that I knew what it was and she gave me the antibiotics.
>
> Study One, Bella

Overall, women's illness perceptions about UTIs in pregnancy and their conceptualisation of the effects of AMR on personal and societal health contributes to pharmaceuticalisation in pregnancy. The uncertainties and risks associated with experiencing an infection, which can affect both their own and their baby's health, resulted in women considering antibiotics as a safe necessity while the health risks of AMR became overshadowed.

Pregnancy as deviation from the norm

Previous research into women's experiences has shown that UTIs can cause painful symptoms that might lead to a significant disruption to women's daily lives (Butler, Hawking, Quigley, & McNulty, 2015; Flower, Bishop, & Lewith, 2014; Malterud & Bærheim, 1999). The research studies presented in this chapter also correspond with the previous research, as women frequently expressed their pain and discomfort if they had a symptomatic UTI. In addition to the unpleasant symptoms, however, women's concern for their child was clearly evident in their frustration and anxiety. Feelings of guilt due to developing an infection which put their unborn baby at risk were a significant difference between experiencing a UTI in pregnancy compared to when not pregnant. Descriptions of the infection in relation to the pregnancy were therefore highly emotive and highlighted the pregnancy as a unique physiological state:

> I don't know why but it makes me feel like such a failure each time the results come back with an infection still present. I get angry with myself that I can't get my body to do its job to fight it and I'm putting my baby at risk. Stupid I know but I can't help it.
>
> Study One, Nadia

The increased anxiety due to the infection, because of the risks of the UTI in pregnancy, also affected how women considered the management of the infection. For example, a number of women described themselves as people who do not like taking antibiotics because of the side effects or because they had concerns about AMR. During pregnancy, however, they felt that it was their only option even if they had concerns about using medicines in pregnancy. The following quote demonstrates the reluctance of a woman to take antibiotics but she changed her mind after communicating with a healthcare professional who convinced her to take them:

> Um, I – I think this is where she [pharmacist] just said, if – you know, if the infection goes from your urinary tract into the womb [sic] that it, it could be very very serious, that it could... it could go wrong very quickly.
>
> Study Two, Participant 9, 43 years

The distinctiveness of pregnancy also highlighted the issue with using any new alternative treatment to antibiotics. Although they might be useful in response to AMR, new treatments might not be an option for pregnant women because of concerns about how they might impact the foetus:

> It's a very good idea, anything that reduces the need for antibiotics. It depends what they are in some respects so if you're talking about probiotics or food supplements or something like that, that's one thing, but if it's a novel drug then you're always concerned about new drugs in pregnancy.
>
> Study Two, Participant 3, 31 years

Women's references to their pregnancy demonstrated that they had a strong maternal attachment that drove them to be concerned about the safe development of their baby. This 'prenatal attachment' to the foetus before its birth has been described in literature and was derived from John Bowlby's Theory of Human Attachment (Bowlby, 1958). Prenatal attachment can be described as 'the extent to which women engage in behaviours that represent an affiliation and interaction with their unborn child' (Cranley, 1981). Research has shown the value of prenatal attachment in promoting health behaviours, as women with higher levels of attachment are more receptive to adopting health protective behaviours (Lindgren, 2001; Magee et al., 2014). Almost all women strongly perceived UTIs to threaten the normal progression of their pregnancy and feared that developing an infection would hinder the normal growth of the foetus and also increase the risk of preterm birth. Their main concern, therefore, arose not from experiencing debilitating symptoms but a fear for the safety of their child, particularly evident by women expressing worry even when they had asymptomatic infections. Prenatal attachment to the baby also led some women to question the use of antibiotics during pregnancy. It was this same attachment and concern for their child, however, that meant they were convinced by healthcare professionals to use the antibiotics because it was in the best interests of their baby. In essence, the research studies highlighted feelings that are deeply emotive, as seen through women's illness perceptions, and conveyed a clear sense of maternal concern for their baby and less focus on the impact of the UTI on their own health. Pregnancy is therefore a state that deviates from the norm in terms of the immediate concerns that a non-pregnant individual affected by ill health might face.

Discussion

Prenatal attachment in competing health priorities

The nature of UTIs in pregnancy is a situation where a relatively common and easy to treat infection affects an individual whose health directly affects the health of another, the developing foetus. Pregnancy, therefore, presents multiple challenges for women as they seek to weigh the risks and benefits to their own health and the developmental health of their baby.

Both studies report women's distress when they develop a UTI during pregnancy because of debilitating symptoms that significantly affect their quality of life. Experiencing symptoms of a UTI at a time when a woman is going through potentially uncomfortable physical changes can be an emotional experience and cause feelings of frustration. At the same time, risks of a UTI such as preterm birth or even miscarriage can be particularly frightening. This is especially true in circumstances where the pregnancy can be classed as 'precious', for example, in cases where women struggled with infertility or a history of miscarriage. The use of pharmaceuticals during pregnancy adds an additional layer of distress for some women. Research on the perceived risks of harm to the foetus has shown that women consider antibiotics to be moderately harmful in pregnancy (Petersen, McCrea, Lupattelli, & Nordeng, 2015). Although most women who participated in our research were quite optimistic about the safety of antibiotics, there was still a small proportion of women who experienced side effects or for whom using an antibiotic while pregnant was a source of anxiety. This was evident in some of the quotes in earlier sections and in the following quote, 'I'm petrified that taking amoxicillin will harm baby!' (Study One, Liza). The well-established risk of AMR that is associated with the use of antibiotics adds further complexity to this mix of issues. Health campaigns on AMR have been targeting the public with the message of conserving antibiotics to ensure they are effective when their need is essential. Faced with these issues, it would appear that women's behaviour is determined through a process of assigning priority to these problems.

The findings from the two studies presented in this chapter show the crucial role of prenatal attachment in women's decision-making about the management of UTIs during pregnancy. In the presence of multiple issues, it is the attachment to the foetus and the desire to protect and ensure its safety that primarily determines women's perceptions and behaviour. Therefore, while maintaining concerns about using antibiotics in pregnancy, women opt to use them to minimise the risks to their pregnancy from UTIs as these are the risks that they are more aware of and consider to be severe. Similarly, while recognising AMR as a risk to societal health, prenatal attachment to the foetus remains the determining factor for mothers' reliance on antibiotics to achieve and maintain health.

Conclusion

This chapter summarises the research from two qualitative studies that explored women's experiences of UTIs during pregnancy and their perceptions of AMR. Women attributed pregnancy as the cause of their UTIs, due to lowered immunity that increased the risk of developing infections. Most considered it harder to get diagnosed and be treated for UTIs in pregnancy compared to when not pregnant. Similarly, they also viewed UTIs to be more serious in pregnancy because of risks such as preterm birth and miscarriage. For these reasons, the majority of women expected and relied on antibiotics when they had symptoms suggestive of a UTI, such as increased frequency of urination, even though these might be normal symptoms of pregnancy. Illness perceptions reflected in a biomedical model reduced self-efficacy and increased pharmaceuticalisation in pregnancy. The women sought medical solutions (external) in favour of behaviour change (internal) that could ease symptoms and prevent infections.

AMR was conceptualised similarly to previous studies and many women were uncertain about how it affects society when it is an individual who is given antibiotics. Most also viewed AMR to be a future threat, with short-term worries about developing UTIs transcending their concern about resistant infections. Some women also expressed confusion about conflicting messages with regards to AMR that resulted in feelings of uncertainty about how this health issue could be tackled by them. The perceptions surrounding AMR also show reduced self-efficacy as women looked towards healthcare professionals for solutions and were uncertain about how they could be involved with tackling AMR.

Both the studies highlighted pregnancy as a unique state and a deviation from the non-pregnant norm in terms of how UTIs affect health. Prenatal attachment to their baby was pivotal in shaping women's decision-making and behaviour. As the UTI not only affected their own health but also the development of the foetus, women had strong maternal feelings and, in some cases, expressed guilt about developing an infection. Since UTIs could result in negative outcomes for the pregnancy, women considered antibiotics to be a better and safer option than avoiding antibiotics, even when they had concerns about using pharmaceuticals during pregnancy. In this way, pregnancy was pharmaceuticalised in response to the high risks associated with a UTI in this population.

The research presented in this chapter demonstrates the complexity of issues that arise when women experience UTIs in pregnancy. Women have to consider their own health as well as the effects of the infection and treatment on their baby. At the same time, the rising risk of AMR requires careful evaluation of antibiotics, which has been the focus of multiple public health campaigns discouraging excessive use. Faced with these competing priorities, women base their decisions on the best interest of their baby because of prenatal attachment. Ultimately, this results in increased pharmaceuticalisation through reliance on antibiotics, as the risks of AMR become eclipsed by the risks of a UTI.

References

Bandura, A. (1986). *Social Foundations of Thought and Action*. Englewood Cliffs: Prentice Hall.

Boltz, M., Rau, H., Williams, P., Rau, H., Williams, P., Upton, J., ... Remaud, A. (2013). Illness cognitions and perceptions. In *Encyclopedia of Behavioral Medicine* (pp. 1027–1030). New York: Springer. doi:10.1007/978-1-4419-1005-9_967.

Bowlby, J. (1958). The Nature of the child's tie to his mother. *The International Journal of Psychoanalysis*, 39, 350–373.

Brookes-Howell, L., Elwyn, G., Hood, K., Wood, F., Cooper, L., Goossens, H., ... Butler, C. C. (2012). "The body gets used to them": Patients' interpretations of antibiotic resistance and the implications for containment strategies. *The Journal of General Internal Medicine*, 27(7), 766–772. https://doi.org/doi:10.1007/s11606-011-1916-1.

Brooks, L., Shaw, A., Sharp, D., & Hay, A. D. (2008). Towards a better understanding of patients' perspectives of antibiotic resistance and MRSA: A qualitative study. *Family Practice*, 25(5), 341–348. https://doi.org/doi:10.1093/fampra/cmn037.

Butler, C. C., Hawking, M. K. D., Quigley, A., & McNulty, C. A. M. (2015). Incidence, severity, help seeking, and management of uncomplicated urinary tract infection: A population-based survey. *British Journal of General Practice*. doi:10.3399/bjgp15X686965.

Cranley, M. S. (1981). Development of a tool for the measurement of maternal attachment during pregnancy. *Nursing Research*, 30(5), 281–284.

Crider, K., Cleves, M., Reefhuis, J., Berry, R., Hobbs, C., & Hu, D. (2009). Antibacterial medication use during pregnancy and risk of birth defects national birth defects prevention study. *Archives of Pediatrics and Adolescent Medicine*, 163(11), 978–985. Retrieved from http://jamanetwork.com/journals/jamapediatrics/fullarticle/382406.

Delzell, J. E. J., & Lefevre, M. L. (2000). Urinary tract infections during pregnancy. *American Family Physician*, 61(3), 713–721.

Flores-Mireles, A. L., Walker, J. N., Caparon, M., & Hultgren, S. J. (2015). Urinary tract infections: Epidemiology, mechanisms of infection and treatment options. *Nature Reviews. Microbiology*, 13(5), 269–284. doi:10.1038/nrmicro3432.

Flower, A., Bishop, F. L., & Lewith, G. (2014). How women manage recurrent urinary tract infections: An analysis of postings on a popular web forum. *BMC Family Practice*, 15, 162. doi:10.1186/1471-2296-15-162.

Ghouri, F., Hollywood, A., & Ryan, K. (2018). A systematic review of non-antibiotic measures for the prevention of urinary tract infections in pregnancy. *BMC Pregnancy and Childbirth*, 18(99), 1–10. https://doi.org/doi:10.1186/s12884-018-1732-2.

Ghouri, F., Hollywood, A., & Ryan, K. (2019). Urinary tract infections and antibiotic use in pregnancy – qualitative analysis of online forum content. *BMC Pregnancy and Childbirth*, 19(1), 289. doi:10.1186/s12884-019-2451-z.

Leventhal, H., Meyer, D., & Nerenz, D. (1980). The common sense representation of illness danger. In *Contributions to Medical Psychology*. (Rachman S., Ed.), (Vol. 2). New York: Pergamon.

Lindgren, K. (2001). Relationships among maternal-fetal attachment, prenatal depression, and health practices in pregnancy. *Research in Nursing & Health*, 24(3), 203–217. doi:10.1002/nur.1023.

Luszczynska, A., & Schwarzer, R. (2015). Social cognitive theory. In *Predicting and Changing Health Behaviour: Research and Practice with Social Cognition Models*. 3rd ed. (M. Conner & P. Norman, Eds.). Maidenhead, UK: Open University Press.

Magee, S. R., Bublitz, M. H., Orazine, C., Brush, B., Salisbury, A., Niaura, R., & Stroud, L. R. (2014). The relationship between maternal-fetal attachment and cigarette smoking over pregnancy. *Maternal and Child Health Journal, 18*(4), 1017–1022. doi:10.1007/s10995-013-1330-x.

Malterud, K., & Bærheim, A. (1999). Peeing barbed wire: Symptom experiences in women with lower urinary tract infection. *Scandinavian Journal of Primary Health Care, 17*(1), 49–53. doi:10.1080/028134399750002908.

Matuszkiewicz-Rowińska, J., Małyszko, J., & Wieliczko, M. (2015). Urinary tract infections in pregnancy: Old and new unresolved diagnostic and therapeutic problems. *Archives of Medical Science, 11*(1), 67–77. doi:10.5114/aoms.2013.39202.

McNulty, C. A. M., & Johnson, A. P. (2008). The European antibiotic awareness day. *Journal of Antimicrobial Chemotherapy.* doi:10.1093/jac/dkn410.

McNulty, C. A. M., Nichols, T., Boyle, P. J., Woodhead, M., & Davey, P. (2010). The English antibiotic awareness campaigns: Did they change the public's knowledge of and attitudes to antibiotic use? *Journal of Antimicrobial Chemotherapy, 65*(7), 1526–1533. doi:10.1093/jac/dkq126.

Mumsnet Census. (2009). Mumsnet Census. Retrieved May 25, 2017, from https://www.mumsnet.com/info/census-2009.

Norris, P., Chamberlain, K., Dew, K., Gabe, J., Hodgetts, D., & Madden, H. (2013). Public beliefs about antibiotics, infection and resistance: A qualitative study. *Antibiotics, 2*(4), 465–476. doi:10.3390/antibiotics2040465.

Ogden, Jane. (2012). *Health Psychology: A textbook*, 5th edition. Maidenhead: Open University Press.

Ogden, J., Boden, J., Caird, R., Chor, C.., Flynn, M., Hunt, M., … Thapur, V. (1999). You're depressed, no I'm not': GPs and patients different models of depression. *British Journal of General Practice, 49*, 123–124.

Ogden, Jane, Bandara, I., Cohen, H., Farmer, D., Hardie, J., Minas, H., … Whitehead, M.-A. (2001). General practitioners' and patients' models of obesity: Whose problem is it? *Patient Education and Counseling, 44*(3), 227–233. doi:10.1016/S0738-3991(00)00192-0.

Petersen, I., McCrea, R. L., Lupattelli, A., & Nordeng, H. (2015). Women's perception of risks of adverse fetal pregnancy outcomes: A large-scale multinational survey. *BMJ Open, 5*(6), e007390–e007390. doi:10.1136/bmjopen-2014-007390.

Rizvi, M., Khan, F., Shukla, I., Malik, A., & Shaheen. (2011). Rising prevalence of antimicrobial resistance in urinary tract infections during pregnancy: Necessity for exploring newer treatment options. *Journal of Laboratory Physicians, 3*(2), 98–103. doi:10.4103/0974-2727.86842.

UK National Screening Committee. (2017). *Antenatal screening for asymptomatic bacteriuria.* Retrieved October 4, 2018, from https://legacyscreening.phe.org.uk/asymptomaticbacteriuria.

6 'What the medications do is that lovely four-lettered word – hope'

A phenomenological investigation of older people's lived experiences of medication use following cancer diagnosis

Adam Pattison Rathbone

Introduction

Cancer has high morbidity and mortality in the United Kingdom (Smittenaar, Petersen, Stewart, & Moitt, 2016), with breast, prostate, lung and bowel cancer accounting for over half of the malignant cancers in England (Office for National Statistics, 2015). Oral and non-oral pharmaceuticals are key parts of treatment to optimise health outcomes (Claros, Messa, & Garcia-Perdomo, 2019; Puts et al., 2014). Indeed, the emotional, cognitive and physical impact of pharmaceutical use in cancer treatment is well documented (Burbridge et al., 2019; Claros et al., 2019; Ellingson & Borofka, 2020; Raijmakers et al., 2013). For cancers such as prostate and breast cancer, which largely affect older populations (Cinar & Tas, 2015), oral anticancer medications (i.e., tablets and capsules, rather than non-oral formulations like infusions and injections) are widely available and thought to improve the likelihood that a patient will use treatment (Iacorossi et al., 2018, 2019). Rates of medication use, however, are low, between 14% and 60%, suggesting some people with these cancers do not to use medications as prescribed (Simon, Latreille, Matte, Desjardins, & Bergeron, 2014; Wu et al., 2014). This is particularly problematic for older people with cancer, where the burden of managing medications for existing co-morbidities (Puts et al., 2013, 2014) may contribute to negative experiences of medication use, leading to treatment discontinuation and suboptimal health outcomes. Understanding the phenomenology of cancer medication use, what happens when patients use medications, the work involved and how it feels to use cancer medications may provide insights to support patients to continue treatment.

Reducing the work involved in medication use is thought to improve the likelihood a patient will continue treatment (Iacorossi et al., 2018). This includes both the physical work of administration, such as taking medication from the cupboard and swallowing it, as well as the cognitive work of keeping track of medications and monitoring side effects (Kampf, 2010; Twigg, Wolkowitz, Cohen, & Nettleton, 2011). Patients are thought to be motivated to complete the work involved in medication use when they hope that their medications are special (Cohen, McCubbin, Collin, & Pérodeau, 2001; Eliott & Olver, 2002). Medications are thought to take on special meanings due to interactions with healthcare professionals, whose professional and authoritative status may be transferred to (non-oral) pharmaceuticals as they are administered following diagnosis (Cohen et al., 2001). It has been suggested, however, that the growing predominance of self-administered, oral medications for the treatment of cancers that largely impact older people – as opposed to infusions or injections administered by health professionals – might make these pharmaceuticals less special (Wood, 2012). Exploring experiences of using medications may help to expand our understanding of treatment continuation (and therefore discontinuation) in older people with cancer.

Merleau-Ponty (1982) theorised that human experience can be 'prereflective' or 'perceptive'. Prereflective experiences are intuitive or natural responses based on expectations. For example, a cancer diagnosis might induce fear so that a person's first inclination is to take medication provided as prescribed. This response may be modified over time as a result of people's 'perceptive' experiences – moments of physical awareness where information is drawn from the environment to understand the situation and create a response. Nascimento et al. (2017) suggested medication use was a 'perceptive' experience, rather than a 'prereflective' response, as people become physically aware of the effects (and side effects) of medication use and draw on information around them to assess the risks and benefits of treatment. For older people with cancer, however, there is little empirical evidence to illuminate whether medication use (rather than discontinuation or non-use) is due to a 'prereflective' response or the 'perceptive' experience of using medications. Exploring the lived experiences of older people using medications following a cancer diagnosis might help to illuminate how people experience this phenomenon.

The aim of this chapter is to examine older people's lived experiences of medication use following cancer diagnosis.

Methods

A transcendental phenomenological approach was adopted to identify the essence of the lived experience (Moustakas, 1994). Essences are made up of objects (e.g., physical objects, ideas) and their subjective characteristics (e.g., feelings, thoughts, memories and emotions). The essence of a phenomenon describes both the noema, 'what is experienced', and the noesis, 'how it is experienced'. The noema refers to the objective, physical aspects of the experience, for example, what medications are used, or what happens physically when medications are used (or not). The noesis refers to the internal context of experiencing something, for example, feeling scared to take medications or using medications as part of a routine. To uncover the essence of a phenomenon, researchers must pursue experiential data of those who have lived experience of the phenomenon itself that can tell us what happens and how it happens (Moustakas, 1994).

Phenomenologists 'bracket' their presuppositions in an effort to reduce bias (Moustakas, 1994). I did this in preparation for this investigation of medication use in older people with cancer. As a clinical pharmacist, I expected people with cancer to be reluctant to use medications due to anticipated negative side effects. As a healthcare professional, I practice evidence-based medicine (i.e., using research from clinical trials, case reports and regulatory bodies to construct my knowledge and practice). I believed that chemotherapy, hormonal and adjuvant anticancer treatments were particularly toxic, more than medications for other diseases, acting both as a poison and a cure (Martin, 2006). I believed that these side effects, in addition to the burden of using medications for other co-morbidities, contribute to poor medication use for older people with cancer. I believed my role was to encourage patients to tolerate these side effects and to use treatments as they were prescribed to achieve optimal outcomes of their cancer treatment. In other words, my primary role was to instruct, guide and encourage patients to use pharmaceuticals to treat their cancer – so as to minimise the risk of death from the disease. Reflecting on these previously held beliefs raised questions about patients' experiences of using medications for cancer and how these pharmaceuticals and the side effects they create fit into patients' everyday lives.

A convenience sample of participants was recruited from four general practices in North East England, United Kingdom, between April and June 2014. General practices were selected to include areas of low (n = 1), intermediate (n = 2) and high levels of deprivation (n = 1) using the Index of Multiple Deprivation (McLennan et al., 2011), to include a diversity of socioeconomic experiences. To support recruitment, general practices displayed posters that read 'Have you had cancer? We are trying to find out about patient experiences of treatment. Ask your GP for more information'. General practices screened expressions of interest and forwarded contact details of people who met the inclusion criteria: adults over 55 years old with a previous diagnosis of any type of cancer, who had past or current experience of receiving treatment for cancer, who were conversant in English and had capacity to consent to take part in research. A limitation of this recruitment strategy is it may have inadvertently excluded people who had experiences of declining, discontinuing or not using cancer treatments following their cancer diagnosis.

Participants were given an information sheet that explained the project was being completed by a doctoral student and included my post-nominals (MRPharmS) that enabled participants to identify that I was a pharmacist. I then made contact to arrange the interview. To prevent my identity as a pharmacist influencing data collection, prior to each interview participants were informed that, although I had pharmacy training, I could not offer any clinical advice during the interview, would not share anything they disclosed with their usual care team and wanted to know both about using and not using medications for cancer as prescribed (see Rathbone and Jamie, 2016, for more information about the ethico-legal tension this raised). In taking this approach, I hoped to motivate participants to provide honest and open accounts of their experiences, rather than sharing what they expected a pharmacist would want to hear, such as positive stories of medication use as prescribed (Brenner & DeLamater, 2016). Originally the aim was to recruit 15 participants based on theoretical data saturation (Crotty, 1998; Moustakas, 1994); however, once data collection had started, it became apparent that much smaller numbers, approximately five participants, were adequate to reach saturation. A small number of additional interviews, in this case three, were conducted to confirm saturation had been reached (Crotty, 1998). See Table 6.1 for demographic data.

Data collection included a single in-depth, semistructured interview with each participant. Participants were interviewed at home for between 68 and 115 minutes, with a mean interview length of 90 minutes. Data were collected between May 2014 and June 2015 using a topic guide, which included three open-ended questions:

(i) 'what was it like being prescribed medicines?'
(ii) 'what are your experiences of taking your medicines as prescribed?'
(iii) 'what are your experiences of not taking your medicines as prescribed?'

These questions were open and, initially, did not specifically focus on cancer, as I wanted the participants to frame their experiences in their own way. Further probing relevant to their cancer diagnosis included determining the medications used for cancer and how each participant felt about using them. Interviews were audio recorded and additional notes, as relevant, were made regarding emphasis, gestures and how participants interacted with their medications during the interview.

Interviews were transcribed verbatim and anonymised by the interviewer (APR). Transcripts were quality checked by a postgraduate research associate in the same research group. Data were thematically analysed via manual coding followed by computer coding using NVivo. Coding was conducted inductively and iteratively by a single author and verified by supervisors and postgraduate research associates during data discussion group meetings between interviews and following the completion of all interviews. Codes were generated, deconstructed and merged until dominant themes were clarified. This approach was guided by the works of Crotty (1998), Moustakas (1994) and Halldorsdottir (2000).

The study received approval from institutional and national ethics committees.

Findings

Findings are presented below describing the noema (what happened) and the noesis (how it happened). The noema includes what medications were used and physical experiences of symptom control and side effects. The noesis describes how participants initially interpreted cancer medication use as a natural response to being diagnosed with cancer and then challenged this response over time, drawing on information around them to make decisions to continue or discontinue treatment. At the time of interviews, participants were all currently using their cancer medications as prescribed. Interview excerpts illustrate participants' experiences in their own words. Each quote is identified according to a participant's number (1–8), age (55–75), gender (F/M) and cancer type (breast, bowel, lung, prostate).

Table 6.1 Participant demographics

ID	Age	Sex	Occupation	Cancer	Time since diagnosis	Surgery	Radio-therapy	Chemo-therapy	Hormone	Adjuvant	Deprivation Level	Co-morbid disease
1	63	M	Retired	Prostate	10 years	Yes	No	Yes	Yes	Yes	Intermediate	Yes
2	55	M	Manager	Bowel	4 years	Yes	No	Yes	No	Yes	Low	No
3	75	M	Retired	Prostate	1 year	Yes	Yes	No	Yes	Yes	Low	Yes
4	65	F	Retired	Breast	5 years	Yes	Yes	Yes	Yes	Yes	High	No
5	67	F	Retired	Breast	2 years	Yes	Yes	No	Yes	Yes	Low	No
6	57	F	Nursing Assistant	Breast	3 years	Yes	No	Yes	Yes	Yes	Intermediate	Yes
7	70	M	Retired	Prostate	7 years	Yes	No	No	Yes	Yes	Low	Yes
8	61	F	Retired	Bowel & Lung	8 years	Yes	No	Yes	No	Yes	Low	No

The noema (what happened)

Participants shared descriptive experiences of 'what happened', including what medications were used (see Figure 6.1) and what happened physically when medications were used (and not used) including symptom control and side effects.

Following diagnosis, participants were exposed to a range of pharmaceuticals that they identified as 'cancer medications' including chemotherapy, hormonal and additional treatments that were supplied. This included infusions and injections as well as tablets, creams and gels:

> When I was diagnosed with cancer the cancer medication entered my life in a rather bigger way.
> [Interviewer What do you mean by cancer medication?]
> Well the whole lot of them. You get given all sorts of medications for cancer.... Each time I go I get a bag full of them, creams for this and that and then the nausea [tablets].
>
> Participant 8, aged 61, female, bowel+lung

> They give you plenty. They have a whole load of stuff to take. They gave me the anaesthetic, obviously for the operation to get it out, then when I'd pulled myself round they did give me co-codamol and antibiotics... then you get a bundle of stuff to take home in a little bag that's full of all kinds, so they're all part of the anti-cancer group of pills and potions and pricks you get once you've got cancer.
>
> Participant 6, aged 57, female, breast

What happened when cancer medications were used as prescribed related to the claimed or perceived pharmaceutical effect on the disease, that is, stopping cancer recurrence or slowing down cancer growth:

> The medication can't remove [the cancer] from the body, it can only slow the growth down.
>
> Participant 7, aged 70, male, prostate

> [Cancer medication] shrinks the cancer that is there but also goes around and catches any little bits of cancer that are trying to spread, so it stops it spreading and stops the bits they can't cut out from getting bigger, it fights the tumour, so to speak.
>
> Participant 2, aged 55, male, bowel

Using cancer medications, however, also led to physical side effects.

> My hands have swollen, and I've seen the consultant and he said 'lymphedema', and that is a side effect of [the cancer medication]
>
> Participant 6, aged 57, female, breast

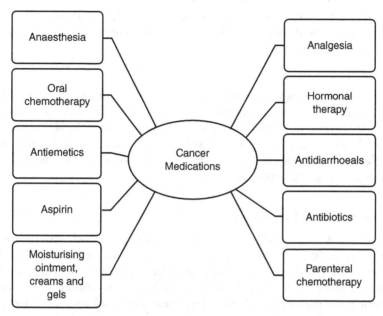

Figure 6.1 What participants described as cancer medication.

My feet and my fingers, the ends of the extremities, I still can't feel my toes... my fingers were all cracked and my toes were all cracked, I could hardly walk, and that was with using all the creams and gels they'd given me that I was putting on.

Participant 2, aged 55, male, bowel

Conversely, experiences of not using medications as prescribed were perceived to have caused the return of symptoms that were linked to cancer:

If I do miss one... I've had a few bouts of when I've went to the toilet or I haven't went to the toilet I've just felt like [I needed to], it's just a trickle, and I've been up all night and when you want to you just can't, it's horrible, you just, I wouldn't wish it on anybody... you just feel like you want a wee all the time and you're sat on the toilet and nothing is coming, and if it gets really bad, you've got to go to A&E... and they put a catheter in for you.

Participant 1, aged 63, male, prostate

When medications were restarted, symptoms associated with cancer were perceived to be under control.

If I forget to take them, I feel as though… my body is aching… and when I do go back on them I feel as though I'm all right again, so I can feel [physically] when I come off them.

Participant 6, aged 57, female, breast

What happened to these participants following diagnosis included exposure to a wide range of different pharmaceuticals that were identified as 'cancer medications'. Medication use was characterised by users in terms of the physical effects of the pharmaceuticals on the cancer as well as side effects on participants' bodies. Not using medications was also described as producing physical effects in that cancer symptoms returned.

The noesis (how it happened)

This section describes how participants experienced using medication as part of their everyday life, initially accepting using cancer medication as an expected response to diagnosis and then challenging this approach by drawing on information around them to make decisions to continue or discontinue treatment.

Participants initially experienced using cancer medications as an automatic, prereflective response, that is, it was 'just done' in response to diagnosis.

I had just simply taken [the cancer medications] because that's what you do when you get told you have cancer.

Participant 8, aged 61, female, bowel+lung

You know, you've got to take them, so you do it.

Participant 2, aged 55, male, bowel

It's just something you do. It feels right and you don't question why, you just do it.

Participant 4, aged 65, female, breast

Some participants readily adopted specific procedures for medication use that were similar to other routine self-care activities, such as washing and eating.

I've got a little procedure I do, and I just do it, it's just a couple of tablets per day, as I say it's like cleaning your teeth when you get up in the morning and going to bed in the night.

Participant 7, aged 70, male, prostate

Participants who had used medications for co-morbidities previously felt they were already in the frame of mind to manage the routine work required to use cancer medications.

I was [so] used to taking a tablet first thing in the morning, because when I was on HRT, I used to take that first thing on a morning, when I'd cleaned my teeth, I could take it straight away, you know your routine, when I was at work, you'd get up, have your breakfast, have your shower and clean your teeth and tablet, that was when I was on the HRT, so I was in that mind set of taking a tablet first thing in the morning so I just continued, it was just an orange tablet instead of a white one.

Participant 4, aged 65, female, breast

Indeed, for some participants, using medication was a natural response for any condition and part of their everyday life, prior to their cancer diagnosis.

I mean I used to take pain killers for headaches and things like that when I needed them and such like. I don't have any qualms taking medications… if I was given medicine, I took it. I didn't think about it, I just took it.

Participant 5, aged 67, female, breast

While some participants indicated they generally avoided using medications, the 'scary' and 'life changing' experience of the cancer diagnosis and the belief that cancer medications enhance survival meant that cancer medications were special:

When you're told you have cancer, it's like, it's like nothing else, your life changes, you know they say this and that information and you take it, then they give you information about something else and you take it, but I was feeling so strange, you don't think, you just accept it, they give you the medication and you just take it, and then you read the leaflets, about side effects, you can get with them, it doesn't really matter because I suppose, although with other medications you have the option to think about it, there isn't really an option with the cancer… if you want to, in other words it's like saying if you want to live then take it, if you don't want to live then don't bother, but there isn't anything else so you know, sort your affairs out, so you just do it.

Participant 3, aged 75, male, prostate

Another participant reported that cancer diagnosis changed his identity, from someone who rejected using medications to someone older, who accepted using them:

I never took any medicines you know all my life… because I still felt like a young man and the idea that I have to take medications… collect my prescription and take it every day and have side effects and all that kit and caboodle, it's old man stuff that I thought was a long way off. But… when they tell you you've got cancer, your time's come, your whole idea about who you think you are… all that changes in an instant, you go from being, you know, normal, to this older, kind of, less, less, I suppose… you're just completely different you know, you are one of the crowd who got ill, you're one of them [emphasis on them, slight grimace on his face] now, so you have to try and rebuild your life after the diagnosis and that life, obviously, includes taking medications, going to the doctor, going to the pharmacy, having check-ups and all that, so you just sort of take the medications and everything else they give you without thinking despite the stigma… that goes with it, because you end up being one of them, in the queue at the pharmacy, with the oldies, fighting to get to the front [laughing] but you don't think about it, it just happens to you.

Participant 1, aged 63, male, prostate

That using medications following a cancer diagnosis naturally 'felt right' was reflected in participants' distress when medications were missed or in low supply. One participant described her experience of missing parenteral chemotherapy:

I discovered, when the tube hadn't been unlocked and the drug wasn't in me… I felt terrible… I was fed up about it, I was flattened, I didn't feel well… disappointed. I was really, very angry with myself, with the equipment, with the chemotherapy for not doing its job, because for the whole week the cancer had just been ticking along without anything in me to fight it, so I was scared and I think that made me more angry. I did lash out and I said some terrible things [to the people around me].

Participant 8, aged 61, female, bowel+lung

This also applied to oral formulations that could not be missed.

I think with the other two medications, the lisinopril and statin, they're preventers rather than maintainers, so with that if I did go three or four days without them, I don't think it would be a life or death thing… I don't think it would be a killer, not to have them… but with the cancer pill… I would probably run into trouble quite quickly, probably after a day or so, so… I couldn't bring myself to miss it, it would disrupt my life too much in the long run.

Participant 7, aged 70, male, prostate

One participant reported she made exceptional effort to ensure the supply of her cancer medication, as compared to medication for other conditions.

I do get quite panicky about missing them or if the number of tablets is getting a bit low, because I'm terrified the cancer would come back, I mean if that one [holds up hypothyroidism medication] if I was that bothered about running out I could just borrow from one of my friends but that one [holds up cancer medication] I don't think anyone would borrow [sic] me to be honest [laughing] we all need our own little magic pill so they wouldn't want to miss it and neither would I and I wouldn't want them to have to miss it for me either, to be honest. [So, if I'm running out] I'll phone the doctors up and get a prescription straight away for that one [holds up cancer medication], I don't rest until they agree [to supply it] I make such a fuss… they sort it out.

Participant 6, aged 57, female, breast

Undertaking the 'hard work' of tolerating side effects was accepted as 'part of' using cancer medications.

I had to go into the chemotherapy treatment ward, at the hospital, for them to dispense my chemotherapy, and I'd see all these other poor people, with all these other problems and it reminded me so much but you've got to go and do it, it's a bit like going to work on a Sunday, you don't want to do it but you've got to. [Chemotherapy] was a regimen that you get into. Erm, collecting tablets, getting check-ups and taking my tablets on a daily basis but you had campaigns, ten days of hard work, because it knocks the stuffing out of you like, and at the end of it you're weak but it's just part of it.

Participant 2, aged 55, male, bowel

These excerpts indicate that using cancer medications was 'special' due the life threatening and identity-changing experience of cancer diagnosis. As using cancer medications following diagnosis 'felt right' and missing medication was distressing, participants prereflectively completed the additional work (such as maintaining supply and tolerating side effects) involved in using cancer medications on top of medications for existing comorbidities. Over time, however, missing treatment became less distressing.

I think I've probably forgot to take it maybe once or twice and panicked in the beginning, I thought 'oh my god, I've forgotten to take my tablet, I'm going to get another lump'… 'oh my god, has it come back again' but as time passes, you get to be a little bit more [aware and able to] calm yourself down a little bit, missing one tablet isn't going to make any difference [laughing].

Participant 4, aged 65, female, breast

Participants reported (perceptive) experiences of reflecting, evaluating and negotiating how they felt about continued medication use over time:

Sometimes you contemplate why you're taking these terrible pills because, really in the beginning you just take them because someone told you to, but then after a while, you get to know them for yourself and think things over a bit.

Participant 8, aged 61, female, bowel+lung

This included feeling suspicious about the motives of healthcare professionals and uncertainty about the long-term impact of the medication itself:

> There is an element that people are trying to sell you their idea aren't they? Like the doctor wants you to take it so that you don't get ill and go back isn't it, so they want you to take it and the chemists they want you to take it because that's their money isn't it?... they say this is good but actually until you take it you don't know..., you just don't know what it's doing in there you know, if it's going to give you a cancer later on or a heart attack in ten years?
>
> Participant 6, aged 57, female, breast

Participants negotiated unknowns about medication use by drawing on information around them. This included discussions with other older people as well as using information from the television and newspapers, learning about their medications and weighing up the pros and cons of using them:

> Like lots of old men that I spoke to said they wouldn't want to take a female hormone but if you look into it and discuss it with people, like I have done, you realise that actually it's only a very small amount of a female hormone, so it's not like you're going to grow breasts and start carrying a handbag, but... the doctors can only tell you so much and then the rest comes from reading the papers or watching the doctor on the TV, talking to other people in the waiting rooms and things like that, that's really what gives you the information and helps you decide to stick to taking these things.
>
> Participant 3, aged 75, male, prostate

One participant reported that hearing positive things about his cancer medications from the people around him helped balance out negative experiences of side effects and supported treatment continuation:

> When it gets tough physically, you need people to keep saying good stuff about these pills because the pills they can be nasty, give you awful side effects, so you need the people to tell you they're nice, to balance it all out. I mean it's sad that some people, that they don't have people around them to push themselves to take it.
>
> Participant 2, aged 55, male, bowel

Participants also used information about how their bodies responded when cancer medications were taken by monitoring blood test and scan results or the presence or reduction in symptoms they associated with their cancer:

> So that one [holds up cancer tablet packet] has brought the PSA down, right down, you know very low, [and controls my symptoms] so I still have cancer but it's under control, so when you think about it on the days you're dwelling on whether to take it or not, it's doing the job now and that's good

and if it turns on me down the line then that won't be so good, but you've got to accept some risk to balance the benefits, nothing comes for nothing.

Participant 1, aged 63, male, prostate

Perceiving this information during periods of reflection supported decision-making to continue (or discontinue) treatment:

Then after a while, you get to know them for yourself and think things over a bit, and so I made my own decision, that… [if] the scans [CT and MRI] didn't show the cancer was pushed back, then I would stop at that point.

Participant 8, aged 61, female, bowel+lung

When you've got cancer and you've been given all these [points to anti-cancer medication kit] to use, at the end of the day, when you've thought about it, and read about it, and talked about it with everyone and their aunt… what the medications do is that lovely four lettered word – hope. They give you hope… you've got some [emphasis on some] hope that you can go on, and get a new life [so you keep taking them].

Participant 2, aged 55, male, bowel

Well after you've had some experience of using these cancer tablets, and you know what's going on, you just feel like, like it's a little miracle isn't it really? A little tiny pill that stops that awful c-word from taking everything away again. So, it's worth taking it… because at least you're here.

Participant 6, aged 57, female, breast

The data show how participants started using medications for cancer automatically following their diagnoses but then gradually challenged their initial, prereflective acceptance of medication use over time. Participants reflected and evaluated their experiences by perceiving information from the people around them, the television and newspapers as well as information about their own bodies monitored with blood tests and scan results. 'Getting to know' their cancer medications in this way minimised distress when cancer medications were missed and facilitated decisions to continue and discontinue treatment. Overwhelmingly, participants in this study continued their cancer treatment, thus while the findings do not advance our understanding of cancer medication discontinuation, they do provide insight into participant perceptions of these pharmaceuticals as givers of hope and new life.

Discussion

The findings cover people's use of a broad range of pharmaceuticals including chemotherapy and hormonal treatments as well as analgesics, antiemetics, anaesthetics and antibiotics that participants identified as 'cancer medications'. Experiences of life-changing cancer diagnoses meant medications for cancer were initially used prereflectively, as an automatic response to diagnosis.

This included the additional work to use cancer medications on top of existing medications for comorbidities, such as maintaining supplies as well as learning how to tolerate side effects. Over time, however, participants perceived the pros and cons of medication use, drawing on their physical experiences of symptoms, information from tests and scan results and knowledge from people around them, in newspapers and on the television to make decisions about treatment continuation. The essence of the experience of using cancer medications for these participants was the opposite of cancer diagnosis; just as the latter was 'life-taking', 'scary' and associated with 'death', the former was 'life-giving', 'hopeful' and associated with 'life'.

Merleau-Ponty's (1982) notion of 'prereflective responses' is captured here in participants' descriptions of their initial approaches to medications following their cancer diagnosis. After being given a cancer diagnosis, participants' natural responses were to use medications without question. This seemed to be a normal response to cancer diagnosis, even by participants who typically avoid using medications. The 'special status' of cancer as a life-threatening condition and the significance of diagnosis related to the high mortality and negative health outcomes associated with cancer (Smittenaar et al., 2016) appeared to confer upon cancer medications a 'special status' too, as 'life givers', 'little miracles', and givers of 'hope' for these participants. This raises questions beyond the scope of cancer medications, about the relationship between medication use and disease severity more generally. For example, are older people more likely to use medications for more severe or debilitating conditions than ailments that are less so? The findings also raise questions about patients who actively decide not to use cancer mediations, as the participants in this study only reported not using cancer medications as prescribed accidentally (e.g., forgetting occasionally or running out) rather than declining or discontinuing treatment. Only one participant, P8, reported feeling that she would discontinue treatment if her scan results indicated her chemotherapy was not 'pushing back' the cancer. However, her scan results did show her cancer was shrinking, so although she had considered discontinuing treatment, she did not. Future work might explore this tipping point, where patients have decided to discontinue treatment but then reverse this decision and pursue treatment based on their (perceptive) experiences.

Existing research suggests oral cancer medications may be considered as less special than non-oral formulations (Wood, 2012). The data in this study suggested that both non-oral and oral cancer medications had special meaning compared to medications for other co-morbidities. As suggested by Eliott & Olver (2002), the special status of cancer medications as givers of 'hope', supports and motivates the action and work required (Nguyen, Ako, Niamba, Sylla, & Tiendrébéogo, 2007; Twigg et al., 2011) for adherence. The findings do show, however, that participants' experiences changed over time, as they perceived the physical effects (and side effects) of using cancer medications and learned about using medications from the environment around them, as Nascimento et al. (2017) suggested. Although not seen in this study, perceptive experiences may contribute to the high rates of cancer treatment discontinuation reported in the literature. Further work is needed to explore the relationship between perceptive experiences and medication use and discontinuation by older people with cancer.

Overwhelmingly, participants in this study made decisions to continue – rather than to discontinue cancer treatment – the latter being a phenomenon of concern as reported in the literature (and seen in my clinical practice). The positive experiences reported by these participants may be due to a selection bias at the point of recruitment or because of my identity as a pharmacist. Although I did bracket my presuppositions, asked participants for honest accounts, and managed my tone of voice and body language during interviews, participants might have expected that, as a pharmacist, I would want to hear positive experiences of medication use. To draw again on Merlaeu-Ponty's work, participants might have had prereflective responses to being asked about how they use medication by a pharmacist (even a pharmacist in a research setting), to automatically provide positively orientated medication use stories to appear prosocial (Brenner & DeLamater, 2016). Further work should explore the impact of researcher identity in studies exploring medication use in older people.

Conspicuous by absence in the data was the role of healthcare professionals and pharmacists in providing special meaning to cancer medications. The only mention of pharmacists was related to suspicion about remuneration for supplying cancer medications. I expected participants would share stories about pharmacists supporting them to tolerate side effects, by providing information and advice; that pharmacists would make the medications 'special' (Cohen et al., 2001). Instead, participants referred to support, information and advice from television, newspapers and other patients in waiting rooms – not from pharmacists! Although not the primary focus of this study, the data suggest that rather than providing information to support patients to deal with side effects, as I expected, simply by supplying cancer medications in close temporal proximity to diagnosis, pharmacists are part of a broader system that confers upon pharmaceuticals the 'life giving' properties that make side effects tolerable. Pharmacists working with cancer patients should consider carefully how they contribute to peoples' experiences of cancer medication use, what they do and how they do it, to critically examine their own contribution to the prereflective and perceptive use of medications.

Conclusions

This study explored older people's lived experiences of medication use following a cancer diagnosis. The findings showed the moment of diagnosis as significant and life-changing and that this meaning was transferred to cancer medications themselves, which also became special and life-changing. Cancer medications opposed cancer diagnosis; the latter was perceived to take life away, the former as life giving. This is surprising, as the side effects of these medicines were expected to lead to negative experiences and treatment discontinuation. In this study, however, participants elevated their cancer medications to a status well above medications used for other co-morbidities; they accepted the physical side effects of medicines because of their assumed 'life giving' properties.

References

Brenner, P. S., & DeLamater, J. (2016). Lies, damned lies, and survey self-reports? identity as a cause of measurement bias. *Social Psychology Quarterly*, 79(4), 333–354. doi:10.1177/0190272516628298.

Burbridge, C., Randall, J. A., Lawson, J., Symonds, T., Dearden, L., Lopez-Gitlitz, A.,… McQuarrie, K. (2019). Understanding symptomatic experience, impact, and emotional response in recently diagnosed metastatic castration-resistant prostate cancer: A qualitative study. *Supportive Care in Cancer*. doi:10.1007/s00520-019-05079-3.

Cinar, D., & Tas, D. (2015). Cancer in the elderly. *Northern Clinics of Istanbul*, 2(1), 73–80. doi:10.14744/nci.2015.72691.

Claros, M. P., Messa, C. V. M., & Garcia-Perdomo, H. A. (2019). Adherence to oral pharmacological treatment in cancer patients: Systematic review. *Oncology Reviews*, 13(1), 49–53. doi:10.4081/oncol.2019.402.

Cohen, D., McCubbin, M., Collin, J., & Pérodeau, G. (2001). Medications as social phenomena. *Health*, 5(4), 441–469.

Crotty, M. (1998). *The Foundations of Social Research: Meaning and Perspective in the Research Process*. Sydney: SAGE Publications Ltd.

Eliott, J., & Olver, I. (2002). The discursive properties of "Hope": A qualitative analysis of cancer patients' speech. *Qualitative Health Research*, 12(2), 173–193. doi:10.1177/104973230201200204.

Ellingson, L. L., & Borofka, K. G. E. (2020). Long-term cancer survivors' everyday embodiment. *Health Communication*, 35(2), 180–191. doi:10.1080/10410236.2018.1550470.

Halldorsdottir, S. (2000). The Vancouver School of doing phenomenology. in: Fridlund, B., & Hildingh, C., eds. *Qualitative Research Methods in the Service of Health*. Lund, Sweden. pp. 47–81. ISBN 9144012489.

Iacorossi, L., Gambalunga, F., De Domenico, R., Serra, V., Marzo, C., & Carlini, P. (2019). Qualitative study of patients with metastatic prostate cancer to adherence of hormone therapy. *European Journal of Oncology Nursing*, 38, 8–12. doi:10.1016/j.ejon.2018.11.004.

Iacorossi, L., Gambalunga, F., Fabi, A., Giannarelli, D., Marchetti, A., Piredda, M., & De Marinis, M. G. (2018). Adherence to oral administration of endocrine treatment in patients with breast cancer: A qualitative study. *Cancer Nursing*, 41(1), E57–E63. doi:10.1097/ncc.0000000000000452.

Kampf, A. (2010). "The risk of age"? Early detection test, prostate cancer and practices of self. *Journal of Aging Studies*, 24(4), 325–334. doi:10.1016/j.jaging.2010.08.002.

Martin, E. (2006). The pharmaceutical person. *BioSocieties*, 1(3), 273–287. doi:10.1017/s1745855206003012.

McLennan, D., Barnes, H., Noble, M., Davies, J., Garratt, E., & Dibben, C. (2011). *The English Indices of Deprivation 2010*. London, UK: Department for Communities and Local Government.

Merleau-Ponty, M. (1982). *Phenomenology of Perception*. London, UK: Routledge.

Moustakas, C. (1994). *Phenomenological Research Methods*. London: Sage Publications Ltd.

Nascimento, Y. A., Filardi, A. F. R., Abath, A. J., Silva, L. D., & Ramalho-de-Oliveira, D. (2017). The phenomenology of Merleau-Ponty in investigations about medication use: Constructing a methodological cascade. *Revista da Escola de Enfermagem da USP*, 51, e03296. doi:10.1590/s1980-220x2017017603296.

Nguyen, V. K., Ako, C. Y., Niamba, P., Sylla, A., & Tiendrébéogo, I. (2007). Adherence as therapeutic citizenship: Impact of the history of access to antiretroviral drugs on adherence to treatment. *Aids*, 21(5), S31–S35. doi:10.1097/01.aids.0000298100.48990.58.

Office for National Statistics. (2015). *Cancer Registration Statistics, England, 2013*. Retrieved from http://www.ons.gov.uk/ons/dcp171778_409714.pdf.

Puts, M., Tu, H., Tourangeau, A., Howell, D., Fitch, M., Springall, E., & Alibhai, S. (2014). Factors influencing adherence to cancer treatment in older adults with cancer: A systematic review. *Annals of Oncology*, 25(3), 564–577.

Puts, M., Tu, H. A., Tourangeau, A., Howell, D., Fitch, M., Springall, E., & Alibhai, S. M. H. (2013). A systematic review of factors influencing treatment adherence in older adults with cancer. *Supportive Care in Cancer*, 21, S202–S203. doi:10.1007/s00520-013-1798-3.

Raijmakers, N., van Zuylen, L., Furst, C., Beccaro, M., Maiorana, L., Pilastri, P.,… Costantini, M. (2013). Variation in medication use in cancer patients at the end of life: A cross-sectional analysis. *Supportive Care in Cancer*, 21(4), 1003–1011.

Rathbone, A. P., & Jamie, K. (2016). Transferring from clinical pharmacy practice to qualitative research: Questioning identity, epistemology and ethical frameworks. *Sociological Research Online*, 21(2), 4. Retrieved from http://www.socresonline.org.uk/21/2/4.html.

Simon, R., Latreille, J., Matte, C., Desjardins, P., & Bergeron, E. (2014). Adherence to adjuvant endocrine therapy in estrogen receptor-positive breast cancer patients with regular follow-up. *Canadian Journal of Surgery*, 57(1), 26–32.

Smittenaar, C. R., Petersen, K. A., Stewart, K., & Moitt, N. (2016). Cancer incidence and mortality projections in the UK until 2035. *British Journal of Cancer*, 115(9), 1147–1155. doi:10.1038/bjc.2016.304.

Twigg, J., Wolkowitz, C., Cohen, R. L., & Nettleton, S. (2011). Conceptualising body work in health and social care. *Sociology of Health & Illness*, 33(2), 171–188.

Wood, L. (2012). A review on adherence management in patients on oral cancer therapies. *The European Journal of Oncology Nursing*, 16(4), 432–438. doi:10.1016/j.ejon.2011.10.002.

Wu, S., Chee, D., Ugalde, A., Butow, P., Seymour, J., & Schofield, P. (2014). Lack of congruence between patients 'and health professionals' perspectives of adherence to imatinib therapy in treatment of chronic myeloid leukemia: A qualitative study. *Palliat Support Care*, 1–9. doi:10.1017/s1478951513001260.

7 The paradox of vaccine hesitancy and refusal

Public health and the moral work of motherhood

Alison Thompson

Introduction

Public health, because of its anticipatory and preventive actions, is frequently a victim of its own success. Vaccines are a case in point. The current phenomenon of parents choosing to not vaccinate their children, on non-religious grounds, is in part attributable to the fact that the diseases against which childhood vaccines are given are now rare, thanks to the success of immunisation programs. Or so the thinking goes. This leads parents to believe that the risks of vaccination are now greater than the risks associated with getting the disease (Brown, 2010).

In this chapter, I posit that the decline in parental uptake of childhood vaccines – within the segment of society that is well educated and middle-class – is indeed because of the success of public health. It is, however, not only because of the success of public health in the near eradication of many formally endemic diseases that risk perception among this group of parents has shifted. Neoliberal public health regimes have rendered this group of parents, and mothers in particular, hypervigilant risk managers who place self-and-infant-care above care for the other. This Canadian, narrative study of maternal experiences with vaccines reveals that regardless of whether mothers vaccinate their children fully or not, their experiences are embedded within the construction of the 'good mother' metanarrative. Public health has created the very maternal subjectivities that made the emergence of this form of resistance to public health directives inevitable.

Background

Nowhere is the governance of risk in neoliberal societies more heavily promoted than in the context of childrearing. The retraction of the state from responsibility for health is in keeping with the tenet of minimal government intervention (Ericson et al., 2000) and results in the downloading of responsibility for health onto the individual. According to Ayo, 'this not only benefits the individual, but it is also presumed to work for the good of society as a whole' (Ayo, 2012). Health promotion becomes a primary means of creating 'healthist' subjectivities and many scholars have identified a variety of what Peterson calls, 'new preventive strategies of social administration… that target the 'at risk' individual and utilise the agency of subjects in processes of self-regulation (Petersen, 1996, p. 44).

Crawford describes how the political ideology of neoliberalism, 'situates the problem of health and disease at the level of the individual', (Crawford, 1980, p. 374) and individual responsibility for health has been transformed into a moral imperative to be a 'good and healthy' citizen (Crawford, 1980). This theory fits well with Foucault's notion of governmentality, where individuals wilfully regulate themselves (through self-surveillance) in the best interest of the state (Bunton & Petersen, 1997). The investment of mental and material resources on the part of individuals, particularly those in the middle class, in the pursuit of health is not seen as an obsessive preoccupation with the self (Rose, 1990). Rather, this pursuit is valued by society and is an essential part of being a good citizen. Those who fail to follow the duties and obligations related to the pursuit of health are subject to moral sanction.

The subject position of motherhood within the context of modern public health in neoliberal states has become increasingly the focus of injunctions, duties and obligations to ensure the production of healthy children. This phenomenon has been well studied, and its implications for maternal subjectivities explored (Douglas & Michaels, 2004; Furedi, 2002; Hays, 1996; Henderson et al., 2010; Lee et al., 2014; Lupton, 2011). Mothers are subjected to idealised notions of motherhood that 'insist that mothers acquire professional-level skills such as those of a therapist, paediatrician, consumer products safety inspector, and teacher' (Douglas & Michaels, 2004); essentially they must become hypervigilant risk managers in the effort to avoid harming their offspring (Lee et al., 2014).

The overlapping moral discourses that construct and produce our notions of what it means to be both a good public health citizen (Crawford, 1980; Lupton, 1993; Osborne, 1997; Petersen & Lupton, 1997) and a good mother (Douglas & Michaels, 2004) have given rise to a culture of 'mother-blaming' that 'is ever-present and a powerful influence over moms' feelings of inadequacy and worth' (Henderson et al., 2010). The moral work that women undertake to rationalise what they perceive to be failures to live up to notions of public health citizenship have been the object of study, particularly around breastfeeding (Murphy, 1999; Ryan et al., 2010; Shaw, 2004). As is also the case with healthism, those people who are most susceptible to, and who are the cultivators of, discourses around the 'good mother' are those in the middle class (Greenhalgh & Wessely, 2004; Henderson et al., 2010).

Making the right choice to vaccinate one's child is not just about individual health, but is also a 'duty of citizenship' (Ayo, 2012), and an obligation of good motherhood. Because vaccines are most effective when approximately 95% of the population is immunised, the requirement to contribute to herd immunity is an additional moral obligation of the public health citizen. Because of this, there have been many studies of parental decision-making which seek to understand why parents do and do not vaccinate their children (Brown, 2010; Brunson, 2013; Diekema, 2005; Heininger, 2006; Kennedy et al., 2005; Wilson et al., 2008). The medical discourse frames non-vaccination as an issue of skewed risk perception and bad risk management (Blume, 2006; Shao, 2008). The decision to vaccinate is set up as a binary choice and is decontextualised. There is also a binary view of parents: those whose children are immunised, and those who are under-immunised. Anything less than full immunisation is constructed as problematic, and indeed, as a moral failure to uphold a social contract (Freed et al., 1996), thereby creating the notion that non-vaccinators are 'free riders' on the backs of those who do contribute towards the public good of herd immunity through vaccination (Diekema, 2005; Hershey et al., 1994).

The recent creation of a new category of the 'vaccine hesitant' is indicative of a view of parents as 'moldable' and without agency: empty vessels just waiting to be filled with the 'correct' information (Poland & Jacobson, 2001). The subjectivities created by healthism and New-Momism (Douglas & Michaels, 2004), however, require active management of risks, which entails the consumption and digestion, so to speak, of health information, including public health messaging. Studies show that within the middle-class demographic, people who do not fully immunise their children tend to be well educated and white (Barker et al., 2004; Diekema, 2005; Gust et al., 2008; Jessop, 2010). Ironically, this is the demographic within which consumption of public health messaging, and health goods, is typically done conspicuously (Crawford, 1980; Greenhalgh & Wessely, 2004).

We must question, then, explanations that assume that non-vaccinating parents, and mothers in particular, are ill-informed and suffering from some kind of science deficit. This study asked what a deeper, contextualised understanding of parental experiences with childhood vaccines can tell us about how vaccines fit into their broader views about health, science and risk. Surprisingly, social scientists have largely failed to ask this with some notable exceptions (Hobson-West, 2003, 2007; Lupton, 2011; New & Senior, 1991; Rogers & Pilgrim, 1995). A recent paper which provides a critical review of attitudes to vaccination shows that reasons for vaccine hesitancy are more often cited as having to do with trust than an information deficit, and safety is the most cited concern of vaccine hesitant parents (Yaqub et al., 2014).

Method

This study used a qualitative, narrative methodology to elicit 'medication narratives' (Bissell et al., 2006; Ryan et al., 2007). Fundamental to this approach is the notion of the 'embedded, emplotted nature of medication narratives within wider narratives of health and illness, and within an individual's life story' (Ryan et al., 2007, p. 354). Initially, the intent of this study was to use the public understanding of science's contextual model (Miller, 2001) to examine lay understandings of vaccine science. After only mothers responded to recruitment (see below), however, and after having done several interviews, it became clear that the participants' narratives had more to do with demonstrating the 'moral work' of motherhood (Murphy, 1999; Ryan et al., 2010) than mothers' understandings of risk. It was important, therefore, that the research elicit broader narratives about health as it showed how medications were given meaning within this context. Since the childhood vaccines under examination are preventive, not therapeutic, the aim was to examine how vaccines fit within the health (as opposed to illness) narratives mothers constructed and what role vaccines played in the construction of their subjectivities as public health citizens.

Sample selection and recruitment

Purposive sampling was used to recruit parents who had recent and varied experiences with vaccinating their children. Posters were placed in local coffee shops; children's, maternity and health food stores recruited in a variety of middle-class, downtown Toronto neighbourhoods. Middle-class neighbourhoods were targeted as this is the economic demographic within which non-religious vaccine resistance has been identified (Barker et al., 2004; Diekema, 2005; Gust et al., 2008; Jessop, 2010). A range of parental experiences within this demographic was sought: parents who did vaccinate their children, parents who did vaccinate but wish they had not, and parents who refused vaccines. Additional inclusion criteria were: (1) that the participant be able to be interviewed in English; (2) that they be able to provide informed consent and; (3) that they must have been involved with childhood vaccinations within the past 7 years to ensure that the experiences were not too far in the past, and to ensure that the publicly funded vaccine schedule had not changed too much in Ontario since the parent was faced with the decision to vaccinate their child(ren).

Informed consent was sought in keeping with approval from the University of Toronto Research Ethics Board. All 11 participants had university degrees, and an annual household income over $60,000 CAD. Four participants had vaccinated their children, three had partially vaccinated their children but had stopped after the child experienced what they thought were likely adverse events following vaccination, and four participants had not vaccinated their children at all. The relatively small sample size generated a large amount of data through narrative interviews (Lieblich et al., 1998).

Interviews

Narrative, self-reflective interviews were undertaken between June 2012 and June 2013 in the participants' homes (9) or places of business (2) and lasted between one and two and a half hours. Interviews were audio recorded and transcribed verbatim. Names have been changed to preserve anonymity in the reporting of the results.

Following the methodology of Ryan et al. (2007) participants were asked to talk about how they think about health in general, and the health of their children in particular. After these broader narratives about health were solicited, participants were asked to talk about their experiences with vaccination. Probing questions were kept to a minimum, were used towards the end of the interviews, and included: Do you think your experience with vaccination is unique relative to other parents? How difficult or easy was the decision making around vaccination for you? How do you think your decision affects others in the community? Based on your experiences, what advice would you give another parent about vaccinating their child?

Data analysis

Transcripts were entered into NVivo 10 and subjected to iterative, interpretative thematic analysis using constant comparison to develop descriptive codes that were grounded in the participants' own words (Corbin & Strauss, 2008; Miles et al., 2013). Codes were then collapsed into broader conceptual themes that were 'tightly integrated and tied to supporting data' (Maines, 2004). Crawford's theory of healthism and Foucault's notion of governmentality were used to interrogate the data. A narrative analysis was conducted 'to reveal the personal, social and interactive functions that the narratives perform' (Ryan et al., 2007).

One important facet of narrative methodology is the notion that participant narratives have a purpose. Narratives can be used to achieve some ends, justify actions, establish meaning and construct a sense of self (Ryan et al., 2007). Thus, I also questioned what work was being accomplished by the mothers' narratives.

Findings

Most striking about these findings was how similar the participants' narratives were. They demonstrated how the participants attended to the health of their children, and their developing immune systems. In all participants, there was evidence of an internalisation of broader public health narratives about how to be 'good mothers' but those who did not vaccinate their children or did but now regret it, resisted the idea that vaccines are safe and effective. Even the mothers who did vaccinate described the anxiety over safety issues involved in that decision. These narratives also demonstrated resistance to what some participants identified as 'mom shaming'. There was a corresponding acknowledgement that mothers struggle to know what 'the right thing' to do is, in the context of vaccination.

Infant body 'at risk'

For many participants, the infant body is thought to be in the state of becoming and is therefore vulnerable. Lupton, in research on infant embodiment, found the concept of the 'at risk' infant informed maternal thinking about the vaccination issue (Lupton, 2011). This was a common conceptualisation by participants and was articulated by one mother this way:

> One of my tremendous concerns about vaccinations is that they start when the baby is an infant. The schedule begins when they are a precious two months old... so that's a really, really little baby.
>
> Karen, three children, unvaccinated

The immune system is thought to be developing, and therefore vulnerable. Vulnerability to contaminants thought to be within a vaccine was the primary source of dis-ease in these mothers, even for some who had vaccinated their children:

> ... the risk of an adverse effect from receiving the vaccination, especially because they come in multiple doses and to bombard the immune system with different diseases in one day, for a two-month old, seems insane to me.
>
> Sarah, one child, partially vaccinated

> The thought... of all these foreign things [in the vaccine]: chemicals and bugs and god knows what, going into... his body all at once. You know, that doesn't make me feel great.
>
> Kat, one child, fully vaccinated

All participants were concerned about chemical contaminants entering their children from environmental sources like, for example, 'diesel trains' (Karen, three children, unvaccinated), or 'cleaners' (Sally, one child, unvaccinated), but most especially from food:

> The way I picture it it's like a pyramid: the more things I eat that have pesticides and chemicals and fungicides on them, the farther up the food chain you go, the more concentrated those sources are in your food products... somehow putting the food in *her* turned a switch for me.
>
> Kristy, two children, fully vaccinated

Those who did not vaccinate, or who only partially vaccinated their children, however, feared chemical contaminants more than viral contagion. Many participants expressed concern over what was in the needle and the need to know what was going into the infant body.

> I don't think we should be injecting our kids with chemicals... My look at the way that vaccines work relative to natural immunity tells me actually natural immunity is going to serve them better.
>
> Tina, one child, unvaccinated

One participant commented that not vaccinating was a 'huge risk' (Kat, one child, vaccinated) indicating that her fear of infectious disease was equal to or stronger than her fear of chemicals. For another participant however, overcoming the fear of contamination was an act of reason over emotion:

> I [had] some emotional anxiety when... we had our first immunizations... my brain, my rational side was saying 'I know [the safety concern around vaccines] has been debunked'. I know it's not true. Nonetheless... it did make me a little nervous but my rational side, as is usually the case, won out.
>
> Kristy, two children, fully vaccinated

The fear of contamination from vaccine 'chemicals' was relative to participants' perceptions of how likely their children were to contract a disease. When asked if they would reconsider vaccinating their children if they were to travel to other parts of the world where herd immunity is not prevalent, two of the mothers of under- or unvaccinated children said they would vaccinate.

Immunity/health building practices

The notions of 'building' a child's health, and of the immune system as being in a state of 'becoming' were prevalent in these interviews. All participants spent a large portion of the interview telling the story of how they promoted the health of their children, and their immunity in particular. Vaccination was but a moment in a child-health odyssey in which the immune system was a central character.

For all participants, the 'breast is best' strategy of infant feeding played an important role in what one mother called her 'immune strategy':

> A major piece of our immune strategy in this family is all of my children are breastfed and they're breastfed until they're ready to wean… looking at the science, I trust profoundly in the power of breast milk as an immunological strategy. And I feel it protects them quite a bit.
>
> Karen, three children, unvaccinated

Not all mothers, however, thought breastfeeding was an unmitigated good. In keeping with the concerns over contamination from pollutants, one participant expressed concern while still thinking it was important for immunity:

> I strongly believe breast milk provides [immunity], however, there is a slight concern about being contaminated with my heavy metals… we know that the fat tissue accumulates all the toxins from the environment.
>
> Sally, one child, unvaccinated

There was a widely shared understanding that the microflora of the intestine is important for child immunity:

> Actually our immune system is in our guts; that's where most of the defence mechanism is happening… and so the proper balance [is] very hard to achieve with the food that is commercially available. So a person has to be highly conscious… Every culture, always made sure that they had enough probiotics in their fermented vegetables.
>
> Sally, one child, unvaccinated

Many participants gave their children probiotics, especially after having given them antibiotics. Along with this understanding came a related understanding about the importance of using antibiotics appropriately:

> I do not like to give my kids antibiotics. And it drives me crazy when people get a cold and they run off and their crazy doctor gives them antibiotics. And

he'll do it over the phone. It's crazy because it's the more serious issue, drug resistant diseases, and the overuse of antibiotics, as opposed to vaccination.

Jane, two children, vaccinated

In keeping with Lupton's findings about motherhood and risk management (Lupton, 2011), there was a strong focus on food as a means of promoting the health of the child, indicating a preoccupation with contaminants and with building the healthy infant body. Breast milk was one important way these mothers built immunity in their children. When asked about their health practices in general, all participants mentioned eating habits as an important part of staying healthy:

So, we've been very conscious of eating whole food, and if we're going to buy meats, we try to get organic or at least free range; in terms of chicken and eggs... we try to do as much local foods, seasonal food. We grow our own garden... We really want to cultivate the whole, the 'food comes from the ground'.

Doris, two children, partially vaccinated

Participants expressed numerous other ways that they attended to their own health and the health of their infant, such as home-schooling as a health strategy, the importance of sleep, the use of vitamins and natural health products, and a holistic approach to health including 'being a nice person' (Susan, two children, partially vaccinated and unvaccinated):

Our kids don't go to school... the benefit is that they sleep when they're tired; they eat when they're hungry. It's not possible in a school setting for them to follow those rhythms of their body as closely. And as young children, we really feel like that is a health strategy for them, like that they learn to understand their bodies.

Karen, three children, unvaccinated

I don't see the Western medical model; it's very disease focused. I don't find it's very health focused... my view of health is more holistic, I don't think anything is in isolation. I like to look at everything as a whole, including emotional, mental underpinnings of anything that might be going on.

Tina, one child, unvaccinated

Moral work and the 'Mom Network'

Just as Crawford described the phenomenon of self-care as at once highly individualistic yet reliant on a social group for its promotion and support, these parents described a community of mothers who were like-minded in their self-care and holistic health ethos. One participant called this the 'mom network':

It's the information that gets passed along in a community. 'Cause with word of mouth of moms, we chat so much and information gets passed that way. Depending on what area you are in, I think you receive different information. So lots of like, you know, organic diets, the farmers' market goers, you know very eco-friendly and very environmentally conscious. And I think that goes hand in hand with health consciousness for children when it comes to vaccination.

Doris, two children, partially vaccinated

More than being sources of information, these networks had a moral function, which was discussed by many mothers in the study. Some felt the need to keep their vaccination choices private:

I try not to talk to [other] women… I don't like to talk about it in public, because, you know, people get really defensive and they feel like you're threatening their child.

Susan, two children, one partially vaccinated and
one not vaccinated

A number of the participants whose children were partially vaccinated or unvaccinated talked about a culture of what one participant called 'mom-shaming':

I have a big problem with mom-shaming. I believe that every mother is doing the absolute best that they can for their kid, and if a mother looks at the situation and makes a decision about it, nobody has any business telling that mom that she's doing a bad job.

Sarah, one child, partially vaccinated

This sense that mothers are doing the best they can in a difficult situation was shared by nearly all participants:

And then, part of the whole parent guilt comes in. Especially for moms. You're like 'Oh am I making the right decisions… for my child?' And then you hear other people's stories. And you hear other parental decisions. And you have family of different generations telling you, 'You should do this. You should do that'. So sometimes it's really hard. 'Okay, what is the right thing to do?'

Doris, two children, partially vaccinated

I try to make what's going to be the best decision. Generally, my stance would be 'to each his own'. So, if they don't want to immunize their kids, my feeling is, 'Fine, let them do what they want'.

Lucy, two children, vaccinated

One mother went so far as to express concern about the pressure on mothers to pursue health for themselves and their children and the worry it produces:

Guess what? Pregnancy is not a sickness. And neither is living. Living is not a sickness. We live as though we are constantly afraid of these pathogens in

the society… Like, everything is a pathogen. It's like the onslaught of pathogens and we're so worried constantly.

Karen, three children, unvaccinated

This worry and questioning about the 'right thing to do' indicates that participants view their vaccine decisions as embedded in the broader moral context
of being a 'good mother'. At the same time, they have compassion for other
mothers engaged in the struggle to do the right thing, and for the uncertainty
that can characterise the quest for their child's health. This is demonstrated in
their dislike of 'mom shaming', and their tolerance for others' decisions around
vaccination.

Discussion

In the construction of these narratives, mothers were concerned to demonstrate
that they are 'good mothers' through their discussion of how they promote the
overall health and immune systems of their children, regardless of their choice
around vaccination. What is remarkable in these women's narratives is not their
divergences but the similarities in their stories about the practices they engage
in and the struggles they have over questions about how to keep their children
healthy. For these participants, their children's health and its promotion are central to their notions of what it means to be a 'good mother'. They have demonstrated with their stories, however, that this is not always an easy task, and that
they feel they are subject to moral scrutiny about their choices. The vaccination issue is thus embedded and emplotted in this broader odyssey of health and
motherhood.

All the participants could be characterised as 'healthists' (Crawford, 1980) in
their beliefs around holistic health and their participation in 'mom networks'
that resemble the self-care networks Crawford described. They engaged in
health practices that involve sleep, food, responsible use of drugs, exercise, home
schooling and 'being a nice person' that fit well with Crawford's description of
these movements. It is evident from their singular focus on individual behaviours
regarding health that these practices are thought to be sufficient for achieving
health, and for fostering the development of robust immunity in their offspring.
They have chosen to focus exclusively on the infant body and its 'vulnerable, developing' immune system as a way to fend off contagion, ignoring other
possible points upstream in the causal chain at which their children could be
protected: protection from disease takes place within the infant body, or in the
inter-embodied experience of breastfeeding where antibodies are shared between
mother and child. This is entirely consistent with Crawford's observation that
causation within the phenomenon of healthism is focused solely on psychobiol-
ogism and towards host resistance and adaptation. The social or political determinants of health are not a feature of these narratives.

The infant body is thought to be vulnerable, and the developing immune
system needs to be protected from contamination; for some this meant that it

should only be educated through 'natural' exposure to pathogens. The need to know 'what is in the needle', and the suspicion that it contains 'very strong chemicals' or other toxins, is consistent with Lupton's observation that 'issues of bodily permeability and inter-embodiment are to the fore' (Lupton, 2013, p. 4). More than this, however, is evidence of the imperative to make informed decisions that are required by healthism. The construction of the infant body as 'at risk' from contamination, yet for some mothers, strong enough to deal with contagion that it encounters in a 'natural way' no longer seems paradoxical when we consider these beliefs as part and parcel of mothers' subjectivities as 'inter-embodied risk managers' who are part of the holistic health and self-care movements that believe that 'nature is an interactive friend' (Crawford, 1980). All mothers disciplined their own bodies during pregnancy, breastfed their children, and engaged in what Foucault would have called 'technologies of the child' but of course, these health practices are also technologies of the self, since through them mothers constitute themselves as good mothers and good citizens.

From these observations, we can posit that neoliberal 'good motherhood' is itself a form of Crawford's holistic health and self-care, and by extension, childcare. These data show that the framing of vaccination as a problem of personal choice fails to situate it within its broader social and political context. These findings force us to consider shifting away from viewing the issue of vaccine refusal as just another bad lifestyle choice, akin to overeating or smoking, and chalked-up to poor risk assessment and management on the part of the parent. Perhaps the problem is, rather, the neoliberal approach to improving the health of children, through the construction of the atomistic 'good mother' subjectivity. I suggest that uncertainty about vaccination is made possible through the creation of the hypervigilant, risk managing, 'good mother' who fears the risks of contamination as much as, if not more than, the risk of contagion. This is a rational risk calculation made by the informed risk calculator that is the neoliberal mother.

While Crawford maintained that medicalisation has given rise to healthism, he noted its singular focus on individual behaviour that is in keeping with medicalisation's focus on the body, and not the person as a whole, or on society. The focus on health, and its endless pursuit, is entirely in keeping with the moral discourse of public health, which has chosen to prioritise lifestyle factors over addressing the social and political determinants of health. These non-vaccinating parents are revealed to be moral public health citizens. Their subjectivities of 'the good mother' are entirely consistent with public health discourse around parenting, risk management and self-and-infant-surveillance. The paradox is not that these 'good mothers' and good citizens are resistant to vaccination. The real paradox here is that the choice to not vaccinate is at once a means of resisting the social control of governmentality and one made possible by the particular maternal subjectivity it creates.

Participants resisted discourses of 'mom shaming' that public health and other mothers can engage in (Henderson et al., 2010). This is likely the result of the intense forms of (self) surveillance that motherhood entails in neoliberal societies, and the moral scrutiny that comes along with it (Henderson et al., 2010;

Petersen & Lupton, 1997). Participants do demonstrate resistance to the discourse of public health through their hesitance and resistance to immunising their children. This resistance to vaccination, however, is itself shaped by neoliberal public health as it is the logical end point of the neoliberal, hypervigilant and hyperresponsible subjectivity of motherhood. As Hobson-West has found, trusting blindly is not the responsible thing to do as a parent, and is not consistent with critical consumption of health services and products (Hobson-West, 2007). Resistance to moral suasion and vaccination for herd immunity purposes reveals the participants' deep commitment to healthism: if you are 'doing the best that you can' as a mother, you should not be subject to moral scrutiny from others.

That public health has created the very maternal subjectivities that are prone to resist measures such as vaccination that typically have more benefit for the collective than for individuals, raises important questions about public health citizenship in the era of neoliberalism. For healthism gives rise to an elitist morality in which thwe individual is entirely responsible for health, and where health is a super value (Crawford, 1980). This takes place in the context that Starfield et al., described as a narrowing of the view of prevention in public health to a focus on interventions based on managing risks in individual patients, rather than in populations (Starfield et al., 2008). This narrowing has caused us to lose sight of the public health goals of equity and improving overall population health through collective action (Starfield et al., 2008). Scant attention is thus paid to obligations of citizens that obtain when ensuring the health of the population requires collective action.

Successful collective immunisation programs rely at least in part on citizens having duties to the *polis* to contribute to herd immunity. This is because little direct benefit accrues to the individual but herd immunity usually requires very high rates of immunisation for its preservation. Despite this, Dawson has pointed out that 'herd protection is an important public good which is a benefit shared by all individuals' (Dawson, 2004). It is, however, precisely this kind of public good that neoliberalism has systematically obscured and undermined with its singular focus on individual responsibility for health (Ayo, 2012), its focus on the management of risks in individual patients instead of the population (Starfield et al., 2008), and the privatisation of public goods such as water (Prudham, 2004). When a notion of collective responsibility for health is absent, it cannot then be mobilised to motivate people to act in aid of the common good. For some participants, vaccination must provide some direct benefit to the individual to invoke a duty to immunise, as we saw when some were willing to consider vaccination for their children if they were to travel to places where there was a higher risk of catching vaccine preventable disease. And while we can reproduce the neoliberal focus on individual responsibility for health by choosing to frame the moral issue as one of 'free riding' on herd immunity, 'free riding' is itself the logical endpoint of a neoliberal notion of citizenship. Instead, we need to be asking important ethical questions about the responsibility that neoliberal public health has for creating the very subjectivities that are primed to reject its dictates.

The fact that the antivaccine movement is on the rise may not be a result, then, of a subset of middle-class parents who are bad risk managers, ill-informed or prone to take medical advice from celebrities like former Playboy Bunny, Jenny McCarthy. The rise might be due to the successful internalisation of public health norms around how to be a 'good mother', who is intensely focused on her vulnerable child's body, and actively fostering the development of a robust immune system through the practice of numerous health promoting behaviours. We must consider the possibility that public health itself shares some of the responsibility for creating hypervigilant, self-and-infant-surveillant mothers who are concerned about contamination from toxins like pesticides, diesel fuel, mercury and other 'mystery' contaminants and who are focused on the ingress and egress of substances from the infant body. For if we continue to focus so closely on the individual body as the locus of health, assign sole responsibility for health to the individual and make public health issues about individual choices, we should not be surprised when the instinct to protect the herd is absent.

References

Ayo, N. (2012). Understanding health promotion in a neoliberal climate and the making of health conscious citizens. *Critical Public Health*, 22(1), 99–105. doi:10.1080/095815 96.2010.520692.

Barker, L. E., Chu, S. Y., & Smith, P. J. (2004). Children who have received no vaccines: Who are they and where do they live? *Pediatrics*, 114(1), 187–195.

Bissell, P., Ryan, K., & Morecroft, C. (2006). Narratives about illness and medication: A neglected theme/new methodology within pharmacy practice research. Part I: conceptual framework. *Pharmacy World & Science: PWS*, 28(2), 54–60. doi:10.1007/s11096-006-9005-y.

Blume, S. (2006). Anti-vaccination movements and their interpretations. *Social Science & Medicine*, 62(3), 628–642.

Brown, K. F. (2010). Factors underlying parental decisions about combination childhood vaccinations including MMR: A systematic review. *Vaccine*, 28(26), 4235–4248.

Brunson, E. K. (2013). The impact of social networks on parents' vaccination decisions. *Pediatrics*, 131(5), e1397–e1404. doi:10.1542/peds.2012-2452.

Bunton, R., & Petersen, A. (1997). *Foucault, Health and Medicine*. London: Routledge.

Corbin, J., & Strauss, A. (2008). *Basis of Qualitative Research: Techniques and Procedures for Developing Grounded Theory* (3rd ed.). London: Sage Publications Inc.

Crawford, R. (1980). Healthism and the medicalization of everyday life. *International Journal of Health Services*, 10(3), 365–388. doi:10.2190/3H2H-3XJN-3KAY-G9NY.

Dawson, A. (2004). Vaccination and the prevention problem. *Bioethics*, 18(6), 515–530.

Diekema, D. S. (2005). Responding to parental refusals of immunization of children. *Pediatrics*, 115(5), 1428–1431. doi:10.1542/peds.2005-0316.

Douglas, S., & Michaels, M. (2004). *The Mommy Myth: The Idealization of Motherhood and How it has Undermined All Women*. New York: Free Press.

Ericson, R., Barry, D., & Doyle, A. (2000). The moral hazards of neo-liberalism: Lessons from the private insurance industry. *Economy and Society*, 29(4), 532–558. doi:10.1080/03085140050174778.

Freed, G. L., Katz, S. L., & Clark, S. J. (1996). Safety of vaccinations: Miss America, the media, and public health. *JAMA*, 276(23), 1869–1872. doi:10.1001/jama.1996.03540230019013.

Furedi, F. (2002). *Paranoid Parenting: Why Ignoring the Experts May be Best for Your Child.* Chicago, IL: Chicago Review Press.

Greenhalgh, T., & Wessely, S. (2004). 'Health for me': A sociocultural analysis of healthism in the middle classes. *British Medical Bulletin, 69*(1), 197–213. doi:10.1093/bmb/ldh013.

Gust, D. A., Darling, N., Kennedy, A., & Schwartz, B. (2008). Parents with doubts about vaccines: Which vaccines and reasons why. *Pediatrics, 122*(4), 718–725. doi:10.1542/peds.2007-0538.

Hays, S. (1996). *The Cultural Contradictions of Motherhood.* Bloomsbury, London, UK: Yale University Press.

Heininger, U. (2006). An internet-based survey on parental attitudes towards immunization. *Vaccine, 24*(37–39), 6351–6355. doi:10.1016/j.vaccine.2006.05.029.

Henderson, A. C., Harmon, S. M., & Houser, J. (2010). A new state of surveillance? An application of Michel Foucault to modern motherhood. *Surveillance & Society, 7*(3/4), 231–247.

Hershey, J. C., Asch, D. A., Thumasathit, T., Meszaros, J., & Waters, V. V. (1994). The roles of altruism, free riding, and bandwagoning in vaccination decisions. *Organizational Behavior and Human Decision Processes, 59*(2), 177–187. doi:10.1006/obhd.1994.1055.

Hobson-West, P. (2003). Understanding vaccination resistance: Moving beyond risk. *Health, Risk and Society, 5*(3), 273–283. doi:10.1080/13698570310001606978.

Hobson-West, P. (2007). "Trusting blindly can be the biggest risk of all": Organised resistance to childhood vaccination in the UK. *Sociology of Health & Illness, 29*(2), 198–215. doi:10.1111/j.1467-9566.2007.00544.x.

Jessop, L. J. (2010). Socio-demographic and health-related predictors of uptake of first MMR immunisation in the Lifeways Cohort Study. *Vaccine, 28*(38), 6338–6343.

Kennedy, A. M., Brown, C. J., & Gust, D. A. (2005). Vaccine beliefs of parents who oppose compulsory vaccination. *Public Health Reports, 120*(3), 252.

Lee, E., Bristow, J., Faircloth, C., & Macvarish, J. (2014). *Parenting Culture Studies.* Camden, UK: Palgrave Macmillan.

Lieblich, A., Tuval-Mashiach, R., & Zilber, T. (1998). *Narrative Research: Reading, Analysis, and Interpretation* (Vol. 47). Londin, UK: SAGE Publications, Inc.

Lupton, D. (1993). Risk as moral danger: The social and political functions of risk discourse in public health. *International Journal of Health Services: Planning, Administration, Evaluation, 23*(3), 425–435. doi:10.2190/16AY-E2GC-DFLD-51X2.

Lupton, D. (2011). 'The best thing for the baby': Mothers' concepts and experiences related to promoting their infants' health and development. *Health, Risk and Society, 13*(7–8), 637–651. doi:10.1080/13698575.2011.624179.

Lupton, D. (2013). Infant embodiment and interembodiment: A review of sociocultural perspectives. *Childhood, 20*(1), 37–50. doi:10.1177/0907568212447244.

Maines, D. (2004). Theoretical sampling. In M. Lewis-Beck, A. Bryman, & T. F. Liao (Eds.), *The SAGE Encyclopedia of Social Science Research Methods* (pp. 1122–1123). London, UK: SAGE Publications, Inc.

Miles, M., Huberman, M., & Saldana, J. (2013). *Qualitative Data Analysis* (3rd ed.). SAGE Publications. https://us.sagepub.com/en-us/nam/qualitative-data-analysis/book246128.

Miller, S. (2001). Public understanding of science at the crossroads. *Public Understanding of Science, 10*, 115–120.

Murphy, E. (1999). 'Breast is best': Infant feeding decisions and maternal deviance. *Sociology of Health & Illness, 21*(2), 187–208. doi:10.1111/1467-9566.00149.

New, S. J., & Senior, M. L. (1991). "I don't believe in needles": Qualitative aspects of a study into the uptake of infant immunisation in two English health authorities. *Social Science & Medicine, 33*(4), 509–518. doi:10.1016/0277-9536(91)90333-8.

Osborne, T. (1997). Of health and statecraft. In A. Petersen & R. Bunton (Eds.), *Foucault, Health and Medicine* (pp. 173–188). London, UK: Routledge.

Petersen, A. R. (1996). Risk and the regulated self: The discourse of health promotion as politics of uncertainty. *The Australian and New Zealand Journal of Sociology, 32*(1), 44–57. doi:10.1177/144078339603200105.

Petersen, A.R., & Lupton, D. (1997). *The New Public Health: Health and Self in the Age of Risk* (1st ed.). London, UK: Sage Publications Inc.

Poland, G. A., & Jacobson, R. M. (2001). Understanding those who do not understand: A brief review of the anti-vaccine movement. *Vaccine, 19*(17–19), 2440–2445. doi:10.1016/S0264-410X(00)00469-2.

Prudham, S. (2004). Poisoning the well: Neoliberalism and the contamination of municipal water in Walkerton, Ontario. *Geoforum, 35*(3), 343–359.

Rogers, A., & Pilgrim, D. (1995). The risk of resistance: perspectives on the mass childhood immunisation programme. In: Gabe, J. (ed.) *Medicine, health and risk: sociological approaches*. Oxford: Blackwell. pp. 73–90.

Rose, N. (1990). *Governing the Soul: The Shaping of the Private Self* (Vol. xiv). Milton Park, Oxfordshire: Taylor & Frances Group/Routledge.

Ryan, K., Bissell, P., & Alexander, J. (2010). Moral work in women's narratives of breastfeeding. *Social Science & Medicine (1982), 70*(6), 951–958. doi:10.1016/j.socscimed.2009.11.023.

Ryan, K., Bissell, P., & Morecroft, C. (2007). Narratives about illness and medication: A neglected theme/new methodology within pharmacy practice research. Part II: medication narratives in practice. *Pharmacy World & Science, 29*(4), 353–360. doi:10.1007/s11096-006-9017-7.

Shao, J.-Y. (2008). To MMR or not MMR: Is that the Question? MSc Dissertation. University of Toronto, Toronto, Canada.

Shaw, R. (2004). Performing breastfeeding: Embodiment, ethics and the maternal subject. *Feminist Review, 78*(1), 99–116. doi:10.1057/palgrave.fr.9400186.

Starfield, B., Hyde, J., Gervas, J., & Heath, J. (2008). The concept of prevention: A good idea gone bad? *Journal of Epidemiology and Community Health, 62*, 580–583.

Wilson, K., Barakat, M., Vohra, S., Ritvo, P., & Boon, H. (2008). Parental views on pediatric vaccination: The impact of competing advocacy coalitions. *Public Understanding of Science, 17*(2), 231–243. doi:10.1177/0963662506067662.

Yaqub, O., Castle-Clarke, S., Sevdalis, N., & Chataway, J. (2014). Attitudes to vaccination: A critical review. *Social Science & Medicine, 112*, 1–11. doi:10.1016/j.socscimed.2014.04.018.

8 The pharmaceutical imaginary of heart disease

Pleasant futures and problematic present[1]

Sofie Rosenlund Lau, Bjarke Oxlund and Anna Birna Almarsdóttir

Introduction and background

Since the 1950s, an increasing focus of many nations has been on preventing cardiovascular disease (CVD), the global leading cause of death. Subsequently, the market for pharmaceuticals to prevent CVD has exploded and today statins (cholesterol-lowering drugs) are the most sold class of pharmaceuticals in many western countries (Weintraub, 2017). Statins are used both as secondary prophylaxis among people with manifested CVD and as primary prophylaxis among heart healthy individuals. The treatment strategy is widely acknowledged as rational and is perceived as a cornerstone for the management of CVD (Stroes et al., 2015; Collins et al., 2016). At the same time, the effectiveness and safety of statins, especially among heart-healthy individuals, is subject to intense debate (Abramson, Rosenberg, Jewell & Wright, 2013; Godlee, 2016; Petursson, 2012) and critical voices against a *statinisation* of populations have been raised (Khanna, Emerick & Lewis, 2013). The widespread use of statins is both a matter of course and a matter of concern. This makes the utilisation of statins an interesting lens through which to explore contemporary notions of health and disease (Lau, 2018). In this chapter, we focus on the role of pharmaceutical prevention in the lives of individuals with elevated cholesterol who have been offered statin treatment. As such, we explore how subjectivity shapes and is shaped by statin treatment, by asking: Why do so many subscribe to statins for prevention of heart disease? How does the routinisation of statins influence the individual experience of being at risk? And how does statin use impact the sense of self?

Healthy living in the 21st century

There is a growing body of literature that looks at the experience of being at risk, including how pharmaceuticals influence the perception and management of 'at risk states' (Greene, 2007; Clarke, Shim, Mamo, Fosket & Fishman, 2010; Dumit, 2012). Greene (2007) describes a new form of health care emerging in the 20th century where masses of people are treated with preventive medicines based on numerical deviations rather than symptoms. This approach to health care is defined by epidemiological measures of risk rather than individual experiences of illness, and the pharmaceutical treatment aims to reduce the risk rather than to treat the disease (Greene, 2007; Aronowitz, 2009; Dumit, 2012). Today, public health regimes in relation to the prevention of CVD are founded on the principle of early risk reduction attached to everyday practices. Specifically, the awareness of heart healthy diets, restriction on alcohol consumption, smoking cessation and the importance of daily exercise are widely recommended. Arguably, health has become a moral imperative (Crawford, 1980; Lupton, 1995) and obtaining a healthy body an individual responsibility (Rose, 2007). To be healthy is no longer just about treating illness, it is also about keeping future disease at bay by engaging in anticipatory practices in the present (Adams, Murphy & Clarke, 2009). Adams, Murphy, and Clarke (2009), p. 247 offer an understanding of preventive health as a practice of anticipation that makes possible futures into a highly present *affective state*. 'As an affective state', they argue, 'anticipation is not just a reaction, but a way of actively orienting oneself temporally'. Screening for elevated blood cholesterol and taking statins can thus be interpreted as ways of managing uncertain health futures through the means of biotechnologies available here and now. In that sense, knowing your cholesterol and preventing heart disease with statins are practical ways of adapting to the unknown, of actively reorienting possible future lives towards what seems to be safe and healthy trajectories.

Selves and imageries of statins

Heart disease as a global health threat has already been subject to pharmaceuticalisation (Abraham, 2010), since pharmaceuticals have been defined as the main way to decrease mortality and morbidity from CVD. Inspired by the work of Foucault (1997) and Rose (2007), one could say that statins have become a technology of the self to govern the health of populations. Yet, pharmaceuticals also have social lives, as argued by Whyte, van der Geest & Hardon (2002); '[Medicines] have power, in the hands of humans, to transform bodies, minds, situations and modes of understanding' (Whyte et al., 2002, p. 5). At a more structural level, Williams, Martin & Gabe (2011) argue for the need to 'explore the broader way in which pharmaceutical futures are shaping how we think about innovation, policy and the very meaning of health and illness, therapy and enhancement.' (Williams, Martin & Gabe, 2011, p. 730). In other words, how do we attribute power and trust to pharmaceuticals, and how does the pharmaceutical imaginary influence how we anticipate possible futures and manage contemporary problems in our individual lives and local environments? Jenkins (2010) applies the concept of *pharmaceutical self* and *pharmaceutical imaginary* to account for the reciprocal relationship between the individual experience and the cultural or structural context of medicine use. Jenkins depicts the pharmaceutical self as the aspect of the self that is oriented by and towards pharmaceuticals (Jenkins, 2010, p. 23), and the pharmaceutical imaginary (while referring to Castoriadis' take on the imaginary, 1987) as the global shaping of consumption – 'the region of the imaginary in which pharmaceuticals play an increasingly critical role' (Jenkins, 2010, p. 6). With the dual concept of self/imaginary, Jenkins' point is that subjective experiences of pharmaceuticals are tightly linked to the social and cultural conundrums of pharmaceuticals' local and global lives.

The pharmaceutical self/imaginary has mainly been used to study psychopharmacology (Jenkins, 2010; Schlosser & Hoffer, 2012), in which symptomatic conditions and suffering are pronounced. In this chapter, however, we use the dual concept as a tool to analyse the ways in which the routinisation of pharmaceutical prevention of CVD in Denmark shapes imaginaries of futures without heart disease, and how these imaginaries translate into people's everyday lives. By following individuals with elevated cholesterol, we zoom in on the pharmaceutical self as the self that is oriented by statin use and towards the possibilities (and problems) that statins offer in everyday life now and in the future.

The question becomes: what does anticipation entail from the perspective of individual statin users? Borrowing from the terminology developed by Adams, Murphy & Clarke (2009), we argue that the pharmaceutical imaginary of statins turns the pharmaceutical self into one that is morally obliged to be oriented towards *optimising* the future and one that is in a constant mode of *bioprepared-ness*. Through this framework, statin use can be understood as *abductive* work; as a way of moving back and forth between uncertain futures and (potentially unpleasant) presents.

Methodology

The analysis is based on ethnographic fieldwork carried out in the capital region of Denmark in 2013–2014 by the first author.[2] High cholesterol was studied as an object in order to understand how the condition is produced, governed and managed, and what role pharmaceuticals play in risk reduction. High cholesterol is neither stable nor easily captured as a coherent whole, and the fieldwork thus spread across a variety of physical sites and actors. 'Ethnographic assemblage' methodology (Wahlberg 2018) was used as a way to capture how juridical, medical, social, economic, cultural and institutional processes came together to produce the condition: high cholesterol (see also Lau, 2018).

The fieldwork consisted of participant observation at work-place health checks and at a national health fair, where opportunistic health screenings and blood tests were offered. It involved participant observation at a lipid clinic and in a so-called Heart Café organised by a local branch of the Danish Heart Foundation. Visits were paid to five GP clinics, while participation was exercised in a heart rehabilitation program. In-depth interviews were conducted with 15 former and current statin users (eight males and seven females) spanning 28–79 years with a mean age of 62 years. Furthermore, the empirical material includes semi-structured interviews with eleven health care professionals and several informal conversations with healthcare professionals and other experts. The fieldwork has solicited a variety of perceptions of and experiences with statins and allows for an analysis of the links between individual and larger sociocultural aspects of pharmaceutical prevention of CVD.

The interviews were conducted in Danish and were transcribed verbatim. All quotes used in this article have been translated into English by the first author.

In Denmark, qualitative studies do not undergo official research ethics approval (cf. Danish Act on Research Ethics Review of Health Research Projects), but the study is registered with the Committee of Health Research Ethics and has been conducted in accordance with the regulations of the Danish Data Protection Agency. The article makes use of pseudonyms for all interlocutors quoted.

Findings

Optimising the future

In the pharmaceutical imaginary, the main effect of statins is to keep coronary heart disease at bay. In that sense, statin use can be interpreted as a mode of optimisation or 'the effort to secure one's own, one's family's, one's group's, or even one's population's "best possible future"' (Adams et al., 2009, p. 256). In the pharmaceutical imaginary of statins, anticipated futures do not necessarily link to any prior discomfort. Only two of the participants in the study did not consider themselves to be healthy and well, which means that to most of the participants the diagnosis of elevated cholesterol came unexpectedly. Many had not even thought about the possibility of being at risk of CVD before their blood was tested and the testing was often opportunistic. For instance, Thomas (aged 51) found out he was at risk of CVD during a health check offered at his workplace. Karen (aged 57) found out during an opportunistic screening for osteoporosis, while Bent (aged 68) found out as part of a standardised general health check when he moved to a new general practice. In all three cases, a blood test triggered the at-risk label. Since Thomas, Karen and Bent have not experienced any bodily symptoms they have had difficulties relating to the label. As Thomas explained: 'It [elevated cholesterol] is distant somehow, because I do not experience any problems. I have no symptoms. It is just something written on a piece of paper.' In one way, elevated cholesterol resembles an illness in the sense that the condition is medically defined as a deviation from a 'normal', healthy body. On the other hand, the condition is asymptomatic, leaving no traces or phenomenological experiences besides a deviant number from a blood test.

It is characteristic of medicine in the 21st century that individuals who are otherwise healthy are epidemiologically constructed as 'subjects at risk' (Langdridge, 2017). While the participants did not feel at risk, many still perceived the test as a good way to keep their health in check. Bent explained:

> I think, as with many other preventive measures, it is good to do a test like that. You can't see if your cholesterol is high, right? It is not something that you feel – you are not conscious about it at all. So if they hadn't done the blood test, then I wouldn't have known. And maybe I would have been told that it was nothing, but I think it is nice to know, and nice to know that you can do something about it.

Apparently, Bent found it reasonable and appropriate to have the blood test, because it was the only way for him to know about his cholesterol. Screenings and health checks have become an ordinary and highly integrated part of health-care. As such, the blood test is a concrete example of what Adams, Murphy & Clarke (2009) term 'technologies of anticipation'. The blood sample functions as a way to ' [push back CVD] to predictive 'virtual pathologies' identified as diag-nostic risk signs probabilistically linked to symptoms that are made real in the predictive moment of now' (Adams et al., 2009, p. 251). Keeping your health in check via screening and tests now equals good citizenship, since it improves the prospects of living long healthy lives (Lupton, 1995; Gillespie, 2012; Schwen-nesen & Koch, 2012). This is one of the reasons opportunistic health checks have become popular in Denmark despite limited evidence on the efficacy of these assessments (Krogsbøll, Jørgensen & Gøtzsche, 2011). Participants in the study were quite appreciative of health checks, when they said: 'It is nice to be at the forefront of things' (Tom, 60) and 'I am really glad that I am a part of the system – that someone is keeping an eye on me' (Bodil, 61). Since health checks have become a routinised part of clinical encounters, and since they are regularly offered by health insurers and employers, they are in general positively evaluated.

The screening experience is not attractive to all, though. To Karen, the knowledge about elevated cholesterol triggered a shock reaction: 'I kind of pan-icked. I thought it was terrible.' While many of the other participants were not worried by their at-risk status, Karen began to think of elevated cholesterol as a serious disease. She pondered: 'Well, it's fat in the blood, right. And it makes the arteries smaller, I mean, the fat aggregates on the inside, making the arteries smaller, so that you can easier [sic] suffer from a blood clot.' This imagery of fat accumulating in the veins is not something that Karen had made up on her own, but rather the reproduction of the standardised pathology of atherosclerosis (Greene, 2007). Despite the on-going academic dispute on whether cholesterol is in fact a risk factor for CVD, this pharmaceutical imaginary of the drugs effec-tively reducing the blocking of the veins works as a powerful promoter of the screening and subsequent pharmaceutical management of elevated cholesterol. At the same time, the pathology of atherosclerosis also works on another level. Karen's experience of being told that she had elevated cholesterol resembled the experience of being told that she suffered from a serious disease. As such, the pharmaceutical imaginary promotes elevated cholesterol as a disease in itself. As noticed by Aronowitz, 'the risk state itself has become more embodied and, in other ways, more disease-like' (Aronowitz, 2009, p. 419). In that sense, the pos-sibility of risk assessments to forecast future illnesses potentially induces fear and anxiety in the present (Adams et al., 2009; Aronowitz, 2009; Rosenberg, 2009). Although the cholesterol number is just a surrogate marker for potential future illness, to be told that 'you are at risk' easily translates into prospects of CVD. It fosters a need to optimise future health.

Being (bio)prepared

In interviews, the screening for elevated cholesterol and the statin use often melted together as mutual strategies for controlling risk. Most participants per-ceived both as a matter of actively being prepared for what might come. Thomas said: 'It's not like it keeps me awake at night. Neither does the risk. I see it more like when you take your car in for service to prevent future problems.' The analogy of the service check surfaces many times in the interviews. In fact, many of the healthcare professionals also referred to the standardised health check as a '10,000 km service'. The logic of prevention is persuasive since it offers control and certainty for risks that are otherwise hidden. Adams and colleagues (2009, p. 258) use another analogy, namely that of military pre-emptive strike. They argue that 'anticipation authorizes pre-emptive actions… in the name of an anticipated future danger'. Most of the participants talked of someone who had died from CVD and were thus keenly aware of the dangers that may lie ahead. In the anticipatory regime, both screening for elevated cholesterol and statin treatment function as a 'pre-emptive strike' against this danger. As 'safety pills', statins become a way of actively lowering blood cholesterol and keeping the danger at bay. In short, statins provide an easy and tangible way of changing problematic futures.

Tom (aged 60) stated bluntly: 'I think it's a good and easy solution to the problem of getting the number down.' The pills easily become a mundane part of everyday living, as Bodil expressed: 'Honestly, I don't give it much thought. It has become part of my everyday routine, one of those things you just do, like brushing your teeth. One of those ordinary practices' (Bodil, 61).

Statin use is just a small part of the anticipatory regime that is already making up our daily living. We are not in doubt that we should fasten our seatbelt, brush our teeth or insure our bodies. In comparison with other kinds of biopreparedness such as immunisation, cancer screenings, and prenatal screenings, it is easy to take a pill. To most, it does not raise much of a concern.

Yet, the need for preparedness may still be interpreted as a moral failure by the individual. This was the case for Kirsten (77) who called her GP to ask for a general health check. Everything turned out to be normal except the cholesterol. The GP thus prescribed statins, but the use of pills conflicted with Kirsten's notion of a 'morally good' life. This was clearly evidenced by the way she talked of her own mother: 'I would rather be without the medicines. I can tell you, my old mother died at the age of 82. And the day she was admitted to the hospital, the nurse asked her to remember to bring her pills. "Pills? I do not take any pills!"' In sharing this story, Kirsten seemed to convey that having to take statins on a daily basis does not cohere with her ideal self.

Several scholars have written about the moral discourses embedded in the use of medicine (Eborall & Will, 2011; Dew, Norris, Gabe, Chamberlain & Hodgetts, 2015; Polak, 2017). For instance, Polak (2017) describes how statin users fear being identified as lazy or irresponsible in view of health promotion discourses insisting that a healthy lifestyle can reduce cholesterol and prevent CVD. A failing health equals a failing person, seems to be the equation here, and so Kirsten experienced her dependency on pharmaceuticals as a moral failure. As Dew et al. (2015) argue: 'Pharmaceuticals are tied to our identity, what we want to show of ourselves, and what sort of world we see ourselves living in.' (p. 272). What Kirsten's case shows is that actions that one takes to pre-empt the future may affect one's understanding of self in the present.

Statin use may not only have individual consequences. They can also be social. In one interview, Tom, who has taken statins for almost 10 years, explained how he has organised for his two sons (aged 19 and 24) to be tested for elevated cholesterol. The youngest son is pursuing a career as a professional football player, and Tom wants to be reassured that his heart is flawless. The eldest son has gained weight, which makes Tom suspect that his risk of CVD has increased:

> He used to be so handsome and slim, but in the past two years he has become a bit chubby. He found this girlfriend, you know, who cooks traditional Danish food, heavy and greasy. And he used to play a lot of football, but he doesn't do that anymore. So now he spends most of his time in front of his computer at work, sitting still.

The blood tests of both sons revealed slightly elevated cholesterol, yet the GP did not want to prescribe medication. As Tom explained: 'My doctor says that they will not start medication at age 24, not if it is below seven or eight. And obviously, they would first and foremost tell him to lose weight and start exercising.'

Likewise, the recommendation for his younger son was just to 'keep an eye on it.' To Tom, it was a relief to know the numbers and to be able to act on his concern:

> I had to push my doctor a bit to make her do the blood tests, especially on my youngest son, because she doesn't think that you should medicalize people. And there is of course something to that. But I just thought it was nice to know.

In the study, many other participants had urged family members to go for screenings, and several had started statin use on the recommendation of someone in the family. What is clear from Tom's case is that the moral obligation to optimise and being prepared may extend to the future health of relatives. As such, it is an example of how the pharmaceutical imaginary moves beyond the self and into the social lives of families constituting what we might call a social imaginary of pharmaceuticals, since it shows the management of risk and care are also embedded in social relations.

Abduction and the sense of being off-time

Will and Weiner argue that we need to understand healthy living practices as something less coherent and calculated than rational choice (Will & Weiner, 2014). Likewise, Polak and Green ask us to rethink the processes of decision-making about statins purely as a cognitive practice and towards integrated material practices in the conceptualisation of choice (Polak & Green, 2020). When thinking of statin use as an anticipatory practice, these thoughts align. Adams and colleagues (2009, p. 255) suggest that we consider the actual practices of acting towards anticipation as matters of abduction: 'Abduction is the process of considering more precisely *how* to anticipate in actual practice. How is the present abducted by the future? What kind of preventive actions will be pursued? Which interventions are most appropriate?'.

Although statins have often been cast as 'the easy option in a busy life' (Kørner, 2019), statins are not the preferred solution. Even though statin use is heavily promoted in Denmark (Bagge & Hansen, 2011), the Danish clinical practice guidelines still recommend lifestyle changes before pharmacology in moderate cases (Danish Health Authority, ; Sundhedsstyrelsen, 2012). The participants in the current study all expressed a desire to manage their blood cholesterol without drugs. To their disappointment, most of them did not succeed. One example is Thomas, who tried to lower his cholesterol by focusing on his diet. He ate more vegetables and consumed less fat, but the changes were not enough to lower his cholesterol. Even as an ultramarathon runner, who runs 70–100 km per week, it took statins for Thomas to lower his cholesterol number. In his own words, he stated:

> I am of the opinion, that if you can change something through your lifestyle, it is definitely worth it, compared to taking medicines. Medication should always be secondary. Indeed, it can be an easy and convenient solution, but I would rather be without it, because it comes with the risk of side effects. And I think it is best if the body can do what it's designed to. But in this case it can't... I had to realize that eating more vegetables and exercising more did not change anything. The solution had to be found somewhere else. We cannot all be perfect.

The use of statins was the last option in Thomas' attempt to abduct the future. Submitting to statin treatment was to him equivalent to admitting that his body was dysfunctional, which amounted to a moral failure reminiscent of Kirsten. The failure was nicely captured in his sum-up: 'we cannot all be perfect'.

Other participants had also adjusted their lifestyle after receiving information about their elevated cholesterol. Karen had started on a new diet with fewer carbohydrates and more vegetables. She used a vocabulary of discipline and sacrifice when telling about it: 'In the summertime my husband and I love to make barbecue. I just love a roasted chicken. But I don't eat the skin. Not that I don't like it, it tastes so damn good but there is just no reason to stuff yourself with things like that.'

Others too talked about adjusting their eating practices and how vegetables and plant oils had replaced big steaks and butter.

In his study of statin users, Dumit argued that 'many patients consume pharmaceuticals as a means of maintaining rather than changing a lifestyle' (Dumit, 2012, p. 192). This is not the case for participants in this study, but none of them eventually managed to truly lower their blood cholesterol level on their own. Perhaps this is why there seems to be agreement among statin users and clinicians that statins are much more efficient than dietary changes. This assumption was verbalised during a health fair, where a cardiology nurse explained that: 'Quitting smoking and starting exercising might help some. But it is really the medicines that make the difference.' According to the pharmaceutical imaginary, statins are the most efficient and safe way to manage elevated cholesterol. The pharmaceutical self is torn between wanting to avoid medicines on the one hand and wanting to stay safe on the other. By considering statin use as a process of abduction, of navigating practices, obligations and future health, we are left with an understanding of 'choice' that is much more nuanced than the framing of statins as a quick fix.

This raises another important question: what happens when the safety strategy fails, for instance, when people experience deteriorating side effects from statins? The fieldwork revealed that when statins are prescribed in the clinic, side effects are rarely mentioned and most physicians believe that side effects of statins are rare and reversible. The assumption that side effects of statins are minimal makes it easier to leave them out in clinical encounters. Some GPs in the study held that patients prefer not to know about the risks associated with statins. This was to some extent confirmed in interviews with statin users. Those who had actually discussed side effects with their GPs, had only done so because they experienced discomfort. Some even expressed a sense of alienation when it came to knowledge of side effects. Kirsten thus explained how an assistant at her local pharmacy had urged her to read the packet insert, to which she responded: 'Do you know what, if I read that, then I don't even dare take the pills, because then I will die from them! So no, I have not read it.'

In the pharmaceutical imaginary of statins, side effects exist as an uncommon and hence irrelevant risk. However, to some statin users, side effects are very real. Bent (aged 68) had suffered from erectile dysfunction after starting statin use about six months before our first interview. Together with his GP, he decided to discontinue statins. He reflected: 'So, time will tell if I have to take it again. Maybe there is an alternative that does not cause me these inconveniences. I don't know. But it is also a choice from my side, do I want one thing or another. … So that is the question: do you want a good life one way or another?' Stopping statin treatment presented Bent with a dilemma about 'the good life': was it about anticipating the future by taking statins and accepting the side effect of a troubled sex life, or was it worrying about the future, while enjoying an active sex life now. Bent repeatedly emphasised that his cholesterol was only 'slightly elevated,' which justified his choice to temporarily stop statin therapy. Still, he worried about the risk of CVD: 'I know that high cholesterol can cause strokes and heart attacks, so I was certain that I wanted to start statin treatment when my doctor recommended it. Now I don't really know.'

The case shows that once a person identifies with the label 'at risk,' it is difficult to let go of that label. As Gifford (1986) explains: 'For the patient, risk becomes a lived or experienced state of ill-health and a symptom of future illness. To the patient, risk is rarely an objective concept. Rather, it is internalized and experienced as a state of being' (p. 215). The depiction of elevated cholesterol as a disease, together with the ability of statins to 'treat it', makes the rejection of statins equivalent to an acceptance of future suffering due to CVD. Here, the work inherent in anticipating futures without CVD is entangled with the desire for living a preferred life in the present. This ambiguity is even more apparent in Karen's case.

For almost 7 years, Karen (aged 57) had been taking a small statin pill with a glass of water every night. This constituted an insignificant event in her daily routine. During a standard health check-up, her GP suddenly decided to discontinue the drug, since he found that Karen's cholesterol had fallen below the threshold. Karen explained: 'He showed me different tables and measurements, and how I had jumped from the red to the green zone'. To Karen's surprise, the discontinuation of statins did away with the chronic pain she had been experiencing in her joints: 'I had so much pain in my elbow joints that sometimes I couldn't move them. And now, since I stopped taking the pills, I feel nothing! It is completely gone'. Both Karen and her GP were convinced that the pain was caused by statins. But just as in Bent's case, the discontinuation of statins brought with it a feeling of risk and vulnerability in Karen:

> My GP says that too many people are taking these drugs. That they are over-prescribed. And he showed me this table on the Internet where you can calculate your risk. And sure, I get that. It is just, in the back of my head I feel like, uh-oh, what now? What if I suddenly die of a heart attack? What if there is not enough room or free passage in my veins for my blood to flow freely?

Karen now found herself in the ambiguous situation of having to choose between living with chronic pain from statins and feeling safe versus worrying about possible futures with heart disease while enjoying freedom from pain. Where Bent represents the typical temporal experience of side effects (statins made him feel uncomfortable), Karen was unaware of the side effects of statins until she discontinued treatment and let go of the pain. This reveals the profound capacity of the pharmaceutical imaginary to mediate experiences of effects. The representation of statins as safe trumped the actual experience of side effects, and did so to an extent that Karen wonders whether she should resume statin treatment: 'It is still a thought in the back of my head... I am really not sure I can manage without them. But right now I do not take them.' Both examples highlight the way in which biological side effects may translate into questions and ambiguities about which preventive actions to take. Neither Karen nor Bent is sure they want to discontinue treatment. Hence, statin use as a practice of abduction becomes an embodied feeling of wresting of the present with alien futures (Adams et al., 2009, p. 255).

Concluding remarks

In this chapter we prefer to ask *what* it means to live with preventive pharmaceuticals rather than *whether or not* one should live with preventive pharmaceuticals. We have focused on the individual experiences of taking statins to lower blood cholesterol and reduce the risk of CVD. Using the theoretical framework of Adams et al. (2009), we have shown that statin use can be interpreted as a way of anticipating futures without CVD. In that sense, testing for high cholesterol and taking statins becomes a way of *optimising* life through the effort to secure one's future and *preparing* the body by changing biomechanisms that might or might not cause future disease. Yet, the work associated with optimisation and preparedness is not always simple. Pharmaceutical prevention may affect the way we see ourselves and the way we live our lives. In some instances, statin use becomes a moral failure because it is indicative of a dysfunctional body and unmanageable health. In other cases, optimisation and preparedness result in actions imposed on or by others. We have thus shown that the preventive work is never just about taking a pill. It also includes daily moral contestation over food and medicine and about living life the 'right' way.

We have also demonstrated that the abductive work of navigating possible futures in the present comes to the fore when statins have side effects and cause discomfort. Statin users who experience side effects thus have to choose between the prevention of possible unwanted futures and living well in the present. As such, pharmaceutical prevention is an affective state that brings the future into the now. In that sense, managing elevated cholesterol is an anticipatory mode that 'enable[s] the production of possible futures that are *lived and felt* as inevitable in the present' (Adams et al., 2009, p. 248).

The production of possible futures is not something entirely connected to the self. It is something that is brought forward by the pharmaceutical imaginary of statins, that is, the belief in the risk of CVD as something that is caused by high cholesterol and which can be managed by taking statins. This imaginary is anchored in global and local interpretations of pharmaceuticals as technologies of both care and control (Petryna, Lakoff & Kleinman, 2006; Greene, 2007; Dumit, 2012). What matters to statin users is not so much the treatment of risk as such, but rather how to stay healthy (Lau, 2018; Jauho, 2019). As long as the pharmaceutical imaginary determines the prospects of controlling CVD through screening and pill-taking, the pharmaceutical self has to navigate between a pleasant future and a problematic present.

Note

1 A version of this paper was presented at the International Social Pharmacy Workshop Symposium "Living Pharmaceutical Lives" Leuven, Belgium, July 23–26, 2018.

2 This study is a part of the interdisciplinary research project, LIFESTAT (Living with Statins), which combines approaches and knowledge from health sciences, the humanities and social sciences to analyze the impact of statin use on health, lifestyle and well-being among Danish citizens (Christensen et al., 2016). Furthermore, it forms part of Sofie Rosenlund Lau's PhD entitled *A Matter of Course – An Ethnographic Assemblage of the Routinization of Pharmaceutical Prevention with Statins in Denmark* (Lau, 2018).

References

Abraham, J. (2010). Pharmaceuticalization of society in context: Theoretical, empirical and health dimensions. *Sociology*, 44(4), 603–622. doi: 10.1177/0038038510369368.

Abramson, J. D., Rosenberg, H.G., Jewell, N., & Wright, J.M. (2013). Should people at low risk of cardiovascular disease take a statin?.*BMJ*, 347, f6123. doi: 10.1136/bmj. f6123.

114   *Sofie Rosenlund Lau et al.*

Adams, V., Murphy, M., & Clarke, A. E. (2009). Anticipation: Technoscience, life, affect, temporality. *Subjectivity, 28*(1), 246–265. doi: 10.1057/sub.2009.18.

Aronowitz, R. A. (2009). The converged experience of risk and disease. *Milbank Quarterly, 417*, 422. doi: 10.1111/j.1468-0009.2009.00563.x.

Bagge, T., & Hansen, H. L. (2011). *Bekæmp Kolesterolen Med Statiner*. BT. Retrieved from http://www.bt.dk/sundhed/7-bekaemp-kolesterolen-med-statiner.

Castoriadis, C. (1987). *The Imaginary Institution of Society. Translation*. Cambridge: Polity in association with Basil Blackwell.

Christensen, C. L., Helge, J.W., Krasnik, A., Kriegbaum, M., Rasmussen, L.J., Hickson, I.D., ... Dela, F. (2016). LIFESTAT – Living with statins: An interdisciplinary project on the use of statins as a cholesterol-lowering treatment and for cardiovascular risk reduction. *Scandinavian Journal of Public Health, 44*(5), 534–539. doi: 10.1177/1403494816636304.

Clarke, A. E., Shim, J., Mamo, L., Fosket, J. & Fishman, J. (2010). Biomedicalization: Technoscientific transformations of health. In Adele E. Clarke, Laura Mamo, Jennifer Ruth Fosket, Jennifer R. Fishman, & Janet K. Shim (Eds) *Illness, and U.S. Biomedicine.* Durham, North Caroline, USA: Duke University Press.

Collins, R., Reith, C., Emberson, J., Armitage, J., Baginet, C., Blackwell, L., ... Blumenthal, R. (2016). Interpretation of the evidence for the efficacy and safety of statin therapy. *Lancet, 388*(10059), 2532–2561. doi: 10.1016/S0140-6736(16)31357-5.

Crawford, R. (1980). Healthism and the medicalization of everyday life. *International Journal of Health Services, 10*(3), 365–388. doi: 10.2190/3H2H-3XJN-3KAY-G9NY.

Danish Health Authority. (2012). Fokusrapport - Viden om forbrug og bivirkninger ved behandling med statiner. [Focus Report - Knowledge on usage and side effects of statin treatment]. October 22. Copenhagen. Available at : https://laegemiddelstyrelsen.dk/~/media/B678C7B81BD44157A133F96A936B8B95.ashx.

Dew, K., Norris, P., Gabe, J., Chamberlain, K., & Hodgetts, D. (2015). Moral discourses and pharmaceuticalised governance in households. *Social Science & Medicine, 131,* 272–279. doi: 10.1016/J.SOCSCIMED.2014.03.006.

Dumit, J. (2012). *Drugs for Life: How Pharmaceutical Companies Define Our Health*. London: Duke University Press.

Eborall, H. C., & Will, C. M. (2011). Prevention is better than cure, but ...: Preventive medication as a risk to ordinariness?. *Health, Risk & Society, 13*(7–8), 653–668. doi: 10.1080/13698575.2011.624177.

Foucault, M. (1997). Technologies of the self. In Rabinow, P. (ed.) *Ethics, Subjectivity and Truth.* (pp. 225–251). New York: The New Press.

Gifford, S. M. (1986). The meaning of lumps: A case study of the ambiguities of risk. In Janes, C. R., Stall, R., and Gifford, S. M. (eds.), *Anthropology and Epidemiology.* (pp. 213–246). Dordrecht: Springer Netherlands. doi: 10.1007/978-94-009-3723-9.

Gillespie, C. (2012). The experience of risk as "measured vulnerability": Health screening and lay uses of numerical risk. *Sociology of Health & Illness, 34*(2), 194–207. doi: 10.1111/j.1467-9566.2011.01381.x.

Godlee, F. (2016). Statins: We need an independent review. *British Medical Journal, 354,* i4992.

Greene, J. A. (2007). *Prescribing by Numbers. Drugs and the Definition of Disease.* Baltimore: The Johns Hopkins University Press.

Jauho, M. (2019). Patients-in-waiting or chronically healthy individuals? People with elevated cholesterol talk about risk. *Sociology of Health & Illness, 41*(5), 867–881. doi: 10.1111/1467-9566.12866.

Jenkins, J. H. (2010). *Pharmaceutical Self – The Global Shaping of Experience in An Age of Psychopharmacology. Sante Fe: School for Advanced Research Press.*

Khanna, V., Emerick, T., & Lewis, A. (2013). *The statinization of America, The Health Care Blog*. Retrieved from https://thehealthcareblog.com/blog/2013/11/14/the-statinization-of-america/.

Kørner, L. (2019). Tager vi medicin, vi ikke behøver?. *Samvirke, 9,* 45–47.

Krogsbøll, L., Jørgensen, K., & Gøtzsche, P. (2011). General health checks for reducing morbidity and mortality from disease. *Intervention, 2.* doi: 10.1002/14651858.CD009009.

Langdridge, D. (2017). Recovery from heart attack, biomedicalization, and the production of a contingent health citizenship. *Qualitative Health Research, 27*(9), 1391–1401. doi: 10.1177/1049732316668818.

Lau, S. R. (2018). *A matter of course. An ethnographic assemblage of the routinization of statins in Denmark.* Copenhagen, Denmark: University of Copenhagen.

Lupton, D. (1995). *The Imperative of Health: Public Health and thr Regulated Body*, London, Thousand Oaks, New Delhi: Sage Publications.

Petryna, A., Lakoff, A., & Kleinman, A. (2006). *Global Pharmaceuticals: Ethics, Markets, Practices*. Durham and London: Duke University Press.

Petursson, H., Sigurdsson, J. A., Bengtsson, C., Nilsen, T. I. L., & Getz, L. (2012). Is the use of cholesterol in mortality risk algorithms in clinical guidelines valid? Ten years prospective data from the Norwegian HUNT 2 study. *Journal of Evaluation in Clinical Practice, 18,* 159–168.

Polak, L. (2017). What is wrong with "being a pill-taker"? The special case of statins. *Sociology of Health & Illness, 39*(4), 599–613. doi: 10.1111/1467-9566.12509.

Polak, L., & Green, J. (2020). Rethinking decision-making in the context of preventive medication: How taking statins becomes "the right thing to do". *Social Science and Medicine, 247,* 112797. doi: 10.1016/j.socscimed.2020.112797.

Rose, N. (2007). *The Politics of Life Itself: Biomedicine, Power, and Subjectivity in the Twenty-First Century.* Princeton, NJ: Princeton University Press.

Rosenberg, C. (2009) .Managed fear. *The Lancet, 373*(9666), 802–803. doi: 10.1016/S0140 6736(09)60467-0.

Schlosser, A. V., & Hoffer, L. D. (2012). The psychotropic self/imaginary: Subjectivity and psychopharmaceutical use among heroin users with co-occurring mental illness. *Culture, Medicine, and Psychiatry, 36*(1), 26–50. doi: 10.1007/s11013-011-9244-9.

Schwennesen, N., & Koch, L. (2012). Representing and intervening: "Doing" good care in first trimester prenatal knowledge production and decision-making. *Sociology of Health & Illness, 34*(2), 283–298. doi: 10.1111/j.1467-9566.2011.01414.x.

Stroes, E. S., Thompson, P., Corsini, A., Vladutiu, G., Raal, F., Ray, K., … Wiklund, O.(2015). Statin associated muscle symptoms: Impact on statin therapy – European Atherosclerosis Society consensus panel statement on assessment, aetiology and management. *European Heart Journal, 36*(17), 1012–1022. doi: 10.1093/eurheartj/ehv043.

Wahlberg, A. (2018). *Good Quality – The Routinization of Sperm Banking in China.* Berkeley: University of California Press.

Weintraub, W. S. (2017). Perspective on trends in statin use. *JAMA Cardiology, 2*(1), 11–12. doi: 10.1001/jamacardio.2016.4710.

Whyte, S. R., van der Geest, S. and Hardon, A. (2002). *Social Lives of Medicines.* Cambridge: Cambridge University Press.

Will, C. M., & Weiner, K. (2014). Sustained multiplicity in everyday cholesterol reduction: Repertoires and practices in talk about "healthy living". *Sociology of Health and Illness, 36*(2), 291–304. doi: 10.1111/1467-9566.12070.

Williams, S. J., Martin, P., & Gabe, J. (2011). Evolving sociological analyses of "Pharmaceuticalisation": A reply to Abraham. *Sociology of Health and Illness, 33*(5), 729–730. doi: 10.1111/j.1467-9566.2011.01396.x.

9 A shot in the dark?

Ontario girls, informed consent and HPV vaccination[1]

Michele J. McIntosh

Introduction and background

In Ontario, girls have the right to informed consent (or informed refusal) of the human papilloma virus (HPV) vaccination independent of their parents. The provincial Health Care Consent Act (1996) determines the requirements for informed consent, namely capacity for autonomy, not age. Indeed, there is no minimum age for consent to treatment in Ontario. The appeal to the development of autonomy is one of the pillars of the ethical justification of this legislation (Agrawal & Morain, 2018). The capacity for autonomy requires two elements: liberty (freedom from controlling influence) and agency (capacity for self-rule) (Beauchamp & Childress, 2001). Although this capacity is emergent during adolescence, there is evidence regarding brain development and cognitive processing that supports the ability of teens to demonstrate adult-like decision-making, particularly in low risk, low stress situations, such as one-to-one conversations with health professionals in clinical settings (Steinberg, 2013; Agrawal & Morain, 2018). A full description of the ethical justification for the right of minors to consent is beyond the scope of this paper; I am less concerned with presenting *why* girls ought to have the right to consent, than *how* that right is governmentally constructed and individually experienced. Despite Ontarian girls having the right to autonomous consent (or refusal) of the HPV vaccination, there is little opportunity for them to exercise this right. This chapter presents an analysis of both the top-down institutional implementation of the HPV vaccination program, and girls' experiences of it, particularly as it pertains to their right to consent, and the consequences of this usurpation to their health, and to their lives.

Following Health Canada's approval of the quadrivalent recombinant HPV vaccine Gardasil (Gardasil™, 2008) in 2006, the National Advisory Committee on Immunization (NACI) recommended this vaccine for women aged 9–26 (NACI, 2007). In March 2007, the federal government designated CAD$300 million dollars over 3 years to support provincial and territorial HPV vaccine programs (Department of Finance Canada, 2007). Beginning in the fall, 2007, several of the Canadian provinces, including Ontario, used these federal funds to introduce publicly funded school-based HPV vaccine programs for girls. Schools had become the customary platform for the delivery of vaccination programs to school-aged children and were considered the optimal means for reaching the target population. School-based HPV vaccination programs, however, posed serious ethical challenges regarding consent and authorisation processes, as described below.

First, girls' right to consent was discounted or token. Concomitant with the tradition of school-based vaccine programs is the schools' requirement or request for parental consent and parents' expectation to provide consent for childhood and adolescent immunisations (Wilson, Karas, Crowcroft, Bontovics & Deeks, 2012). Local health units develop the informed consent materials for the schools; students are then asked to deliver these written documents to their parents or legal guardians and to return completed consent/authorisation forms to the school prior to the student receiving the vaccine (Cawley, Hull, & Rousculp, 2010). Only a few Ontario health units (5/36) provide an additional line for the girls' signature on the consent form. But what happens in cases of discrepancy between parental and child wishes? Only some (14/36) provide the vaccine to girls judged capable of providing consent and requesting it, in the absence of parental consent (Wilson et al., 2012) and then only at their own facility, not at the school. Finally, there are reports of vaccine administration at school in the absence of girls' consent: at a conference where this topic was being discussed a spouse of a nurse approached us to relay the moral distress that plagued his wife when she was required to immunise the child against her wishes because the parents had consented (S. Dykeman, Personal Communication, September 2016).

The second ethical challenge was that the informed consent process is reduced to a form. Informed consent is intended to be an interpersonal process wherein information is shared, and questions and concerns expressed and addressed (Peppin, 2007). Only 8/36 schools have specific information sessions for students regarding the HPV vaccination (Wilson et al., 2012).

Third, consent is not informed. An essential component of consent is knowledge regarding risk and benefit. For consent to be legally valid, all material risks must be disclosed (Peppin, 2007). Steenbeek, Macdonald, Downie, Appleton, and Baylis (2012) undertook a study to compare the physical risk disclosures among documents prepared by the various jurisdictions, and against documents prepared by the vaccine manufacturer (Merck Frosst Canada), the NACI, the Society of Obstetricians and Gynecologists of Canada (SOGC), and a 2007 article in Maclean's magazine, a Canadian national current affairs magazine. They found that the communication of risk in materials available to parents, legal guardians and girls was inaccurate, incomplete and inconsistent: 'No jurisdiction provided the same list of vaccine-related physical risks as other jurisdictions. Major discrepancies were identified' (Steenbeek et al., 2012, p. 71). Given that the NACI undertook the evidence-based review of the HPV vaccine, and that they are mandated to set the national standard on vaccine use, this governmental agency could have ensured clear, consistent, plain language and multilanguage document distribution across all public health units. In the absence of full disclosure of the nature and probability of risks, the legal validity of any consent obtained is questionable (Steenbeek et al., 2012). In addition, the vaccination is marketed as an anticancer vaccine rather than a sexually transmitted infection vaccine. This misrepresentation of its purpose prevents a precise understanding of any benefit it may confer upon those vaccinated.

In sum, therefore, school-based vaccination programs have been documented to usurp girls' rights to autonomously consent or refuse the HPV vaccine. There is no mechanism within the school-based programs to ensure girls have either the knowledge or the opportunity to exercise their right.

Methods

We sought to ascertain girls' decision-making experiences regarding HPV vaccination. In particular, we were interested to assess girls' capacity for informed consent; that is, whether making any decision was volitional, and whether it was informed. In-depth interviews and semistructured interviews were the methods selected. In-depth interviews are appropriate for the discovery of new knowledge such as girls' decision-making experiences about the vaccine; semistructured interviews are appropriate when there is sufficient objective knowledge about an experience or phenomenon but the subjective knowledge is lacking (Merton & Kendall 1946; Richards & Morse, 2007). The grand tour question for the in-depth interviews was, 'Please share with me what deciding to get Gardasil was like for you'. The semistructured interview schedule (Table 9.1) was comprised of key components of informed consent: volition, risks, benefits, and alternatives. A literature search was conducted for each component as it pertained to HPV and HPV vaccination; from this search emerged the question stems and probes. For example, 'Do you feel you were capable of making this decision on your own?' or, 'Please tell me what you understand about the benefits of Gardasil?' Although the questions were structured, the girls' responses were not. They were free to refute, correct, or elaborate upon each question. Thus, this type of semistructured interview was interpretive (McIntosh & Morse, 2015).

Purposeful recruitment occurred through distributing posters and handbills around the Peterborough, Ontario region. These promotional materials were also distributed through agencies with youth groups and via email list serves for related interest groups, including the Peterborough Youth Council, Trent University and the Ontario Women's Health Network. Social media was used through promotion on Facebook and Twitter by sharing study information with youth groups and organisations. Recruitment was also done through snowball sampling and in person at a national nursing student conference.

Prospective participants were directed to a website (www.girlstalkaboutgardasil.com) designed for this research project where participant eligibility criteria and study information were listed. Participant eligibility criteria included that the participant be a female who lived in Ontario and had been offered the Gardasil vaccine between the ages of 9 and 17, irrespective of their vaccination choice. After reviewing participant information, prospective participants were able to schedule themselves, via an online form, to be interviewed. Interviews were conducted in-person or over the phone, audio-taped, transcribed, and analysed: the in-depth interviews were thematically analysed, the semistructured interviews were analysed per item. Seventeen (17) young women were

Table 9.1 Interview schedule

Domain	Item	Question (Prompts in italics)	Reference from the literature
Agency in Decision	1	You were/not vaccinated. Who made this decision? *Prompt: Were you involved in the decision?*	Ogilvie et al. (2007), Mishra & Graham (2012)
Agency in Decision	2	Do you feel you were capable of making the decision on your own?	Ford et al. (2014), Polzer & Knabe (2012), Manucso & Polzer (2010)
Agency in Decision	3	Do you feel you had enough knowledge to make the decision on your own?	Herman et al. (2019)
Agency in Decision	4	Did you feel you were free to make this decision for yourself? *Prompt: Did you feel pressure or strong influence in this decision?*	Wilson et al. (2012)
Agency in Decision	5	Was there a consent form for you to get this vaccination? *Prompt: Who signed it? Did you sign it?*	Wilson et al. (2012)
Knowledge pertaining to HPV	6	Please tell me what you know about HPV? *Did you have this knowledge at the time of the vaccination decision or has it changed? Prompt: Can you tell me what it stands for? How is it transmitted?*	Mastrolorenzo, Supuran, & Zuccati (2007)
Knowledge pertaining to HPV	7	Please tell me what you know about the risks of HPV. *Did you know this at the time of the decision?*	Canadian Women's Health Network (2007), Mastrolorenzo, Supuran, & Zuccati (2007)
Knowledge pertaining to HPV	8	Can you tell me ways that can reduce the risk of getting HPV? *Did you know these at the time of the decision?*	
Knowledge pertaining to HPV	9	Do you consider yourself to be at risk for HPV? *Did you consider yourself to be at risk at the time of the decision? Prompt: Elaborate on why/not?*	Thompson (2013)
Knowledge pertaining to HPV vaccination/Gardasil	10	Please tell me what you know about the purpose of HPV (Gardasil) vaccination? *Did you know this at the time of the decision? Prompt: Prevention? How effective is it at achieving this purpose?*	Ogilvie et al. (2007), Mishra & Graham (2012)

(Continued)

Table 9.1 (Continued)

Domain	Item	Question (Prompts in italics)	Reference from the literature
Knowledge pertaining to HPV vaccination/Gardasil	11	Please tell me what you understand about the benefits of Gardasil? *Do you recall these being explained to you? By whom? Has your understanding of these changed since then? What was the catalyst for this change?*	Abdelmutt, & Hoffman-Goetz (2009)
Knowledge pertaining to HPV vaccination/Gardasil	12	Does the HPV vaccination prevent AIDS?	Dell et al. (2000)
Knowledge pertaining to HPV vaccination/Gardasil	13	Please tell me your understanding of any risks of HPV (Gardasil) vaccination? *Prompt: Do you recall these being explained to you? By whom? Has your understanding of these changed since then? What was the catalyst for this change?*	Harris et al. (2014), Torrecilla et al. (2011)
Knowledge pertaining to HPV vaccination/Gardasil	14	Please tell me your understanding of any alternatives to being vaccinated to preventing HPV related consequences? *Do you recall these being explained to you? By whom? Has your understanding of these changed since then?*	Harris et al. (2014)
Knowledge pertaining to HPV vaccination/Gardasil	15	Do you believe the school-based vaccination program for Gardasil is mandatory? *Prompt: Can the school impose consequences if you don't get this vaccination?*	Wilson et al. (2013)
Knowledge pertaining to HPV vaccination/Gardasil	16	How has the decision to be vaccinated or not affected your sexual health practices?	Reiter et al. (2009)
Knowledge pertaining to HPV vaccination/Gardasil	17	What are pap smears? *Prompt: what are they for?*	Mastrolorenzo, Supuran, & Zuccati (2007)
Vaccine Suitability/Public Policy	18	Would making a different decision have been problematic for you?	
Vaccine Suitability/Public Policy	19	Would you make the same decision about vaccination today? *Prompt: If no, why has this decision changed?*	
Vaccine Suitability/Public Policy	20	Were you sexually active before the vaccination? *Since then?*	Canadian Women's Health Network (2007)

interviewed in total; all participated in the semistructured interview and 8 additionally elected to share longer narratives in the in-depth interview. See Table 9.2 for sample characteristics. It is important to note that the women we interviewed were university students who provided retrospective accounts of their vaccination decision-making experiences. This may be considered a limitation of this study. Ethics approval for the study was obtained from the Trent University Research Ethics Board.

Findings

Volition

In this section, findings related to girls' awareness of their right to decide whether or not to receive the HPV vaccine, who made the decision on their behalf, if they felt they were capable of making the decision on their own, if they felt coerced or free to make the decision and if they felt they had enough information with which to decide. Our findings indicate that, in general, girls were entirely unaware of the (Ontario) Health Care Consent Act that authorises their right to give or deny consent.

Despite the fact that in Ontario there is no minimal age to consent to medical treatment, many girls referred to age as a prerequisite for consent. Two participants who did not get the vaccine in Grade 8 (age 13), received it once they turned 18:

> So, at that time I was legal, so I just went to the clinic and got it. It was just like show up and bring your health card and whatever. I remember there was a form to print off and sign for your parents if you were under-age.
>
> Participant 1

Another participant reflected upon how she was treated differently by her physician once she was 18, reinforcing the assumption that age was presumptive of capacity:

> And so, I brushed it off for like, I don't know, a number of years. It must have been Grade 9, Grade 9, 10, 11, 12. Probably like five years! Until this summer, I don't know what changed, but I guess because as soon as I was 18… my mom wasn't there… I think it was a bit of a switch for me when I turned 18 to all of a sudden just have these pressures and have these differences in the way that you're treated.
>
> Participant 3

As evidenced by these quotes, increased age, especially the age of 18 was associated with a notion of being 'legal' and thus being able to, and perhaps expected to, make health care decisions by oneself.

Girls accepted the authority of the school in determining vaccination. After all, the school-based vaccination programs were the usual platform for the vaccination of middle-school children. Two participants assumed it was

Table 9.2 Participant details

Participant	Had in-depth interview	Had semistructured interview	Age when first offered the vaccine	Location first offered vaccine	Vaccinated	Age received vaccine	Location of vaccination
1	Y	Y	13	In school	Y	21	Public health 'catch-up' clinic
2	Y	Y	13	In school	Y	13	In school
3	Y	Y	13	In school	N – not all doses completed	18	Family physician office
4	N	Y	19	In school	Y	19	Family physician office
5	N	Y	13	In school	Y	13	In school
6	Y	Y	13	In school	N	N/A	N/A
7	N	Y	13	In school	Y	13	In school
8	Y	Y	13	In school	Y	13	In school
9	N	Y	13	In school	Y	13	In school
10	Y	Y	13	In school	Y	13	In school
11	Y	Y	13	In school	Y	13	In school
12	Y	Y	13	In school	Y	13	In school
13	N	Y	13	In school	Y	13	In school
14	N	Y	13	In school	Y	13	In school
15	N	Y	13	In school	Y	13	In school
16	N	Y	13	In school	Y	13	In school
17	N	Y	13	In school	Y	13	In school

mandatory that schools had the authority to suspend students who failed to receive the vaccinations.

> So, there wasn't much of a decision, the school just said you have to get this, or you will be suspended.
>
> Participant 13

> Back then I just thought 'Oh, everyone is getting it and it's probably one of the routine vaccines I need to stay in school', you know?
>
> Participant 16

When asked who made the decision to be vaccinated, one participant said,

> My school board I think? I can't remember if I got a consent form for my parents or not. But I remember going to school one day and they were just like you're getting a vaccination with the other girls and that was it.
>
> Participant 16

Another commented:

> Um, I mean I don't think there was really any asking if you wanted to do this, it was just kind of like 'okay, this is what's going to happen' and when you're twelve you're kind of just kind of like 'okay' and do what everyone, the teachers, are telling you to do.
>
> Participant 12

One participant recalled that the school's vaccination program implied consent:

> The school sent out the information that said we were going to be vaccinated on these three days and then I think you were automatically put into it and then parents could opt out. So, I don't know who made that decision, but I didn't opt out.
>
> Participant 12

Participants believed and accepted that parents had the right to consent on their behalf, and they had limited involvement in the decision made between the school and their parents:

> Ya, at school, or at least the school I went to, you had to have parental consent or something like that in order to get the vaccination.
>
> Participant 14

Girls recalled the process of getting parental authorisation:

> So, they [the school] sent home the consent form that has some information to show our parents. And they needed that to be signed. So, I got that signed and brought it back.
>
> Participant 2

Even when they had decided for themselves about the vaccine, several girls conveyed that their decision was not autonomous:

> I'm pretty sure I mentioned it to my parents, 'Oh, I want to get this' and then... [pause]... it just never happened.
>
> Participant 13

> I mean back then I didn't have the same kind of concept of personal autonomy regarding my health care as I do now.
>
> Participant 16

When asked who made the decision to be vaccinated, approximately half of the girls indicated that their mothers made the decision, not them. Examples provided by the participants included the situation where they did not want the vaccination, but their mothers insisted they receive it, and conversely, mothers refused to permit vaccinations their daughters wanted.

> If I had said no, I think my mom would have said, 'You need to get it'.
>
> Participant 8

> I'm not getting it. My mom doesn't know enough about it.
>
> Participant 9

When asked if they felt capable of making the decision on their own, many participants responded affirmatively. One participant responded:

> Yes [very firm]. I also made the decision to get the Hep B vaccine. Oh, I guess it is true that I also got consent from my parents, but I was like, yes, I want to get this.
>
> Participant 1

Some participants explicitly referenced capacity over age:

> I think, like at that age, children now they mature faster. I think I was really mature with sexual health and stuff. I did really well in school, and it was something that really interested me even though I didn't want to have it at the time at all, so I just thought it was a good idea at the time.
>
> Participant 2

Conversely, another participant opined,

> I think that Grade 8 was too young for girls to be making the decisions and I think that it was the moms that were making the decision... I wish I wasn't so young so maybe I would have had a better understanding about it before I made a decision.
>
> Participant 3

Many participants indicated that they felt they would have been capable had they been given more information, but most felt they were not adequately informed to make a decision:

> I would say [I wasn't capable] because I still didn't know information about it. So, I think had I known information, I would have been capable of making that decision but because I didn't know I still wasn't capable, regardless of age.
>
> Participant 3

> I just wanted to say that the one thing that I found interesting when I learned about this study and started thinking about my experience getting the Gardasil vaccine it was just so funny how I didn't know [what] I was getting, I didn't know what it was for. Like all the stuff now when I think about providing care to people and you have to provide them with the risks and benefits for things before they can give consent, I don't remember any of that happening. It was interesting reflecting on that because it really is malpractice. You don't think of that really happening here or you think 'that wouldn't happen to me'. But it does happen and it's interesting thinking about that.
>
> Participant 16

One participant reflected upon her lack of understanding about the vaccination she received in Grade 8:

> I didn't really make an active decision, so I wouldn't have gone about it the same way today. I would be more informed. I would make sure my care provider would inform me of the risks and benefits before I got a vaccine. I would still make the same decision I just would have liked to have been informed.
>
> Participant 16

Girls whose parents refused the vaccination in Grade 8 got vaccinated when they were able to do so autonomously. In one participant's case, she saw an advertisement by Public Health for a 'catch-up' clinic. She actively engaged her mother in driving her to the clinic and actively engaged her sisters in getting it also. A key catalyst for getting the vaccine was knowledge:

> I didn't get the school-based one and that was my mom's choice. I didn't have any information on it then… and then a couple of years ago when I figured out what it really was just before I started university, I got a prescription for it.
>
> Participant 11

Sexual activity may have been another catalyst, increasing the relevance of the vaccination to their lives. The girls who received the vaccine later acknowledged they were sexually active at the time they sought Gardasil, though they were not in Grade 8:

> I had already been sexually active for a few years. I think I decided I wanted it. And then my mom was like 'Yeah, it's a good idea'.
>
> Participant 4

The fact that girls independently sought and received the vaccination subsequent to their parents' initial refusal is evidence of their ability to make independent vaccine decisions. When asked if they would make the same vaccination decision today, most girls responded affirmatively, however, a few did not:

> I wouldn't get it. I would do research about it. Know the risks, know the cases of bad things going on. What are the percentages of effectiveness, and I didn't know any of that. And I wish I would have. It would have helped in making a better decision… but I just wish there was more information about it given to girls so that we can ultimately make a decision for ourselves and not be pressured.
>
> Participant 3

Many said they would make the same decision, however, they would be more informed.

Knowledge: Human papilloma virus

Informed decision-making regarding vaccination to prevent HPV infection requires an understanding of HPV itself. Girls were asked to tell us what they know about HPV, how it is transmitted, its risks, and reducing risks. Most girls' knowledge about the virus itself was vague:

> Some sort of… I don't think it's a bacteria. I think it's a virus. And it's somewhere in the women's reproductive system. Like maybe uterus, I'm thinking. If I remember correctly. Other than that, I don't really know.
>
> Participant 8

Some girls misconstrued the role that different strains of HPV play, that is, some strains cause warts and other strains are involved in the pathogenesis of cancer:

> It's a virus that causes genital warts that can also go on to cause cervical cancer in the future.
>
> Participant 1

Girls were asked what they knew about the risks posed by HPV. Most correctly identified that HPV was linked to cancer, however, they also identified other risks unassociated with HPV specifically:

Ya, cancer and not being able to get pregnant I'm pretty sure.

Participant 12

I keep thinking that it's cancer and it will affect your, um, your nervous system if that's the right word.

Participant 11

Cervical cancer. I do know that. Also throat cancer, because, also what was his name? Michael Douglas – I think said he got oral cancer from it. That's mainly what I know about it. I don't know what symptoms you would have if you had HPV, but it could eventually cause cancer.

Participant 2

Many girls regarded HPV infection as life threatening, and one participant conflated HPV with HIV:

My doctor kind of said it could be associated with cancers, like cancers down there. And like AIDS.

Participant 6

Conversely, other participants, nursing students who had recently taken a class that addressed HPV, were more knowledgeable. However, they acknowledged this was because of the course. There were still gaps in their knowledge, however:

I know it's a virus. Human Papilloma Virus and it is transmitted mostly through sexual activities and it's what brings on genital warts, cervical cancer, and vaginal cancer. A lot of what I learned was this year in nursing. I think it can also be transmitted through blood? Or is it mostly just sexual?

Participant 14

It's sexually transmitted and causes cervical cancer.

Participant 15

I know that it is an infection. But it is very common and usually goes away by itself. They don't even test for it when you get a STD [sexually transmitted disease] test.

Participant 4

This participant's use of the term STD illustrates her lack of knowledge: sexually transmitted infections, for example, HPV may become sexually transmitted diseases, for example, cancer.

When asked how risk of HPV could be reduced, girls primarily cited condom use and getting vaccinated. Condoms are ineffective in preventing HPV infection that is not sexually transmitted, for example, skin-to-skin. Vaccinations are partially protective against certain strains of HPV. Girls did not mention delaying first intercourse, taking folic acid to boost the immune system's ability

to eliminate the virus, and not smoking, a potentiator of virulence. No girl mentioned pap smears as a secondary preventative strategy to prevent cervical cancer.

Knowledge: Gardasil vaccination – risks, benefits, alternatives

Critical to informed consent is knowledge of the risks, benefits and alternatives
to the intervention itself. Girls had significant knowledge gaps about the purpose
of the Gardasil vaccination. Girls recalled believing the vaccination was to prevent cervical cancer; they were less aware of its actual role in preventing specific
strains of HPV associated with 70% of cervical cancers and genital warts.

> No, I didn't even know it was for HPV. I just knew it was for cervical cancer
> which I didn't know was caused by HPV at the time.
>
> Participant 14

> I knew it prevented HPV but I didn't know what that meant.
>
> Participant 17

With one exception, few could cite any risks of the vaccination itself such as
local risks (injection site), or major (myalgia) or minor (fainting) systemic risks,
respectively:

> What is your understanding of any risk of the HPV vaccination?
> Un ya, I read about them recently (laughs), but not any big risks that really
> stood out to me that I can remember reading.

And do you remember any of them being explained to you at the time?

> No [laughs].
>
> Participant 17

One participant described fainting after her second dose and how this was
not attributed to the vaccine even though it is listed on the manufacturer's
vaccine-related risks:

> I got the second dosage and I actually fainted from it. And [the] physician
> kind of brushed it off, like 'You're just scared of needles'.
>
> Participant 3

This participant also described how others fainted too and how students who had
'bad reactions' did so in front of their classmates:

> And we were doing this in the teacher's lounge, lining up… Like quite lit-
> erally they did it in front of the entire girls in our entire grade and ya. There
> were such bad reactions and me and my friend were first and did it in front
> of everybody.
>
> Participant 13

Some participants discussed reading about adverse vaccine reactions on the internet:

> [I had] one of my friend's parents [on Facebook] and she has teenage daughters who are a couple years younger than me. And she started posting stories about people. Like linked articles about some girls who had got it and had these severe problems and were hospitalized and are now impaired for the rest of their lives.
>
> Participant 6

Participants frequently discussed being concerned but not having the knowledge or skills to critically examine the information and assess the veracity of the stories. Although Papanicolaou (Pap) testing is not literally an alternative to vaccination, 'everyone agrees that HPV vaccination must be conducted in conjunction with screening and treatment programs' (Maine, Hurlburt & Greeson, 2011, p. 1552). HPV vaccination prevents HPV infection, pap tests screen for HPV infection. Therefore, it is critical that girls understand the pap smear, its purpose, what it tests for and what it does not, and what the test results mean. In this study, girls evidenced significant gaps in knowledge regarding pap testing. For example, few girls could accurately describe the pap test:

> Can't [laughs]. Sorry.
>
> Participant 13

> I have no idea.
>
> Participant 11

> I don't feel confident explaining what it is.
>
> Participant 5

> [It is] a vaginal exam that involves two different types of swabs. One swab is of the vaginal wall. The second swab is the one that actually goes into the cervix [sic]. Just to swab any abnormal cells that come up in either.
>
> Participant 8

While a few girls correctly identified pap smears as a screening test for cervical changes that could lead to cervical cancer, several girls conflated the pap test with other types of testing for sexually transmitted infections:

> Like you go to the doctor and you sit in the stirrups and they take a part of your cervix and they test it for STIs. That's all I know so far but I still have to get one of those.
>
> Participant 2

> Yeah, they also test for cells that are different, or whatever, for cervical cancer. I think they also test for other STDs.
>
> Participant 4

> I do know that it tests you for HPV, AIDS and all that stuff.
>
> Participant 3

Girls evidenced significant gaps in knowledge regarding HPV, HPV vaccination and HPV screening (pap smears).

Discussion

Girls' decision-making experiences regarding HPV vaccination were characterised by the usurpation of their legal right to informed consent, the assigning of the decision-making authority to others despite the law, lack of voluntariness including little opportunity to express agency, as well as coercion and external pressure, undermining of autonomy and withholding of information. In addition, vaccination clinics undermined girls' right to privacy of personal information, their body and space.

Consent

The right of our study participants to consent to (or refuse) the Gardasil vaccination was usurped; no participant was informed of this right nor were they assessed for capacity but all were apparently deemed to lack capacity presumably because of age or school-board tradition of obtaining parental consent. This marginalisation of young adolescents from the vaccine decision-making process is echoed in other jurisdictions (Herman et al., 2019). Many of our study participants, however, felt capable of making the decision, despite age, except in those cases where they lacked the information to decide. Many indicated their willingness to be involved in the decision-making process with their parents, although there was (typically) no formal or consistent mechanism to acknowledge their perspectives. Although almost all participants reported that they would not change the decision about vaccination, a few students received the vaccination against their expressed desire, and other girls' parents refused to consent to the vaccination despite their expressed desire for it.

Voluntariness

Furthermore, voluntariness was compromised; many girls felt coerced by their school boards or felt pressured by peers or strongly influenced by teachers, their parents, and in some cases, their doctors. Many participants thought this coercion or external pressure was unethical.

Privacy and confidentiality

Study participants identified peer pressure as a significant factor in the vaccination program. Given the public nature of the vaccination clinics themselves, girls were aware of those who had consented versus those who had not. Furthermore, girls reported fainting in public view and witnessing the vaccination responses of others.

Information provision

The girls were also deprived of the information with which to make an informed decision. They were not told of all the material risks inherent in the vaccination, or of its benefits, drawbacks or the risks of not being vaccinated. The study participants emphasised that they were not given sufficient information about the HPV virus, nor the HPV vaccination to be able to make an informed decision. The deprivation of information was what girls found most distressing about the vaccination program. One participant considered this 'malpractice' and implied that a breach of trust had occurred. The thwarting of the girls' right to informed consent is consequential, resulting in harm as discussed below.

Harm

Many ethical arguments in favour of minors having consent focus upon their emergent autonomy and the opportunity for its development through decision-making processes. (Agrawal & Morain, 2018). Indeed, free and informed consent is the hallmark of autonomy (Keatings & Smith, 2010). Usurping girls' right to informed consent deprives them of their right to self-determination in their sexual and reproductive lives. Indeed, in this respect, girls have already been (albeit unintentionally) harmed.

Girls' have experienced physical harm as a result of a change in clinical guidelines for pap smear scheduling which followed on the heels of the introduction of the HPV vaccination initiative. This harm was exacerbated by girls' lack of comprehensive sexual health knowledge including HPV, HPV vaccination and pap smear screening specifically.

HPV vaccination was never intended to be a stand-alone effort in the prevention and control of HPV but was intended to be delivered in concert with cervical cancer screening and treatment (WHO, 2013). The development of cervical cancer is still possible despite HPV vaccination for myriad reasons. Although the HPV vaccines target specific serotypes most associated with cervical cancer, not all serotypes are covered. Furthermore, there is some question regarding whether the serotypes not covered become more virulent with the suppression of others (Kahn et al., 2012). In addition, the vaccination schedule may not have been adhered to, girls may have missed injections or stopped them altogether therefore missing the complete immunisation schedule. Perhaps the vaccinations were not given at the optimal time, that is, presexual initiation. Therefore, screening for cervical changes resulting from HPV infection is still required.

There are several screening approaches (Maine et al., 2011). In Ontario, the pap smear is the recommended screening method (Lees, Erickson, & Warner, 2016; Murphy et al., 2012). Prior to 2012, women were advised to begin having pap tests when they became sexually active and annually thereafter. In May 2012, concomitant with the introduction of the HPV vaccination, Cancer Care Ontario released new guidelines that recommended initiation of screening at age 21 for women who are or who have ever been sexually active and to screen every 3 years thereafter in the context of normal results (Murphy et al., 2012). This change in clinical guidelines was iatrogenic: a significant unintended and harmful consequence of these updated guidelines was a dramatic (60%) decrease in pap testing and a 50% decrease in sexually transmitted infection testing in the primary care setting (Bogler et al., 2015). Indeed, screening for chlamydia, gonorrhea, syphilis and hepatitis C decreased significantly in 2013 (Bogler et al., 2015). There was also a decrease in HIV screening that was 'potentially of clinical significance' (Bogler et al., 2015, p. 463). Correspondingly, the rates of STIs increased exponentially:

> Our findings merit concern considering that Canadian rates of chlamydia and gonorrhea rose by 72% and 53.4%, respectively, during the past decade. These infections, especially chlamydia, disproportionately affect younger women, further underscoring the risk imposed in this population by the effect the updated guidelines have on STI screening.
>
> (Bogler et al., 2015, p. 465)

Furthermore, since 2012 syphilis rates in women have tripled, HIV rates are highest among women and are 20% higher in 2018 compared to 2012 (Public Health Ontario, 2019; Choudry, Miller, Sandhu, Leon & Aho, 2018). These sexually transmitted infections can become sexually transmitted diseases including pelvic inflammatory disease, cause significant morbidity such as ectopic pregnancy, neonatal illness and infertility (Naimer et al., 2017). The population most affected is girls between the ages of 15 and 21 who no longer have a routine, annual pap test (often accompanied by STI testing) and in whom most STIs are asymptomatic. The change in screening guidelines is exacerbated by the inadequate knowledge imparted to girls with which they can advocate for themselves, and access services.

This harm becomes even more pernicious when we consider it in light of the potential benefit the vaccination may confer upon recipients. Cervical cancer is more pervasive and lethal globally than it is in Canada (Maine et al., 2011). Indeed, relatively few women in Canada die from cervical cancer (Brenner et al., 2020), and these women are socially disadvantaged and have not had good access to screening, diagnosis or treatment (Ng, Wilkins, Fung & Berthelot, 2010). School girls may not be the most at-risk population in this regard (Thompson, 2013). Though most girls will become infected, most infections will spontaneously resolve (Lees et al., 2016). Cervical cancer is slow growing and precancerous changes can be successfully treated at many points along its slow trajectory (Massad et al., 2013). Therefore, most of the girls receiving the vaccination will not derive benefit from it, although they may still be harmed by the change in pap smear scheduling.

In their article *Missed Connections, Unintended Consequences of Updated Cervical Cancer Screening Guidelines on Screening Rates for Sexually Transmitted Infections*, the authors attempt to explain the unanticipated negative effects and 'unintended consequences' of changes to clinical guidelines (Bogler et al., 2015). Although the change in the pap smear guideline is consistent with better understanding of the development of disease (Lees et al., 2016) the effect it would have on adolescent girls was clearly missed. Inadvertent as this may have been (though it is unfathomable how this could not have been predicted), adolescent girls are uniquely bearing the costs.

Girls' experiences of decision-making regarding HPV vaccination was situated within the conflictual terrain of competing ideas (despite the law the idea that girls ought not have the right to consent prevailed), interests (girls versus their parents for example), and institutions (School Boards, the Federal Government, Public Health Units - what Hawkes and colleagues refer to as the 'classic triad of policy-making' (Hawkes, Kismodi, Larson & Buse, 2014, p. 1611)). Girls have been harmed within this context; indeed, their human rights have been abrogated.

Conclusion

Human rights laws and principles apply directly in the provision of HPV vaccines (Hawkes et al., 2014). Beyond ethical challenges, the school-based vaccination program in Ontario, Canada, abrogates human rights. Here, I posit recommendations to ensure Ontario's school-based vaccination program affords girls their full human rights.

Hawkes and colleagues, interpreting General comment no. 4 from the Committee on the Rights of the Child (2003) state that:

> By regulating consent to sexual health services, laws and policies should reflect the recognition of the status of people under 18 years of age as rights holders, in accordance with their evolving capacity, age and maturity and their best interest. Even if parental consent is deemed to be necessary because the child's evolving capacity requires further guidance, adolescents should always have a chance to express their views freely and their views should be given due weight.
>
> (Hawkes et al., 2014, p. 1612)

The Ontario Health Care Consent Act reflects these international human rights treaties in theory but not in practice. This must change. Girls' capacity, not age, must determine their right to consent. Girls need to know their rights under these treaties, and the Ontario Health Consent Act specifically. The Grade 8 sexual health curriculum ought to expand the concept of consent covered in primary grades from physical touching to consent to medical treatment. Girls may defer the decision to their parents. In all instances, girls' views ought to be given due weight and formally documented, for example, via their own signature on a consent form. In addition, sex gender-based analysis (Johnson, Greaves & Repta, 2009) ought to be performed on all new clinical guidelines or policies in order to see their prospective impact on this adolescent population.

Furthermore, interpreting General comment no. 15 from The Committee on the Rights of the Child (2003), Hawkes and colleagues state that:

> human rights standards call for the establishment of supportive policies so that children, parents and health workers have adequate rights-based guidance on consent, assent and confidentiality, to ensure that adolescents are not deprived of any sexual and reproductive health information or services.
>
> (Hawkes et al., 2014, p. 1612)

In addition to girls themselves all stakeholders including parents, teachers, nurses, physicians and school boards must be aware of girls' rights to consent and their duty to safeguard confidentiality. Policies must be created to support stakeholders to act in compliance with the law as well as their professional regulatory bodies. School boards must change their traditional practice of obtaining parental consent to align with this provincial legislation and human rights treaty. Schools must also mandate educational sessions pertaining to vaccinations and informed consent. Public health units need to change their consent forms such that they are written to girls as intended recipients and include a line for girls' own signatures. Nurses need to enact their professional ethical obligations pertaining to obtaining informed consent (including assessing capacity), ensuring privacy, safeguarding confidentiality, and patient advocacy (College of Nurses of Ontario, 2009). The Registered Nurses' Association needs to add to their Best Practice Guidelines directives for providing counselling, services and interventions (including vaccination clinics) to adolescents in the absence of parental consent. Public health units need to redesign vaccination clinics to conduct them in accordance with human rights provisions for privacy of body, information and space.

As reported by Hawkes et al. (2014), The Committee on Economic, Social and Cultural Rights, 2000 asserts that 'the right to the highest attainable standard of health requires governments to progressively take steps necessary to make services accessible and available, without discrimination to the maximum of their available resources and to reduce health inequities' (Hawkes et al., 2014, p. 1611). Given the established benefits of HPV vaccines to prevent specific serotypes of HPV associated with cervical and other cancers as well as genital warts, the provincial and federal governments are meeting their responsibilities as stipulated in this human rights document by providing the HPV vaccines to Canadian girls, free of charge, through the schools. However, given that school-aged girls have evidenced the greatest decrease in sexually transmitted infection testing since the pap smear schedule change, it is imperative that these services are prioritised for them. Given the rationale for the vaccination programs that program delivery through the schools optimises accessibility, it follows that schools should offer as many of these services as possible. It is within the registered nurse's scope of practice to administer vaccinations and perform sexually transmitted infection tests including those requiring pelvic examinations, urinalysis and venipuncture. School nurses could provide all of these services on site. These services should also be offered at locations besides the schools and at times compatible with school hours, to ensure accessibility to girls not at school. Furthermore, 'in accordance with their evolving capacities and best interest, children should have access to confidential counselling advice, services and interventions (such as vaccines) without parental or legal guardian consent' (Hawkes et al. 2014, p. 1613).

As reported by Hawkes and colleagues, The UNESCO International Technical Guidance on Sexuality Education (2009) asserts that vaccine delivery must not be a stand-alone effort but supported by engaging young people with comprehensive sexual health education (Hawkes et al., 2014). Here, our findings suggest that school-based vaccination programs profoundly failed the study participants. The school-based vaccination programs must ensure that girls, parents, teachers, nurses, all stakeholders have access to adequate information for informed decision-making around the vaccine, and beyond this, age appropriate sexuality education to enable girls to make informed and responsible choices around their future sexual health (Hawkes et al., 2014). I recommend that this comprehensive sexual health education includes the topic of vaccines generally, informed decision-making (how to ask about risks, benefits, alternatives and the consequences of doing nothing), informed consent, human rights treaties and laws that apply to girls, as well as sexual health counselling and services that they may access. It is critical that girls understand HPV, HPV vaccination and HPV screening (i.e., pap smears) as well as other sexually transmitted infections. It is important that they understand cervical cancer. It is imperative that information is age-appropriate and clear, for example, that HPV vaccinations are not a cancer vaccine per se but a sexually transmitted infection vaccine.

Central to the ethical justification for consent for adolescents is their emerging autonomy; recognition of girls' human and legal rights to informed consent will promote their self-determination in negotiating the fraught terrain of their sexual health.

Note

1 The author gratefully acknowledges the research assistance of Sarah Dykeman and Lauren C. Moore.

References

Abdelmutt, N., & Hoffman-Goetz, L. (2009). Risk messages about HPV, cervical cancer, and the HPV vaccine Gardasil: A content analysis of Canadian and US national newspaper articles. *Women & Health, 49*(5), 422–440.

Agrawal, S., & Morain, S.R. (2018). Who calls the shots? The ethics of adolescent self-consent for HPV vaccination. *Journal of Medical Ethics, (44)*, 531–535. doi:10.1136/medethics-2017-104694.

Beauchamp, T.L., & Childress, J.F. (2001). *Principles of Biomedical Ethics.* 5th ed. Oxford: Oxford University Press.

Bogler, T., Farber, A., Stall, N., Wijayasinghe, S., Slater, M., Guiang, C., & Glazer, R.H. (2015). Missed connections: Unintended consequences of updated cervical cancer screening guidelines on screening rates for sexually transmitted infections. *Canadian Family Physician, 61,* 459–466.

Canadian Women's Health Network. (2007, June 25). *HPV, vaccines, and gender: Policy considerations [PDF].* 1–19. Retrieved from http://www.cwhn.ca/sites/default/files/PDF/CWHN_HPVjuly30.pdf.

Cawley, J., Hull, H.F., & Rousculp, M.D. (2010). Strategies for implementing school-located influenza vaccination of children: A systematic literature review. *Journal of Scholarly Health, 80,* 167–175.

Choudry, Y., Miller, J., Sandhu, J., Leon, A., & Aho, J. (2018). Chlamydia in Canada, 2010–2015. *CCDR, 44*(2), 49–53.

College of Nurses of Ontario (CNO). (2009). *Practice Guideline: Consent*. Retrieved from: http://www.cno.org/Global/docs/policy/41020_consent.pdf.

Committee on the Rights of the Child. (2003). *General Comment No. 4: Adolescent Health and Development in the Context of the Convention on the Rights of the Child*. New York: United Nations committee on the Rights of the Child, 2003. [UN Doc.CRC/ GC/2003/4. Paragraphs, 1, 7, 9, 12, 16, 28, 31, 33, 39 and 40].

Dell, D.L., Chen, H., Ahmed, F., Steward, D.E. (2000). Knowledge about human papillomavirus among adolescents. *Obstet Gynecol*, 96(5, pt.1), 653–656.

Department of Finance Canada. (2007). *The budget plan*, No. F1-23/2007-3E (p. 96). Retrieved from http://www.budget.gc.ca/2007/pdf/bp2007e.pdf.

Ford, C.A., Skiles, M.P., English, A., Cai, J., Agans, R.P., Stokley, S., & Koumans, E.H. (2014). Minor consent and delivery of adolescent vaccines. *Journal of Adolescent Health*, 54(2), 183–189. doi: 10.1016/j.jadohealth.2013.07.028.

Gardasil™. (2008). Quadrivalent Human Papillomavirus (Types 6, 11, 16, 18) Recombinant Vaccine [Monograph].

Harris, T., Williams, D.M., Fediurek, J., Scott, T., & Deeks, S.L. (2014). Adverse events following immunization in Ontario's female school-based HPV program. *Vaccine 32*(9), 1061–1066. doi: 10.1016/j.vaccine.2014.01.004.

Hawkes, S., Kismodi, E., Larson, H., & Buse, K. (2014). Vaccines to promote and protect sexual health: Policy challenges and opportunities. *Vaccine*, 32, 1610–1615.

Health Care Consent Act. 1996, S.O., 1996, c.2, Sched A. Retrieved from http://www. elaws.gov.on.ca/html/statutes_96h02_e.htm.

Herman, R., McNutt, L., Mehta, M., Salmon, D.A., Bednarczyk, R.A., & Shaw, J. (2019). Vaccination perspectives among adolescents and their desired role in the decision-making process. *Human Vaccines and Immunotherapies*, 15(7–8), 1752–1759.

Johnson, J., Greaves, L., & Repta, R. (2009). Better science with sex and gender: Facilitating the use of a sex and gender-based analysis in health research. *International Journal for Equity in Health* 8(14). doi.10.1186/1475-9276-8-14.

Kahn, J.A., Brown, D.R., Ding, L., Widdice, L.E., Shew, M.L., Glynn, S., & Bernstein, D.I. (2012). Vaccine-type human papillomavirus and evidence of herd protection after vaccine introduction. *Pediatrics*, 130(2), e249–e256.

Keatings, M., & Smith, O. (2010). Consent to treatment, Chapter 6, pp. 155–184. In *Ethical & Legal Issues in Canadian Nursing* (3rd ed.) Toronto: Elsevier.

Lees, B.F., Erickson, B.K., & Warner, K.H. (2016). Cervical cancer screening: Evidence behind the guidelines. *American Journal of Obstetrics & Gynecology*, 214(4), 438–443.

Maine, D., Hurlburt, S., & Greeson, D. (2011). Cervical cancer prevention in the 21st century: Cost is not the only issue. *Health Policy and Ethics*, 101(9), 1549–1554.

Manucuso, F., & Polzer, J. (2010). It's your body but…Young women's narratives of declining human papillomavirus (HPV) vaccination. *Canadian Women's Studies*, 28(2/3), 177–181.

Massad, L.S., Einstein, M.H., & Huh, W.K., Katki, H.A., Kinney, W.K., Schiffman, W.K., Solomon, D., Wentzensen, N., Lawson, H.W. (2013). 2012 Updated consensus guidelines for the management of abnormal cervical cancer screening tests and cancer precursors. *The Journal of Lower Genital Tract Disease*, 17(5), S1–S27.

Mastrolorenzo, A., Supuran, C.T., & Zuccati, G. (2007). The sexually transmitted papillomavirus infections: Clinical manifestations current and future therapies. *Expert Opinion on Therapeutic Patents*, 17(2), 172–211. doi:10.1517/etp.2007.17.

McIntosh, M.J., & Morse, J.M. (2015). Situating and constructing diversity in semi-structured interviews. *Global Qualitative Nursing Research*, 2, 1–12. doi: 10.1177/2333393615597674.

Merton, R., & Kendall, P.L. (1946). The focused interview. *American Journal of Sociology*, *51*, 541–557.

Mishra, A., & Graham, J.E. (2012). Risk, choice and the 'girl vaccine': Unpacking human papillomavirus (HPV) immunisation. *Health, Risk & Society*, *14*(1), 57–69. doi:10.1080 /13698575.2011.641524.

Murphy, J., Kennedy, E.B., Dunn, S., McLachlin, C.M., Fung, K., Fung, M., & Gzik, D. (2012). Cervical screening: A guideline for clinical practice in Ontario. *Journal of Obstetrics and Gynaecology Canada*, *34*(5), 453–458.

National Advisory Committee on Immunization. (2007). Statement on human papillomavirus vaccine. *Canadian Communicable Disease Report*. *33*(ACS-2), 1–31. Retrieved from http://www.phac-aspc.gc.ca/publicat/ccdr-rmtc/07pdf/acs33-02.pdf.

Naimer, M.S., Kwong, J.C., Bhatia, D., Moineddin, R., Whelan, M., Campitelli, M.A., … McIsaac, W.J. (2017). The effect of changes in cervical screening guidelines on chlamydia testing. *Annals of Family Medicine*, *15*(4), 329–334.

Ng, E., Wilkins, R., Fung, M.F.K., & Berthelot, J. (2010). Cervical cancer mortality by neighbourhood income in urban Canada from 1971 to 1996. *CMAJ*, *170*(10), 1545–1549.

Ogilvie, G.S., Remple, V.P., Marra, F., McNeil, S.A., Naus, M., Pielak, K.L., … Patrick, D.M. (2007). Parental intention to have daughters receive the human papilloma vaccine. *CMAJ*, *177*(12). doi:10.1503/cmaj.071022.

Polzer, J.C., & Knabe, S.M. (2012). From desire to disease: Human Papillomavirus (HPV) and the medicalization of nascent female sexuality. *Journal of Sex Research*, *49*(4), 344–352. doi:10.1080/00224499.2011.644598.

Peppin, P. (2007). In Informed Consent. J. Downie, T. Caulfield & C.M. Floor (Eds.), *Canadian Health Law and Policy*. Markham, ON: LeisNexis

Public Health Ontario. (2019). *Databases for Sexually Transmitted Infections*. Retrieved from: https://www.publichealthontario.ca/en/search#q=sexual%20transmitted%20 infections&sort=relevancy.

Reiter, P.L., Brewer, N.T., Gottlieb, S.L., McRee, A., & Smith, J.S. (2009). Parents' health beliefs and HPV vaccination of their adolescent daughters. *Social Science & Medicine*, *69*(3), 475–480. doi: 10.1016/j.socscimed.2009.05.024.

Richards, L., & Morse, J.M. (2007). *Readme First for a User's Guide to Qualitative Methods*. Thousand Oaks: Sage.

Steenbeek, A., MacDonald, M.D., Downie, J., Appleton, B.A., & Baylis, F. (2012). Ill-informed consent? A content analysis of physical risk disclosure in school-based HPV vaccine programs. *Public Health Nursing*, *29*(1), 71–79. doi: 10.1111/j.1525-1446.2011.00974.x.

Steinberg, L. (2013). Does recent research on adolescent brain development inform the mature minor doctrine? *Journal of Medical Philosophy*, (38), 256–267.

Thompson, A. (2013). Human papilloma virus, vaccination and social justice: An analysis of a Canadian school-based vaccine program. *Public Health Ethics*, *6*(1), 11–20.

Torrecilla, M.A.R., Gonzales, M.P., Rodriguez, F.G., & Fernandez, J.R. (2011). Adverse effects of the human papillomavirus vaccine. *Atencion Primaria*, *43*(1), 5–9, doi:10.1016/j.aprim.2010.05.007.

UNESCO. (2009). *International Technical Guidance on Sexuality Education*. Paris: United Nations Educational, Scientific and Cultural Organization.

World Health Organization. (2013). *WHO Guidance Note: Comprehensive Cervical Cancer Prevention and Control: A Healthier Future for Girls and Women*. Geneva: World Health Organization.

Wilson, S.E., Karas, E., Crowcroft, N.S., Bontovics, E., & Deeks, S.L. (2012). Ontario's school based HPV immunization program: School board assent and parental consent. *Canadian Journal of Public Health, 103*(1), 34–49.

Wilson, S., Harris, T., Sethi, P., Fediurek, J., Macdonald, L., & Deeks, S.L. (2013). Coverage from Ontario, Canada's school-based HPV vaccine program: The first three years. *Vaccine, 31*(5), 757–762. doi:10.1016/j.vaccine.2012.11.090.

10 Reflections on the use of antiretroviral treatment among HIV+ men who have sex with men (MSM) in Nigeria

Abisola Balogun-Katung, Paul Bissell and Muhammad Saddiq

Introduction

Defined by the World Health Organization as a combination of three or more antiretroviral (ARV) drugs, antiretroviral treatment (ART) suppresses HIV replication, reduces the likelihood of viral resistance, increases the survival of individuals infected with HIV and requires lifetime adherence (World Health Organization, 2016). In the context of HIV, adherence to ART has been long used to describe the 'ability of the person living with HIV/AIDS to be involved in choosing, starting, managing and maintaining a given therapeutic medication regimen to control HIV replication and to improve immune function' (Jana, as cited in Glass & Cavassini, 2014, p. 1). The term 'adherence' is used in this chapter only when the participants have used it explicitly to describe instructions from healthcare providers on how to manage their ART; however, we note that this term may have judgemental connotations, especially as this chapter discusses the lived experiences of men who have sex with men (hereafter referred to as MSM). Therefore, in this chapter, we will simply use 'taking ART optimally' rather than adherence. Taking ART optimally has been demonstrated to be crucial for not just individual but community viral suppression (Holland et al., 2015). Despite this, MSM are known to experience considerable difficulty at multiple levels when taking ART thereby potentially reducing their response to treatment (Graham et al., 2013). Furthermore, in Nigeria, ART is not always readily available or accessible and when available a majority of HIV positive individuals do not access and use it (Charurat et al., 2015). At the time this study was conducted (2014–15), the men who participated obtained their ART from what we refer to as MSM-friendly facilities in Nigeria and were recruited via these facilities. It is important to note, however, that these men also draw on their prior recollections and experiences of obtaining their ART from Nigerian public hospitals. Various challenges have been identified in the literature as shaping sub-optimal use of ART including stigma, discrimination and social isolation of MSM (Graham et al., 2013). Many of these shape the accounts of the participants in this study.

Context: ART program and same-sex criminalisation in Nigeria

Although ART was introduced as the standard of care globally in 1996 (Lange & Ananworanich, 2014), it was not introduced in Nigeria, the context where this study was situated, until the early 2000s. Prior to the introduction of ART in Nigeria, the only available treatment was for opportunistic infections and this often involved palliative care (Daniel et al., 2008). In 2002, the Nigerian government commenced its ART treatment program with $3.5 million dollars' worth of ARVs imported into Nigeria from India. This program was mandated to provide 10,000 HIV infected adults and 5,000 children with ART before 2003 (Shaahu et al., 2008). Generic forms of Nevirapine, Lamivudine and Stavudine were distributed from 25 treatment centres across the six geopolitical zones of Nigeria (Iliyasu et al., 2005). These generic drugs cost approximately $368 per person per year but were subsidised by the government at $7 per person per year (Federal Ministry of Health Nigeria, 2010a).

This ambitious Nigerian ART program was successful until 2004 when patients were left without treatment for up to 3 months due to a supply shortage of ART (Monjok et al., 2010). The ART program resumed after the federal government procured ARV drugs worth $3.8 million dollars. Four years after its inception, a program with the aim of providing patients with ARV drugs at no cost was introduced. This program served 250,000 HIV positive Nigerian citizens at 74 treatment centres spread across Nigeria (Federal Ministry of Health, Nigeria, 2010a). In 2010, the Nigerian ART program was the largest in sub-Saharan Africa and provided 300,000 HIV positive individuals with ARTs. Despite this, approximately 1.5 million eligible patients remained without access to the treatment (Federal Ministry of Health Nigeria, 2010a; Monjok et al., 2010; Oku et al., 2014). Still a long way off from meeting the global target of enrolling 90% of HIV infected individuals on ART, Nigeria has been able to increase treatment access between 2016 and 2017, by enrolling 212,000 additional HIV infected individuals (HIV and AIDS in Nigeria, 2020).

In Nigeria, the Same Sex Marriage Prohibition Act (SSMPA), signed into law in January 2014, criminalises marriage and civil unions between same sex couples (Global Legal Research Centre, 2014). Under this law, any direct or indirect display of affection or marriage contract between individuals of the same sex attracts a sentence of 14 years' imprisonment. In 12 states in Northern Nigeria, where the Islamic Sharia penal code has been extended to cover criminal acts, male same-sex acts are punishable with death by stoning (Global Legal Research Centre, 2014). Although the SSMPA implies criminalisation of same-sex marriage, it goes further to criminalise consensual same-sex sexual activity in both public and private spaces. MSM have been defined as men who have sexual intercourse, either anal or oral, with other men, whether or not they self-identify as homosexual (Ayoola et al., 2013; Wolf et al., 2013; Henry et al., 2010). Because some men in Nigeria who have anal or oral sexual intercourse with other men do not always identify as homosexual but rather as heterosexual, we have adapted the above definition.

The Nigerian socio-political environment has long been hostile and intolerant towards MSM and the passing of the Same Sex Marriage (prohibition) Bill has had additional negative consequences. Numerous cases of arrests and homophobic violence against MSM have been reported (Amnesty UK, 2015) and this has subsequently driven MSM further away from mainstream healthcare services. In 2007, the Federal Ministry of Health of Nigeria commenced surveys aimed at characterising the HIV epidemic in at-risk populations (Federal Ministry of Health Nigeria, 2007). Among the groups categorised as having the highest susceptibility to HIV, the MSM group was the only one that recorded an increase in HIV prevalence from 13.5% in 2007 to 17.2% in 2010 and more recently in 2014, 22.9% (Federal Ministry of Health of Nigeria, 2007, 2010b, 2015). Despite the increase in HIV prevalence among MSM over the years, 2014 data also revealed that only 27.1% of this population accessed HIV and STI treatment from local pharmacies (Federal Ministry of Health Nigeria, 2015). The National Agency for the Control of AIDS (NACA), a federal government agency responsible for the control of HIV/AIDS in the country, released a statement guaranteeing all Nigerian MSM access to HIV treatment (Federal Ministry of Health Nigeria, 2010b). Evidence suggests, however, that many Nigerian MSM remain unable to access the full range of healthcare services with only 18% gaining access to HIV prevention programming in 2010 (Federal Ministry of Health Nigeria, 2010b). It is against these contextual backdrops that the study reported in this chapter was conducted.

Methodology

This study was conducted in two states in Nigeria, Abuja and Lagos. It employed a qualitative research approach to critically explore and describe the lived experiences of HIV positive MSM with taking their ART in the heteronormative context of Nigeria. Qualitative research approaches were deemed appropriate for this study because its focus was on a vulnerable population and issues that can be considered sensitive (Liamputtong and Ezzy, 2006).

An important first step in light of the illegal nature of same sex sexual practices and the associated stigma with researching these issues in Nigeria, was to seek a gatekeeper organisation. Approaching the field with the full backing of a Gatekeeper Organisation (GO) was pertinent to facilitating access to this hard-to-reach and hidden population and the process of rapport building. The three organisations chosen were Heartland Alliance International (HAI), the Population Council (PC) and the International Centre for Advocacy on Rights to Health (ICARH). HAI provides psychosocial support as well as HIV prevention and human rights protection services to Nigeria's most-at-risk-populations, including MSM, using a comprehensive, rights-based approach. The other two organisations, PC and the ICARH provide HIV services including ART to MSM populations. Ethical approval was obtained from the University of Sheffield and also from two research governance bodies in Nigeria, the Federal Capital Territory Health Research Ethics Committee (FCT-REC) and the Lagos State University Teaching Hospital Health Research and Ethics Committee

(LASUTH-REC). A total of 13 in-depth interviews and 3 focus groups were conducted in Abuja. In Lagos, a total of 8 in-depth interviews and 1 focus group were conducted. The interviews and focus groups were transcribed and analysed for emergent themes and some of the principal themes are described here.

Initiating and taking ART

All of the study participants used ART to manage their HIV. The majority of them reported that they had not immediately started using ART upon diagnosis with HIV. In some cases, they had not been able to access ART until many years after diagnosis, when they became seriously ill and were experiencing symptoms of HIV/AIDS or their CD4 count had dropped drastically. The CD4 count refers to a test that measures the number of white blood cells in the blood. The CD4 cell count provides an indication of the health of a person's immune system. Therefore, the higher the CD4 cell count, the healthier the person; a healthy immune system would have a CD4 cell count ranging from 500 to 1,600 cells per cubic millimetre of blood. A person living with HIV can have a cell count over 500, indicating the person is in good health; however, if the person has a CD4 cell count below 200, then they are at high risk of developing life-threatening illnesses. The following quote illustrates the process that occurred before the men initiated their ART:

> Then they told me I wouldn't be placed on drugs yet because my CD4 is still very much high, I was like ok, but I should be taking fruits and I should get Septrin (a drug used to cure pneumonia)… Then after like a month… I think I fell sick, I think, yes, I think I had fever, typhoid and malaria. Then after the typhoid and malaria, I lost some weight, then I was like ok ah, I have to just pick up courage and start taking this medication if not I would start falling ill, what I've been hiding, I don't want anybody to know, to later find out because in our community, whenever somebody is falling sick regularly, regularly, they just conclude, ah he has HIV. So I was like ok I'm ready.
>
> Mustapha, Lagos interview

The above quote highlights the stages participants went through before eventually deciding to start using ART. The Nigerian government in 2010 adopted the World Health Organization 'test and treat' policy, which recommended initiation of therapy for all HIV infected individuals irrespective of CD4 count, but, in Nigeria, HIV positive MSM who had CD4 counts greater than 350 cells/mm^3 were not prescribed ART. Instead, they were counselled on how to maintain good health through diet and if necessary prescribed Septrin, which they said was used in treating bacterial infections. An HIV infected individual was usually not prescribed ART until they began to fall sick consistently.

Once study participants had decided to seek treatment, the next step was to access and obtain ART. Participants expressed that they were reluctant to start using ART for a number of reasons: misconceptions about the treatment and its side effects, fear of others becoming aware of their HIV status, discrimination and marginalisation, and cohabiting with other MSM and non-MSM friends or with family. In a country marked by homophobia these were significant issues. Participants reported that they had to undergo two to three weeks' mandatory 'adherence counselling' so that they would understand the importance of taking ART optimally. They revealed that this mandatory 'adherence counselling' was mainly provided at MSM-friendly clinics.

Participants reported that during 'adherence counselling', they were advised about the basic mechanisms of ART and how to manage their illness with ART. In terms of maintaining good health, participants mentioned that they were advised by healthcare providers to avoid drinking alcohol, smoking cigarettes and using illicit drugs, to use condoms even if their partner is HIV positive as well, to maintain a healthy diet by eating foods high in protein, drinking plenty of water and finally to avoid stress. To use their ART optimally, they had to take their pills at about the same time every day and try not to miss doses. They mentioned that they were informed about possible side effects associated with ART and to expect encountering these side effects until they got used to taking the treatment. After 'adherence counselling', participants were prescribed ART which they used in managing their HIV.

The majority of participants stated that they took their ART once per day and it was usually at night, however, two reported that they took theirs twice a day because they were on a second line treatment regimen. An interviewee who was initially prescribed first-line ART reported that he was placed on a second line treatment regimen when he stopped responding to treatment. He stated:

> When I started... there's this one I take, two in the morning, two in the night, that's how I used to take it but after some, like a year, they said that, I did my CD4 and my viral load... the viral load was increasing, something that supposed to be decreasing because I've been taking drugs, it was increasing... It's either I'm not taking it well or the drug is not working for me, they now had to place me on the second regimen which is the one I'm taking now. And that one is even more stressful, the drugs are very big and you have to take it three in the morning, two in the night with Septrin again making it three in the morning, three in the night... from what they told me, this second line is my last opportunity because if it fails, the third regimen is not in Nigeria, it's either I have to go to abroad and maybe start taking the other one or I'd be ready to die, which I am not ready.
>
> Sule, Abuja interview

In the case above, the number of drugs to be taken daily was an issue and may have caused the participant to stop taking his medicines consistently, which led to the increase in his viral load. He also stated that using second line treatment was even more difficult as there was an even higher pill burden and bigger pills he had to swallow. The difficulties MSM experienced when taking their ART are discussed in more detail in the following section.

Benefits of taking ART

The general consensus among participants was that consistent use of ART offered an abundance of health benefits. All MSM reported that they experienced an overall improvement in their health and wellbeing, and improved CD4 counts and viral loads within a few months of starting their treatment. Some stated that they felt they looked healthier than even those who weren't HIV positive and attributed this to the potency of the treatment.

Feeling and looking healthier as a result of adherence to ART allowed MSM to deal better with stigma. One participant mentioned how he never experienced stigma because there was no physical evidence that he had HIV as a result of using his ART. Common to all MSM in this study was the confidence that they could live longer and normal lives because they were using ART. Participants' responses revealed a high level of self-efficacy and responsibility for their lives and their health and this was one of their motivations for taking their treatment optimally.

Additionally, the feeling that they needed to conceal their HIV positive status from others was one of their major motivations for using ART optimally. On the one hand, without treatment, participants experienced some of the visible side effects of HIV such as drastic weight loss, fever and rashes and there was a possibility of rapid decline to full blown AIDS, which made it impossible to conceal their HIV status. On the other hand, these side effects were also experienced in the initial stages of initiating ART. As a result, participants found it difficult to conceal their HIV positive status from inquisitive family members and friends who often probed into the cause of the side effects. Due to many challenges, predominantly stigma, discrimination and marginalisation, which seemed to envelope their daily lives, many participants in this study struggled with ART, despite their understanding of its numerous benefits.

Challenges to taking ART optimally

Participants reported various challenges of taking their ART that were interlinked and fell into three broad categories including patient-related challenges, nature of the ART and social/structural barriers. It is important to note that the men in this study sometimes experienced these factors at the same time.

Nature of ART

Regarding the aesthetic characteristics and palatability of ART, participants mentioned that the pill bottle, pill size and taste of the pill at times made optimal use difficult. Some of the men mentioned that the pill bottle inhibited their movement, which made adherence difficult especially because MSM in this context are generally highly mobile. The side effects of taking ART were also reported as a reason why they struggled to take their ART. These side effects were especially prominent during the initial weeks and months of commencing treatment. Most recurrent side effects reported were skin rashes, scars, drunken feeling, dizziness, unusual or bad dreams, hot flushes and fever.

One participant mentioned that he experienced visible side effects of using ART and this caused his family members to question him about it:

> When I started the drugs, I did not find it very easy... I had very terrible wounds on my mouth and my eye was like red. That is the reaction of the ART, so my family was like asking me, what is the problem?
>
> Arinze, Abuja interview

These and other visible side effects such as fat redistribution could not be easily hidden from family members and associates, who questioned them about it. There was a concern that revealing that they were HIV positive and taking ART could lead to rejection, stigmatisation and discrimination, which they avoided. Participants who had been on ART for a longer period of time reported that they became used to these side effects and only occasionally experienced the side effects of the treatment.

At the time of the interviews, one participant, Joe, reported that he had not been using ART for almost a year because of the serious side effects he experienced after he had changed to a different brand. Joe was told by healthcare workers to stop using his ART until he had undergone liver function tests because he developed hepatitis and experienced severe symptoms such as weight loss, vomiting and jaundice. He desperately wanted to get back on his treatment as he was uncertain how long he had to live if he did not.

Patient-related challenges

Inability to keep to time

A particular problem for some participants was the difficulty of taking ART at a set time every day for the rest of their lives. The timing of therapy was interrupted by engagements or daily activities or the presence of family or friends when treatment was required. Their inability to keep to the allotted time schedule was enhanced by their high mobility. One focus group participant expressed that the timing requirements made using ART optimally difficult and even impossible:

> Adherence, number one is time taking. You know when you are given the drugs they would tell you that once you start taking it by 9 o'clock, throughout, till you die, till you stop taking it, you must keep taking it at 9 o'clock but I know it's very very hard for us to just get adhere to that kind of thing... I don't think that one is possible getting adhere to time.
>
> Olu, Lagos focus group

In response to Olu's statement, two other focus group participants reported that they were advised by the healthcare workers that once they got accustomed to taking their ART, they could allow more flexibility in the timing.

Forgetfulness

Forgetfulness was another commonly reported challenge to taking ART optimally. Forgetting to take ART was experienced in different ways:

> I think I forgot, I slept off, one of the reason was that I slept off. Like I told you once it 9 o'clock I always feel, naturally once it's 9 o'clock, I always feel like I'm going to sleep as long as I'm not going for a party, I'm not talking or watching anything, so that was the first one. The second one was that I forgot, I was going for a party, it was actually in my pocket, I forgot to take it until when it was 2 o'clock at night, I now remembered that, ah I didn't take this thing. Then the third one was like it was 11:30, I did not take it, I thought maybe once it has passed 10 o'clock I cannot take it again.
>
> Mustapha, Lagos interview

> Taking in the morning maybe you can forget the evening one, if you take it in the evening you can forget the morning one. So that is another one again, those are the challenges.
>
> Boye, Abuja focus group

As shown above, participants reported forgetting to take ART at the scheduled time, forgetting that they had taken it and then double dosing, and forgetting they had ART altogether.

MSM lifestyle

MSM lifestyle in this context describes MSM sexual partnerships and networks as well as their high mobility all of which challenge optimal ART use. Several aspects of the 'MSM lifestyle' impacted participants' ability to adhere to ART. These included clubbing and drinking, inconvenience of carrying pill bottles, drug fatigue and interference with sexual relationships. The most salient struggle related to their lifestyle was perhaps the interference with their sexual relationships. Participants reported that they were unable to take their ART when they were with sexual partners because they feared that their partners would stigmatise them if they found out they were HIV positive. Although this was generally the case, there were a few cases when participants had overcome this fear. Participants who were in a trusting relationship reported that they informed their partners that they were HIV positive and on ART.

Social/structural level challenges

Social or structural level challenges refer to those challenges related to participants' social circumstances including their financial capability to maintain optimal ART use, cohabiting and discrimination and marginalisation.

Lack of financial capital and sustenance

One participant in the study mentioned that his partner was initially reluctant to start taking ART because he was unemployed:

> He was complaining no no no, I wouldn't want to take the drugs, we don't have money now, because as at that time I wasn't working, it's still that volunteer work that I was doing that we were using to feed and the money is still too little so we cannot afford three square meals. So he was telling me that he heard that once you start taking these drugs you need to eat very well and you know we don't have money so how can we eat very well and be taking these drugs? You know there's no money at hand.
>
> Ibrahim, Abuja interview

Lack of financial capital and food insufficiency were key challenges to optimal use of ART among participants in this study. A majority of the participants came from low or middle socioeconomic backgrounds. Some were unable to secure employment, or their income was insufficient to sustain them. The guidance provided by healthcare providers that ART use requires a healthy diet was interpreted as implying that ART could not be commenced in the context of food insufficiency.

Living arrangements

Another challenge to ART use was living with family, non-MSM friends or with other MSM. According to one participant:

> Most MSM are cohabiting… so it makes them miss their drugs often… disclosure is a very big deal in this community. All of you might be on the same issue but you will not know that you are dealing with the same issue, you don't even talk about it.
>
> Peter, Abuja focus group

It was surprising that MSM who were themselves HIV positive could not only hide it from others but also stigmatise other MSM who were HIV positive. This challenged the claim by some participants of being in a close-knit community. Rather, study participants expressed general discomfort and some indicated that they would not take ART when there were others around them:

> So, when they told me I'm HIV positive, it's not immediately I started taking the drugs, why? Because, one, I'm not alone, how can I keep the drugs? That's the first challenge that I have… So, I was afraid to start the drugs, I stayed almost 1 to 2 years before I started taking drugs.
>
> Amaechi, Abuja interview

Then whenever I have visitors in my place, in my room, I would have to do it stealthily, that is trying to take it without being noticed, that is the only barrier.

Ibrahim, Abuja interview

In addition to this, some men in this study revealed that they traded sex for financial benefits and favours. For these men, it was particularly difficult to take their ART when they were with the men they traded sex with:

Me, the only big challenge of that adherence that you said, is that issue of cohabiting, not wanting the person close to you to know that you are taking the drugs… Yeah, you know that would make you miss your drug one day. I know that if you have 'market' and that 'market' would come around at 8 or after 8 and your drug time is 9 o'clock, you understand. You will be trying [to make sure] he no see me carry that bottle.

Peter, Abuja focus group

'Market' according to these men refers to transacting or trading sex. Having clients around when it was time to take treatment was challenging when HIV status had not been disclosed and produced fear of being identified as HIV positive.

It is notable, however, that cohabitation was not only a challenge, but could also facilitate optimal use of ART. Participants who cohabited with trusted lovers or friends, who were in some cases HIV positive as well could remind them when it was time to take their treatment. Participants who lived alone, however, could take ART freely:

I stay alone, I don't really have people that would poke nose and say why am I taking this thing and all that, so it is very free for me.

Kunle, Abuja interview

Living alone meant that participants were able to control disclosure of their HIV positive status.

Stigma and discrimination in everyday life

Salient challenges to taking ART optimally were stigma and discrimination. Experiences of stigma and discrimination permeated every aspect of the daily lived experiences including interaction with healthcare services and the wider society:

As a man who has sex with men I can't go to a public hospital to receive treatment. Number one, it is very notable that a doctor would ask you how come? What is your sexual orientation? They would want to know how come you contracted this virus, how you come in contact with this virus, do I just go there and tell them I am a man who has sex with men? That I'm being penetrated through the ass, you know, I'm going to hide a lot of things.

Olu, Lagos interview

The men in this study experienced stigma and discrimination in various forms: HIV stigma, sexual stigma, stigma of being both HIV positive and MSM, stigma by association, internalised HIV and sexual stigma and finally, anticipated stigma. The most important forms of stigma pertinent to their use of ART were sexual stigma, that is the stigma of being a man having sex with another man, anticipated stigma, as well as the internalisation of sexual stigma. Participants indicated that their response to stigma and discrimination was to conceal their HIV status which frequently meant they were unable to access ART. Where they were able to access ART, the socio-political climate and criminalisation of MSM makes optimal use a secondary concern. Societally, they were often perceived to be possessed by evil spirits and were seen to be more alien than human. Healthcare workers in government hospitals perceived their homosexual practices as sinful and immoral. Participants reported that healthcare workers sometimes threatened to kill anyone they know who engages in homosexual practices, including their children. The men's sexual practices may have been viewed as sinful and immoral because these practices do not conform to the heteronormative expectations of Nigerian society.

Discussion and conclusion

In this chapter, we have explored the experiences of HIV positive MSM living in Nigeria in relation to ART. We discussed the processes of initiating ART as well as challenges and facilitators MSM encounter in their attempt to take their ART optimally. It was revealed that participants understood medical expectations of maintaining optimal adherence to ART regimens. There is a dearth of research on the experiences of ART use in the African MSM population, and this study provides some qualitative data with respect to this problem, although it needs to be acknowledged that the study did not attempt to quantitatively measure ART use.

Taking ART optimally was clearly not without its challenges and these fell into three groups: the nature of ART, patient-related and social/structural level challenges. In terms of the nature of ART, the factors reported by men in this study included those challenges related to the aesthetics and palatability of ART that made its use difficult. These findings are similar to findings in the literature pertaining to aspects of the nature of the drugs as a barrier to taking ART optimally (Mills et al., 2006a; Merten et al., 2010; Bezabhe et al., 2014). Similarly, participants in a study on patient-reported barriers in sub-Saharan Africa revealed adverse reactions as a barrier to taking ART optimally (Weiser et al., 2003; Merten et al., 2010). A study conducted in Botswana reported similar barriers to optimal ART use as those noted here: pill aesthetics (size, taste and overall palatability) as well as drug side effects (Weiser et al., 2003).

Patient related challenges included aspects of the MSM lifestyle and other individual level challenges such as forgetfulness and inability to keep to the recommended schedule. Other studies have also reported patient-related factors that shape the extent to which individuals are able to take ART (van Servellen et al., 2002; Mills et al., 2006a; Uzochukwu et al., 2009). Among these factors are forgetfulness, busy work schedules, financial barriers, mental health problems, and lack of a strong support system (Sanjobo, Frich & Fretheim, 2008; Merten et al., 2010; Musumari et al., 2013; Bezabhe et al., 2014; Portelli et al., 2015). Another aspect of MSM lifestyle is excessive alcohol use, which has previously been cited among factors for 'sub-optimal adherence' to ART in a study conducted in sub-Saharan Africa (Mills et al., 2006b). Furthermore, Chander et al. (2006) provided evidence establishing the deleterious effects of alcohol on both viral suppression and immunological functioning. Alcohol use was also found to be among the main deterrents to taking ART in a review conducted by Heestermans et al. (2016).

Finally, social/structural level challenges included challenges in participants' social circumstances such as income insecurity and living arrangements that made taking ART difficult. A majority of study participants found it difficult to take their ART because they had no steady employment and therefore no income, and they experienced food insecurity. Food access is important given World Health Organization and healthcare worker recommendations that persons on ART maintain a healthy balanced diet to boost their immune system. Financial issues as well as patients' beliefs that ART had to be taken with food have been cited as factors that cause poor uptake of ART in other studies (Nachega et al., 2006; Ramadhani et al., 2007; Rachlis, Mills and Cole, 2011). Studies in similar African contexts have found food insecurity to be a major barrier to taking ART (Weiser et al., 2010; Groh et al., 2011; Musumari et al., 2014). Specifically, participants in Uganda reported that ARV medicines increased their appetite and lack of food exacerbated hunger. In addition, side effects of ART were exacerbated in the absence of food. Users had been counselled on the importance of having a balanced diet when taking ART and competing priorities made them unable to purchase or even use their ART consistently (Weiser et al., 2010). As demonstrated by other findings, living arrangements can impact optimal use of ART (Sanjobo et al., 2008).

Most salient among the aspects of the men's experiences that made it difficult to take their treatment were stigma and discrimination. The socio-political climate in Nigeria is such that same sex relationships are criminalised and as a result, those who are found to engage in same sex relationships are generally stigmatised and discriminated against. Taking ART for these men, therefore, become a secondary concern. These men have to devise methods of adapting to this hostile environment, and in this context where concealment becomes an everyday necessity, a greater openness and awareness about the daily struggles of these men is imperative. It is difficult to underestimate the impact of the wider socio-political climate on the men's experiences of taking ART. In the context of this edited work focused on 'Living Pharmaceutical Lives' it is noted that lives are lived in wider political contexts and these shape both health practices and accounts.

References

Amnesty UK. (2015). *Mapping anti-gay laws in Africa*. Amnesty International UK. Retrieved from: https://www.amnesty.org.uk/lgbti-lgbt-gay-human-rights-law-africa-uganda-kenya-nigeria-cameroon.

Ayoola, O.O., Sekoni, A.O., & Odeyemi, K. (2013). Transactional sex, condom and lubricant use among men who have sex with men in Lagos State Nigeria. *Afr J Reprod Health*, *17*(4), 90–98.

Bezabhe, W.M., Chalmers, L., Bereznicki, L.R., Peterson, G.M., Bimirew, M.A., & Kassie, D.M. (2014). Barriers and facilitators of adherence to antiretroviral drug therapy and retention in care among adult HIV-positive patients: A qualitative study from Ethiopia. *PLoS One*, *9*(5), e97353.

Chander, G., Lau, B., & Moore, R.D. (2006). Hazardous alcohol use: A risk factor for non-adherence and lack of suppression in HIV infection. *JAIDS J Acquir Immune Defic Syndr*, *43*(4), 411–417.

Charurat, M.E., Emmanuel, B., Akolo, C., Keshinro, B., Nowak, R.G., Kennedy, S., ... Blattner, W. (2015). Uptake of treatment as prevention for HIV and continuum of care among HIV-positive men who have sex with men in Nigeria. *J Acquir Immune Defic Syndr*, *68*, S114–S123. doi:10.1097/QAI.0000000000000439.

Daniel, O.J., Oladapo, O.T., Ogundahunsi, O.A., Fagbenro, S., Ogun, S.A., & Odusoga, O.A. (2008). Default from anti-retroviral treatment programme in Sagamu, Nigeria. *African J Biomed Res*, *11*(2), 221–224.

Federal Ministry of Health Nigeria. (2007). *HIV/STI Integrated Biological and Behavioural Surveillance Survey (IBBSS)*. Abuju, Nigeria: Federal Ministry of Health.

Federal Ministry of Health Nigeria. (2010a). National Guidelines for HIV and AIDS Treatment and Care in Adolescents and Adults. *Federal Ministry of Health* 1–67.

Federal Ministry of Health Nigeria. (2010b). *HIV Integrated Biological and Behavioural Surveillance Survey (IBBSS)*. Abuju, Nigeria: Federal Ministry of Health.

Federal Ministry of Health Nigeria. (2015). *Integrated Biological and Behavioural Surveillance Survey (IBBSS) 2014 Report*. https://naca.gov.ng/wp-content/uploads/2016/11/Final-Nigeria-IBBSS-2014-report.pdf. accessed September 28, 2020.

Glass, T., & Cavassini, M. (2014). Asking about adherence – from flipping the coin to strong evidence. *Swiss Med Wkly*, *144*, w14016. doi:10.4414/smw.2014.14016.

Global Legal Research Centre. (2014). *Laws on Homosexuality in African Nations*. Global Legal Research Centre, Washington, DC: The Law Library of Congress. https://www.loc.gov/law/help/criminal-laws-on-homosexuality/homosexuality-laws-in-african-nations.pdf

Graham, S.M., Mugo, P., Gichuru, E., Thiong'o, A., Macharia, M., Okuku, H. S., ... van der Elst, E. (2013). Adherence to antiretroviral therapy and clinical outcomes among young adults reporting high-risk sexual behavior, including men who have sex with men, in coastal Kenya. *AIDS Behav*, *17*(4), 1255–1265. doi:10.1007/s10461-013-0445-9.

Groh, K., Audet, C.M., Baptista, A., Sidat, M., Vergara, A., Vermund, S.H., ... Moon, T. (2011). Barriers to antiretroviral therapy adherence in rural Mozambique. *BMC Public Health*, *11*, 650.

Heestermans, T., Browne, J.L., Aitken, S.C., Vervoort, S.C., & Klipstein-Grobusch, K. (2016). Determinants of adherence to antiretroviral therapy among HIV-positive adults in sub-Saharan Africa: A systematic review. *BMJ Glob Heal*, *1*(4), e000125.

Henry, E., Marcellin, F., Yomb, Y., Fugon, L., Nemande, S., Gueboguo, C., ... Spire, B. (2010). Factors associated with unprotected anal intercourse among men who have sex with men in Douala, Cameroon. *Sex Transm Infect*, *86*(2), 136–140.

HIV and AIDS in Nigeria. (2020). Avert. Retrieved September 29, 2020, from https://www.avert.org/professionals/hiv-around-world/sub-saharan-africa/nigeria.

Holland, C.E., Papworth, E., Billong, S.C., Kassegne, S., Petitbon, F., Mondoleba, V., ... Stefan, D. (2015). Access to HIV services at non-governmental and community-based organizations among men who have sex with men (MSM) in Cameroon: An integrated biological and behavioral surveillance analysis. *PLoS One*, *10*(4), 0122881. doi:10.1371/journal.pone.0122881.

Iliyasu, Z., Kabir, M., Abubakar, I.S., Babashani, M., & Zubair, Z.A. (2005). Compliance to antiretroviral therapy among AIDS patients in Aminu Kano Teaching Hospital, Kano, Nigeria. *Niger J Med*, *14*(3), 290–294.

Lange, J.M.A., & Ananworanich, J. (2014) The discovery and development of antiretroviral agents. *Antivir Ther*, *19*, 5–14.

Liamputtong, P., & Ezzy, D. (2006). Qualitative research methods. *Aust N Z J Public Health*, *30*(2). 375–386.

Merten, S., Kenter, E., McKenzie, O., Musheke, M., Ntalasha, H., & Martin-Hilber, A. (2010). Patient-reported barriers and drivers of adherence to antiretrovirals in sub-Saharan Africa: A meta-ethnography. *Trop Med Int Health*, *15*(1), 16–33.

Mills, E.J., Nachega, J.B., Buchan, I., & Orbinski, J. (2006a). Adherence to antiretroviral therapy in Sub-Saharan Africa and North America. *JAMA*, *296*(6), 679–690.

Mills, E.J., Nachega, J.B., Buchan, I., Orbinski, J., Attaran, A., Singh, S., … Bangsberg, D. (2006b). Adherence to antiretroviral therapy in sub-Saharan Africa and North America: A meta-analysis. *JAMA*, *296*(6), 679–690.

Monjok, E., Smesny, A., Okokon, I.B., Mgbere, O., & Essien, E.J. (2010). Adherence to antiretroviral therapy in Nigeria: An overview of research studies and implications for policy and practice. *HIV/AIDS: Research and Palliative Care*, *2*, 69–76. doi:10.2147/hiv.s9280.

Musumari, P.M., Feldman, M.D., Techasrivichien, T., Wouters, E., Ono-Kihara, M., & Kihara, M. (2013). "If I have nothing to eat, I get angry and push the pills bottle away from me": A qualitative study of patient determinants of adherence to antiretroviral therapy in the Democratic Republic of Congo. *AIDS Care*, *25*(10), 1271–1277.

Musumari, P.M., Wouters, E., Kayembe, P.K., Nzita, K.M., Mbikayi, S.M., Suguimoto, S.P., … Kihara, M. (2014). Food insecurity is associated with increased risk of non-adherence to antiretroviral therapy among HIV-infected adults in the Democratic Republic of Congo: A cross-sectional study. *PLOS ONE*, *9*(1), e85327. doi:10.1371/journal.pone.0085327.

Nachega, J.B., Hislop, M., Dowdy, D.W., Lo, M., Omer, S.B., Regensberg, L., … Maartens, G. (2006). Adherence to highly active antiretroviral therapy assessed by pharmacy claims predicts survival in HIV-infected South African adults. *J Acquir Immune Defic Syndr*, *43*(1), 78–84.

Oku, A.O., Owoaje, E.T., Oku, O.O., & Monjok, E. (2014). Prevalence and determinants of adherence to highly active antiretroviral therapy amongst people living with HIV/AIDS in a rural setting in south-south Nigeria. *Afr J Reprod Health*, *18*(1), 133–143.

Portelli, M.S., Tenni, B., Kounnavong, S., & Chanthivilay, P. (2015). Barriers to and facilitators of adherence to antiretroviral therapy among people living with HIV in Lao PDR: A qualitative study. *Asia-Pacific J Public Heal*, *27*(2), 778–788.

Rachlis, B.S., Mills, E.J., & Cole, D.C. (2011). Livelihood security and adherence to antiretroviral therapy in low and middle income settings: A systematic review. *PLoS One*, *6*(5): e18948.

Ramadhani, H.O., Thielman, N.M., Landman, K.Z., Ndosi, E.M., Gao, F., Kirchherr, J.L., … Krump, J. (2007). Predictors of incomplete adherence, virologic failure, and antiviral drug resistance among HIV-infected adults receiving antiretroviral therapy in Tanzania. *Clin Infect Dis*, *45*(11), 1492–1498.

Sanjobo, N., Frich, J.C., & Fretheim, A. (2008). Barriers and facilitators to patients' adherence to antiretroviral treatment in Zambia: A qualitative study. *Sahara J*, *5*(3), 136–143.

Shaahu, V.N., Lawoyin, T.O., & Sangowawa, A.O. (2008). Adherence to highly active antiretroviral therapy (HAAT) at a Federal Medical Centre. *Afr J Med Med Sci, 37*(1), 29–36.

Uzochukwu, B.S.C., Onwujekwe, O.E., Onoka, A.C., Okoli, C., Uguru, N.P., Chukwuogo, O.I. (2009). Determinants of non-adherence to subsidized anti-retroviral treatment in southeast Nigeria. *Health Policy Plan, 24*(3), 189–196.

van Servellen, G., Chang, B., Garcia, L., & Lombardi, E. (2002). Individual and system level factors associated with treatment nonadherence in human immunodeficiency virus-infected men and women. *AIDS Patient Care STDs, 16*(6), 269–281. doi:10.1089/10872910260066705.

Weiser, S., Wolfe, W., Bangsberg, D., Thior, I., Gilbert, P., Makhema, J., … Marlink, M. (2003). Barriers to antiretroviral adherence for patients living with HIV infection and AIDS in botswana. *JAIDS J Acquir Immune Defic Syndr, 34*(3), 281–288.

Weiser, S.D., Tuller, D.M., Frongillo, E.A., Senkungu, J., Mukiibi, N., & Bangsberg, D.R. (2010). Food insecurity as a barrier to sustained antiretroviral therapy adherence in Uganda. *PLoS One, 5*(4), e10340.

Wolf, R.C., Cheng, A.S., Kapesa, L., & Castor, D. (2013). Building the evidence base for urgent action: HIV epidemiology and innovative programming for men who have sex with men in sub-Saharan Africa. *Journal of the International AIDS Society, 16*(3), 18903. doi: 10.7448/IAS.16.4.18903.

World Health Organization. (2016). Recommendations for a public health approach. In *Consolidated Guidelines On the Use of Antiretroviral Drugs For Treating and Preventing HIV Infection.* (pp. 155). Geneva: World Health Organization.

11 Opioid analgesics, stigma, shame and identity

Richard J. Cooper

Introduction

Opioid analgesics represent a well-recognised class of medicines that have gained increasing notoriety through concerns about their addiction potential (Vowles et al., 2015) increasing prescribing trends (OECD, 2019), and related harms (British Medical Association, 2017) particularly associated with their long-term use such as for chronic pain. The ubiquity of prescribed opioids is reflected in a recent analysis which found that around one in eight adults in England had been prescribed an opioid at least once annually (Marsden et al., 2019). This has been viewed as a significant public health concern and termed an 'opioid epidemic' with a significant risk of harm and mortality. In terms of scale, in the United States during 2017 there were estimated to be around 17,000 deaths related to prescription opioids (Centres for Disease Control and Prevention, 2017), and in the United Kingdom in 2019, there were over 9,000 hospital admissions linked to non-heroin opioids such as codeine and morphine (NHS Digital, 2019). As well as concerns about deaths and overdose, other clinical manifestations arise in relation to loss of therapeutic effect and tolerance over time, hyperalgesia and addiction itself (Deyo et al., 2015). Between 2005 and 2017 in England, there was a 91% increase in presentations of individuals to formal drug and alcohol treatment services where an opioid analgesic only was involved (Public Health England, 2018)

In this chapter, my aim is to move beyond these dominant clinical and public health foci on harm and mortality, to explore the significant psychosocial problems related to the consumption of prescription and over-the-counter (OTC) opioid analgesic medicines. I argue that affected individuals might experience significant stigma and shame through problematic use of opioid medicines themselves. In addition, such medicine use impinges on important aspects of identity, and challenges notions of coping and the management of often chronic conditions. As Eaves notes:

> Consumption of goods, including medications, is a visual and tangible means of communicating social values, performing notions of self and establishing social relationship... Pharmaceutical consumption is part of constructing individual and social identity.

(Eaves, 2015, p. 147)

Issues of stigma, shame and identity have been represented in the literature relating to conditions like chronic pain and associated illness narratives (Åsbring & Närvänen, 2002; Denny, 2017; Frank, 2013; Newton et al., 2013; Werner & Malterud, 2003); however, my aim in this chapter is to show that despite the importance of such studies, they have neglected the additional impact of the consumption of opioid analgesics and its effect on stigma, shame and identity.

Patients and medicines

Much has been written about patients and insights into their illnesses and associated narratives and biographies as part of the 'narrative turn' in recent decades (Polkinghorne, 1988); while the sociological literature in particular has offered important and influential framing of patients and illness in terms of identity, shame and stigma among others, there is a relative lack of corresponding constructs in the more specific area of patients' consumption of medicines. This was recognised more than two decades ago by Vuckovic & Nichter (1997) who recognised the dearth of research and literature that went beyond traditional compliance debates and failed to capture important issues such as 'self-identity'. In an authoritative review of previous research on how individuals use (and more specifically) resist medicines, Pound et al. (2005) suggested that patients were often cautious in the use of medicines, and adopted either active or passive strategies and at times sophisticated lay testing strategies to evaluate medicines. The authors identified key concerns also around identity and stigma and in particular anxieties around dependence and addiction. Of particular note, however, was that this occurred not just for medicines with recognised addiction or tolerance properties – such as opioids – but with other therapeutic groups such as antihypertensives and proton pump inhibitor medicines also. Of note, however, was that identity issues were often not specifically related to addiction fears and arose more in terms of non-acceptance of a medical condition, or associated stigma, that is, preventative asthma medicines were not taken to support patients' denial that they had a significant and chronic illness (Adams et al., 1997) or antiretroviral medicines were not taken regularly as they highlighted a stigmatised condition (Pound et al., 2005).

The role of opioid analgesics in pain

Opioids have been recognised as having an important role in the control of pain for millennia (Rosenblum et al., 2008) initially through naturally occurring opiates found in the opium poppy, to the extraction and identification of morphine and later development of synthetic opioids such as heroin, oxycodone and tramadol. Current clinical guidance (British Medical Association, 2017; Dowell et al., 2016) offers a more conservative understanding of the role of opioids, particularly in the context of chronic pain. This represents the most common presentation for analgesia and is contrasted with pain arising from an acute injury or interventions such as a surgical procedure, or terminal cancer. In chronic pain, opioids are recognised as being one of several pharmaceutical therapies which also include non-opioid analgesics such as paracetamol, non-steroidal anti-inflammatory drugs (NSAIDs), tricyclic antidepressants and most recently gabapentinoids (British Medical Association, 2017). Perhaps most importantly, however, is recognition of a range of non-pharmacological therapies, such as physiotherapy and psychological and cognitive behavioural therapies, which are recognised as having an important place in the overall management of chronic pain. Evidence suggests that opioids often do not have a significant or beneficial effect in the management of chronic pain despite their potency and position in the traditional analgesic ladder, particularly for the most common presentations such as lower back pain (Abdel Shaheed et al., 2016; Ballantyne & Shin, 2008; Deyo et al., 2015; Dowell et al., 2016).

It is tempting to think that such concerns and the lack of evidence of long-term efficacy would have a negative impact on opioid analgesic availability but there has actually been a well-recognised trend towards increasing prescribing of opioids globally (OECD, 2019). Some countries, such as the United States and United Kingdom, have reported more recent reductions in prescribing but concerns remain about, for example, the rise in high strength opioid analgesics (Curtis et al., 2019) and sustained release preparations. Increasing opioid prescribing has not only been attributed to increasingly older patient populations *qua* consumers, for whom chronic musculoskeletal pain is more common, but also to claims of pharmaceuticalisation and the undertreatment of pain (Finestone et al., 2016; Portenoy & Foley, 1986). Pharmaceuticalisation extends the concept of medicalisation (where non-medical problems become medical ones) to include the role of the pharmaceutical industry and activities such as drug marketing and promotion to the public and prescribers (Abraham, 2010). The most well-known example relating to opioid analgesics is that of oxycodone and the pharmaceutical company Purdue who manufactured and marketed it. The company was heavily criticised for overmarketing – particularly their long-acting product Oxycontin – to undertrained primary care doctors in the United States, and also under-representing iatrogenic addiction harms (Finestone et al., 2016; Van Zee, 2009). As Finestone et al., (2016) argue, however, it is not only the inappropriate marketing activities of the pharmaceutical industry but also more systemic failures to provide adequate non-pharmacological services and resources.

Concern about the undertreatment of pain arose in the 1970s and 1980s initially in relation to palliative care (Portenoy & Foley, 1986) and clinicians' litigation concerns regarding iatrogenic addiction. An influential campaign led to pain being considered the 'fifth vital sign' in the United States (Tompkins et al., 2017) which ushered in a trend in increased prescribing in the United States in particular and eventually more widely. Further contributing to the case of under-treatment of pain was the significant problem of framing pain management and to the difficulty of distinguishing between the needs of 'genuine patients' and others using analgesics 'illegitimately' (Bell & Salmon, 2009). Analysing the existing literature, these authors argue that:

> …discourses on pain management and the right to pain relief reify distinctions between the 'deserving pain patient' and the 'undeserving addict',

serving both to further stigmatise people labelled as 'addicts' and delegitimise claims to pain they might voice.

(Bell & Salmon, 2009, p. 170)

Attempts to address concerns about opioid analgesic prescribing and use have
been introduced and a variety of educational, surveillance and regulatory interventions have been attempted (Compton et al., 2015). In the United Kingdom, resources such as *Opioids Aware* (Faculty of Pain Medicine, 2015) were
developed to provide information and advice to both prescribers and patients.
Surveillance has been used particularly in countries such as the United States
through prescription drug monitoring programs and even at the level of individual patient 'doctor shopping' (Compton et al., 2015). A variety of regulatory
changes have been introduced, particularly to limit the supply of opioids. In
Australia, for example, upscheduling has meant that the OTC supply of opioids such as codeine is now prohibited and restricted to prescription supply only
(Roberts & Nielsen, 2018). This resulted from recognition that compound opioid analgesic products may cause significant harm despite being less potent than
prescription medicines (Frei et al., 2010). Changes in prescribing category have
been addressed elsewhere. For example, in the United Kingdom, the synthetic
opioid tramadol was reclassified as a Schedule 3 controlled drug some 20 years
after its introduction, following concerns about increased overdose deaths (Stannard, 2019). Several years earlier, the compound analgesic co-proxamol was
completely withdrawn from the market in the United Kingdom due to fatalities
associated with its use (Hawton et al., 2012). In several countries including the
United Kingdom, OTC opioid packaging was voluntarily changed by manufacturers to carry addiction warning messages and time limited use (Cooper, 2011;
Medicines and Healthcare Products Regulatory Agency, 2009).

An ongoing concern, however, is the lack of long-term evidence of the efficacy of opioid analgesics. Despite concerns, clinical guidelines and subsequent
practice still offer a place for such therapies. Central to the guidance provided to
prescribers and suppliers is the recommendation of punitive surveillance strategies such as urine testing, treatment contracts, and the use of buprenorphine or
take home naloxone when addiction or overdose respectively are considered a
risk (Dowell et al., 2016).

Stigma, shame and identity

In much the same way that patient narratives of illness have neglected the role
of medicines, other health research addressing stigma, and associated shame and
identity have also tended to focus on particular conditions and not on associated
medicine use. Indeed, even in the context of chronic pain and stigma, the significance of medicines has not been captured (Åsbring & Närvänen, 2002; Cohen
et al., 2011; De Ruddere & Craig, 2016). In his seminal work, Goffman (2009)
argued that stigma arises when individuals or groups are perceived to be different
and that this can occur in different ways. Drawing on medical examples, stigma can
arise visibly and most explicitly in *discredited conditions* where it is clear that there

is a deviance from perceived normal behaviour or appearance (such as a disfiguring skin condition or a physical disability, for example). Of particular note, though, is that stigma can also arise in *discreditable conditions*, which also have the *potential* to elicit stigma, such as someone with epilepsy suffering from an epileptic seizure in public which moves a discreditable condition to a discredited one (Scambler, 2009). Central to these accounts is the connection between stigma and identity and the notion of the 'spoiled identity' – one's identity diminished through stigma. One further distinction in relation to stigma arises in the difference between felt (internal) and enacted (external) stigma; the former represents the perceived shame and embarrassment associated with stigma, while the latter relates to the outward experience of being treated differently due to stigma from others (Scambler, 2009). In the context of chronic pain, it has been argued that this is a stigmatising condition (Cohen et al., 2011; Eaves et al., 2015; Jackson, 2005) which is discreditable due to the 'invisible' nature of pain in many cases (Newton et al., 2013). Chronic pain may also be discredited, however, if there is sufficient deviance from expected behaviours and norms and be subject to enacted stigma in such cases. Drug seeking behaviours represent key examples in the context of opioid analgesics where the individual becomes discredited through such actions. Examples of this include increasing the amount of time spent sourcing and using opioids through visiting multiple pharmacies or requesting repeat medicines from prescribers (doctor shopping).

Shame is a term often associated with stigma, sometimes used synonymously or assumed to result from stigma (Lewis, 1998). There have been numerous definitions but central to these are often concerns with a negative evaluative emotion:

> With the experience of shame or its allied effects, we feel or believe that we do not measure up to ideals or standards that we have set for ourselves. We become aware that we are not the kind of persons we think we are, wish to be, or need to be.
>
> (Lazare, 1987, p. 1653)

In the context of healthcare, shame has been regarded as a destructive force which can lead to adverse outcomes including addiction and loss of control (Wiechelt, 2007). It has also been recognised, however, that aspects of health and healthcare can be a cause of shame themselves and lead to chronic shame (Dolezal & Lyons, 2017). The very recognition of any 'defects of body or mind' (Lazare, 1987 p. 1653) by a patient is considered enough to lead to shame, as it involves recognition of a discrepancy and difference. This is potentially further exacerbated through the medical gaze and aspects of the clinical encounter and issues such as lay knowledge. The consumption of opioid analgesics in chronic pain can also constitute a shaming activity and this will be illustrated later in the chapter after considering the final main concept in this chapter, that of identity.

As well as shame, a further concept often referred to when considering stigma is that of identity. While this represents a considerable topic in its own right and is beyond a detailed description in this chapter, in the context of health, medicines and opioid analgesics, identity is an important aspect of how individuals understand themselves and others, and their experiences of health and illness (Britten, 2008; Eaves, 2015; Vuckovic & Nichter, 1997; Whyte et al., 2002). Medicines and identity have in fact been connected previously and this has been linked in particular with the marketing of medicines and claims that medicines can powerfully shape individuals' identities (Eaves, 2015) and as Vuckovic & Nichter (1997, p. 1297) note: 'individuals come to be defined by the medicine which they consume…'. This is illustrated no more so than in the substantial literature relating to addiction recovery narratives and transformational identity; substitution therapies such as methadone and buprenorphine represent important examples of how medicines have been argued to negatively influence identity transformations through their consumption (Doukas, 2011).

Common to this literature is the important presentation of self for those who formerly used illicit substances and of the need to demonstrate recovery and distancing from previous illicit discredited norms (McIntosh & Mckeganey, 2000). Substitution therapies involving methadone and buprenorphine threaten this identity reconstruction work and carry significant stigma through aspects of their supply (visibly in pharmacies and often with supervised consumption) and symbolically (in representing maintenance and not abstinence). In the context of health and related healthcare, issues of stigma, shame and identity have been considered influential ways of framing patient experiences and also applied to chronic conditions that involve pain. The role of medicines such as opioid analgesics, however, has tended to be neglected; in the next section and central to this chapter, examples of where opioid analgesic medicines are explicitly linked to identity, stigma and shame are considered.

Recognising opioid analgesic stigma, shame and identity

At the heart of this chapter is the concern that the use and consumption of medicines such as opioid analgesics does have implications for identity, shame and stigma but has been neglected in the wider literature on illness narratives and chronic pain (Newton et al., 2013), the doctor–patient relationship (Åsbring & Närvänen, 2002; McCrorie et al., 2015; Werner & Malterud, 2003) and issues of diagnosis and legitimacy (Åsbring & Närvänen, 2002). In relation to opioid analgesics more specifically, there have been occasional examples of research that has sought to explore stigma, shame and identity claims and even integrate opioids into illness narratives and these are now considered in turn.

The first example involves a study of 20 patients who attended pain clinics in Melbourne, Australia (Paterson et al., 2016), where it was found that as well as actively resisting opioid analgesic use, patients described concerns linked to identity and stigma which the authors argued were more significant than the chronic pain condition itself:

> [f]or people taking opioids for chronic pain, it is the medicine, more than the illness, which is potentially stigmatizing.
>
> (Paterson et al., 2016, p. 724)

Drawing on Scambler's (2009) distinction between internal (felt) and external (enacted) forms of stigma, the researchers found that patients' felt stigma was linked to shame and fears about being discredited and viewed as undeserving of health care treatment, and that they made active attempts to limit disclosure and communication about their opioid use. Enacted stigma was also apparent in examples of discrediting by allied healthcare professionals such as pharmacists and chiropractors; although such cases were not expanded on further, they appeared to cause significant distress to participants:

> Most examples of enacted stigma, where people were discredited due to taking prescription opioid, were in relation to health professionals. For example, Max described being upset when his pharmacist regularly phoned up and checked his prescription, while he stood in line with 'four guys standing there waiting for their methadone'. Ben described his chiropractor as always 'being very against it' without any explanation or alternative.
>
> (Paterson et al., 2016, p. 724)

Stigma was also linked to perceptions of illicit drug use in this study and another involving OTC codeine and dihydrocodeine misuse (Cooper, 2011, 2013). Paterson et al. also suggested that opioid medicine use was associated with concerns about identity, with examples focused on side effects and more overt embodied aspects of opioid use, related to impaired cognition or tiredness:

> For example, Ruby explained that when she started on opioids in hospital it was 'like my identity wasn't there anymore and I couldn't think straight' which led to her being dependent on others and unable to plan her own recovery.
>
> (Paterson et al., 2016, p.724)

Accounts from the participants in the Paterson et al. study were also analysed separately in a rare example of how opioid analgesics were presented as part of patient illness narratives (Zheng et al., 2013). Drawing on Frank's (2013) influential typology, these authors identified contrasting narratives related to chaos, restitution or quest. Initial accounts were all related to chaos and negative experiences:

> ...all the narratives were at some point, usually near the beginning, chaos narratives i.e., they were characterized by worsening and chaotic pain and/ or opioid related problems and periods of hopelessness.
>
> (Zheng et al., 2013, p. 1830)

The authors noted, however, that while some remained in 'chaos', others appeared to progress and for some this was a partial improvement and recognised as quest narratives while others achieved more stability and were categorised as restitution narratives.

Problems can arise not only with prescription opioids but also with those that can be purchased as OTC medicines from pharmacies and this is illustrated in a second research example where stigma, shame and complex identity issues were identified. Cooper (2011, 2013) explored this with individuals who had self-reported problems with OTC medicines in the United Kingdom, recruited via two online support groups – *Over-count* and *Codeinefreeme*. The majority of participants had experienced problems with their changing use (and subsequent misuse) of codeine or dihydrocodeine following legitimate initial access via prescription. Of note and in contrast to several other studies reported in this chapter, was that chronic pain was not always a feature of their narratives, and their continued consumption of an opioid analgesic extended for some beyond their initial pain. Both felt and enacted stigma were apparent in examples given by participants such as when they both anticipated and experienced detection by staff at the various pharmacies they visited to obtain multiple supplies of opioid medicines. Felt stigma arose also in relation to potentially admitting their problematic use of an opioid analgesic and seeking help and treatment; many participants feared engaging with formal health care providers because of concerns that their addiction would be recorded. Participants also commonly referred to a sense of shame associated with their consumption of OTC opioids and this led to sophisticated attempts to hide their use, and to avoid detection:

> As Ailsa noted, this was bound up in issues of shame about her OTC addiction but, again, fears about identification: 'I was ashamed as well because you don't necessarily want to be identified. I think the people on [an online support group], I think it is more anonymous but then I think that's a trust thing isn't it so you know....'
>
> (Cooper, 2011, p. 57)

Issues of stigma and shame in participant's problematic use of opioid medicines were also bound-up in conflicting identity issues for them. All recognised themselves as being 'addicted' and often explicitly used this term and an associated addicted identity but were clear in distinguishing themselves from illicit drug users. The latter were perceived by participants to be chaotic and different in appearance and in stark contrast to themselves, despite sharing what participants perceived to be a fundamentally similar addicted identity. Participants actively constructed acceptable identity claims about themselves and although recognising their own problematic medicine misuse, presented this as a form of 'respectable addiction' (Cooper, 2011). This was linked to stigma and shame as well as identity and enabled them to simultaneously identify as not only being addicted but also high functioning and socially and economically active within society.

Reinforcing these two examples, research with patients suffering from temporomandibular disorders (TMD) which involves facial pain highlights active attempts by those affected to avoid negative connotations of illness identity associated with the use of opioid analgesics. In one study, participants were selected as they used OTC non-opioid analgesics for TMD and it was found that this was an active strategy in harm reduction in *not* using prescription medicines. Such strategies were directly related to issues of identity and stigma:

> Trade-offs between physical harm reduction and harm justification to one's identity involved narratives of harm justification as chronic pain sufferers described their use as minimal and responsible... Describing medications as 'just over-the-counter' or 'not real pain medication' is social harm reduction. These phrases are uttered with the intention of minimising stigma.... .
>
> (Eaves, 2015, p. 152)

The same participants were also found to undertake sophisticated identity management strategies which were partly linked to medicine use and the perception that consumption of medicines – and in particular prescription analgesics – was a significant threat to their stoic moral identity as someone living with chronic pain. Participants were observed to:

> ...distance themselves from what they perceive to be a stigmatized chronic pain identity associated with medication dependency if not abuse.
>
> (Eaves et al., 2015, p. 163)

Before concluding this section, an associated emerging issue relates to the identification of issues of stigma and identity in the use of medicines used either as alternatives for opioid analgesics when opioid substitution therapy (OST) is initiated, or where overdoses due to a continued opioid analgesic are being prevented (Dowell et al., 2016). In the former case, medicines such as methadone and buprenorphine represent opioids that have been used for many years in the management of illicit drug use (such as heroin for example) but have been increasingly used for patients who have become addicted to opioid analgesics also (Dowell et al., 2016; Independent Expert Working Group, 2017). Of concern in such cases is that it is not just the initial opioid but also the substituted one that can cause problems. As previously noted, this is a recognised issue in terms of stigma and identity reconstruction in illicit substance use (Doukas, 2011) but has also emerged as a specific problem for prescription and OTC opioid analgesic substitution. In the study by Cooper (2013), five of the 25 participants self-reporting addiction to OTC opioid analgesics reported experiences with either methadone or buprenorphine. Although narratives were often associated with positive opioid free outcomes, they remained a contested aspect and were associated with additional stigma and an 'addict' identity (with this term being repeatedly used by participants to describe themselves):

> Treatment options involving specific medicines were also viewed problematically, mainly due to their association with illicit drug treatment or having supervised consumption: 'I was turning up to [the local] drug unit for my daily dose of methadone as though I was a heroin addict... At that stage, I didn't think that methadone was appropriate'.
>
> (Cooper, 2011, p. 57)

Stigma and opioid treatment concerns were also identified in a wider review of literature which found that stigma was linked to the use of OST and also that a sense of blame might prevent individuals seeking treatment, with adverse consequences (Cooper & Nielsen, 2017).

The other aspect related to opioid medicines is the increasing use of approaches to prevent overdose and possible deaths. This often involves naloxone, which is an opioid antagonist that can be administered and even self-administered (hence the term take- home naloxone [THN]) to reverse respiratory depression which is a significant risk if opioids are consumed in excessive amounts. Like OST, THN was originally promoted as a public health initiative among illicit substance users but is increasingly being advocated for people using opioid analgesics legitimately. In a recent study involving 46 adults in Australia who consumed opioids (including 18 who did so primarily for chronic pain), Fomiatti et al. (2020) identified multiple concerns about THN which related to stigma. They identified issues around information provision and perceived risks of overdose and that for those using prescribed (licit) opioid medication, THN was a further source of stigma with negative implications for treatment seeking, like those noted earlier by Cooper & Nielsen (2017):

> The social relations co-produced by prescription opioid consumption are different from those co-produced by illicit opioid consumption, with significant implications for how overdose risk is articulated. For this reason, it is understandable that some consumers articulate take-home naloxone as both irrelevant and stigmatising.
>
> (Fomiatti et al., 2020, p. 16)

Introducing these two additional related perspectives about OST and THN and manifestations of stigma and shame illustrates further complexities in relation to the use of opioid analgesics which go beyond the intended clinical and public health benefits and have been argued to link directly to patient's motivations to seek help.

What role for opioid analgesics?

What has hopefully emerged so far in this chapter is the need to recognise not just the 'complexity of people's lives' but also the 'complexity of opioid therapy' (Esquibel & Borkan, 2014, p. 2581) and in particular, associated issues of stigma, shame and identity disruption. These have been argued to be largely absent in the extant literature relating to illness narratives and particularly those involving chronic pain. Medicines are powerful and complex social phenomena which have been argued to have 'social lives' and indeed 'biographies' that allow them to both imbue and be imbued by different actors with significant – and potentially different – meanings across place and time (Whyte et al., 2002). In one sense, this has been shown in relation to the different settings where opioid medicine-related stigma, shame and identity arise, whether this is in OTC pharmacy encounters, prescribing by doctors, or in online support groups. It is also apparent across time, and in the shifting attitudes towards opioid analgesics from both a public and health care professional perspective. Although Whyte et al. (2002) do not refer specifically to opioids, they argue that all medicines have social lives and are involved in important acts of co-production. Illustrating this subjectivity and providing counter-balance to the negativity of stigma, shame and spoiled identity is the identification of a legitimating role for opioid analgesics. Drawing on qualitative interviews with a sample of patients taking opioid medicines for three months or more in Rhode Island and Massachusetts in the United States, Esquibel & Borkan (2014) identified addiction concerns but importantly contrasting themes of 'validation of pain' and the 'right to pain medicines.' Although issues of stigma, shame and identity did not explicitly arise, in this study – which covered a range of pain-related conditions in the outpatient hospital setting – patients (and also doctors), often referred to opioid analgesics in interviews. It was noted that they:

> ...mention pain medications when describing the pain experience, as if medications were intrinsically tied to the understanding of pain itself.
> (Esquibel & Borkan, 2014, p. 2578)

What this study illustrated and others have sought to do also (McCrorie et al., 2015), is to consider the dyad of both patient and prescriber in relation to pain and opioid analgesics. Important contrasts arose and while opioids were considered important for patients this was not necessarily the case for doctors. Similar themes of legitimation have also been identified among antidepressant users too (Ridge et al., 2015). The example of legitimation is arguably not a dominant one in the literature relating to opioid analgesics, although more widely in terms of pain, legitimation through medical diagnosis is an enduring and dominant theme (Åsbring & Närvänen, 2002; Denny, 2017). The 'social lives' of opioid analgesics are argued to remain contested and often resisted in society (Pound et al., 2005; Britten, 2008). Through the negative associations of different forms of stigma and shame and in association with spoiled identity, opioid analgesics represent potentially destructive forces in relation to chronic pain management in particular.

Presenting these negative consequences has implications for clinical care and management and highlights the need for caution particularly in their initiation but continued use also. Caution is clearly presented in relation to current guidance about chronic pain and opioids in particular (British Medical Association, 2017; Dowell et al., 2016) but at the heart of this chapter is the concern that *additional* psychosocial concerns such as stigma, shame and the potential spoiled identity should also be taken into consideration and are absent from the majority of current discourse. For clinicians, this hopefully offers additional insights and another perspective, and suggests that sensitivity is needed when managing the care of those who use opioid analgesics, to avoid shaming and stigmatisation in clinical encounters (Dolezal & Lyons, 2017; Lazare, 1987). For patients, it provides recognition of further aspects of opioid analgesic use that have hitherto not been widely voiced and may also serve a precautionary function for others.

Facing both these groups – of opioid analgesic prescribers and opioid analgesic consuming patients – is a fundamental dilemma, namely how to optimally control and manage pain but also minimise the use of opioid analgesics. Balancing these two remains a clinical and also public health ideal but is still not supported by robust evidence on the long-term effects of opioid analgesics (British Medical Association, 2017; Juurlink, 2018); arguably, such a dilemma does not help the substantial group of legacy patients already taking an opioid analgesic and for whom issues of stigma, shame and spoiled identity may be all too apparent. Opioid analgesic related stigma, shame and identity issues might exacerbate this enduring conflict between pain relief management and safe, controlled opioid analgesic use.

Conclusion

This chapter has offered novel insights into a highly contested topic and argued that patient narratives about pain have neglected stigma, shame and identity concerns directly related to the use of opioid medicines, and that these must be considered as linked but distinct aspects of overall experiences of pain (Denny, 2017). When considering the arguments in this chapter, caution may be needed in drawing attention to a relatively small body of research literature exploring stigma, shame and identity issues related to opioid analgesic use. Although drawing on exploratory qualitative methodologies that were not intended to be generalisable, it is further argued that more research and evidence is required to understand this issue. A final caution also is that such analysis may inappropriately follow the law of the instrument (Maslow, 1966) and assume that illness and pain narratives and related biographies *must* include the use of medicines as if medicines are the dominant or only treatment. It is important to recognise that although our societal relationship to medicines such as opioid analgesics is long and complex, and involves both negative and positive aspects, non-pharmacological treatments and support – particularly in the context of pain – should not be underestimated.

References

Abdel Shaheed, C., Maher, C. G., Williams, K. A., Day, R., & McLachlan, A. J. (2016). Efficacy, tolerability, and dose-dependent effects of opioid analgesics for low back pain: A systematic review and meta-analysis. *JAMA Internal Medicine, 176*(7), 958–968. doi:10.1001/jamainternmed.2016.1251.

Abraham, J. (2010). Pharmaceuticalization of society in context: Theoretical, empirical and health dimensions. *Sociology, 44*(4), 603–622.

Adams, S., Pill, R., & Jones, A. (1997). Medication, chronic illness and identity: The perspective of people with asthma. *Social Science & Medicine, 45*(2), 189–201.

Åsbring, P., & Närvänen, A.-L. (2002). Women's experiences of stigma in relation to chronic fatigue syndrome and fibromyalgia. *Qualitative Health Research, 12*(2), 148–160.

Ballantyne, J. C., & Shin, N. S. (2008). Efficacy of opioids for chronic pain: A review of the evidence. *The Clinical Journal of Pain, 24.* doi:10.1097/AJP.0b013e31816b2f26.

Bell, K., & Salmon, A. (2009). Pain, physical dependence and pseudoaddiction: Redefining addiction for "nice" people? *The International Journal on Drug Policy, 20*(2), 170–178. doi:10.1016/j.drugpo.2008.06.002.

British Medical Association. (2017). *Chronic Pain: Supporting Safer Prescribing of Analgesics*. March. London, UK: British Medical Association.

Britten, N. (2008). *Medicines and Society Patients, Professionals and the Dominance of Pharmaceuticals*. Basingstoke, UK: Palgrave Macmillan.

Centers for Disease Control and Prevention. (2017). Annual Surveillance Report of Drug-Related Risks and Outcomes — United States, 2017. Surveillance Special Report 1. Centers for Disease Control and Prevention, U.S. Department of Health and Human Services. https://www.cdc.gov/drugoverdose/pdf/pubs/2017-cdc-drug-surveillance-report.pdf

Cohen, M., Quintner, J., Buchanan, D., Nielsen, M., & Guy, L. (2011). Stigmatization of patients with chronic pain: The extinction of empathy. *Pain Medicine, 12*(11), 1637–1643.

Compton, W. M., Boyle, M., & Wargo, E. (2015). Prescription opioid abuse: Problems and responses. *Preventive Medicine, 80*, 5–9. https://doi.org/doi:10.1016/j.ypmed.2015.04.003.

Cooper, R. J. (2011). Respectable Addiction – A qualitative study of over the counter medicine abuse in the UK. In *Pharmacy Practice Research Trust*. https://pharmacyresearchuk.org/wp-content/uploads/2012/11/respectable_addiction_richard_cooper_2011.pdf.

Cooper, R. J. (2013). "I can't be an addict. I am." Over-the-counter medicine abuse: A qualitative study. *BMJ Open, 3*(6). doi:10.1136/bmjopen-2013-002913.

Cooper, S., & Nielsen, S. (2017). Stigma and social support in pharmaceutical opioid treatment populations: A scoping review. *International Journal of Mental Health and Addiction, 15*(2), 452–469. doi:10.1007/s11469-016-9719-6.

Curtis, H. J., Croker, R., Walker, A. J., Richards, G. C., Quinlan, J., & Goldacre, B. (2019). Opioid prescribing trends and geographical variation in England, 1998–2018: A retrospective database study. *The Lancet Psychiatry, 6*(2), 140–150.

De Ruddere, L., & Craig, K. D. (2016). Understanding stigma and chronic pain: A-state-of-the-art review. *Pain, 157*(8), 1607–1610.

Denny, E. (2017). *Pain: A Sociological Introduction*. Hoboken, New Jersey: John Wiley & Sons.

Deyo, R. A., Von Korff, M., & Duhrkoop, D. (2015). Opioids for low back pain. *BMJ (Clinical Research Ed.), 350*, g6380–g6380. doi:10.1136/bmj.g6380.

Dolezal, L., & Lyons, B. (2017). Health-related shame: An affective determinant of health? *Medical Humanities, 43*(4), 257–263.

Doukas, N. (2011). Perceived barriers to identity transformation for people who are prescribed methadone. *Addiction Research & Theory, 19*(5), 408–415.

Dowell, D., Haegerich, T. M., & Chou, R. (2016). CDC guideline for prescribing opioids for chronic pain – United States, 2016. *JAMA, 315*(15). doi:10.1001/jama.2016.1464.

Eaves, E. R. (2015). "Just Advil": Harm reduction and identity construction in the consumption of over-the-counter medication for chronic pain. *Social Science & Medicine, 146*, 147–154.

Eaves, E. R., Nichter, M., Ritenbaugh, C., Sutherland, E., & Dworkin, S. F. (2015). Works of Illness and the challenges of social risk and the specter of pain in the lived experience of TMD. *Medical Anthropology Quarterly, 29*(2), 157–177.

Esquibel, A. Y., & Borkan, J. (2014). Doctors and patients in pain: Conflict and collaboration in opioid prescription in primary care. *PAIN®, 155*(12), 2575–2582.

Faculty of Pain Medicine. (2015). *Opioids Aware: A Resource for Patients and Healthcare Professionals to Support Prescribing of Opioid Medicines for Pain*. The Royal College of Anaesthetists London. https://fpm.ac.uk/opioids-aware.

Finestone, H. M., Juurlink, D. N., Power, B., Gomes, T., & Pimlott, N. (2016). Opioid prescribing is a surrogate for inadequate pain management resources. *Canadian Family Physician*, 62(6), 465.

Fomiatti, R., Farrugia, A., Fraser, S., Dwyer, R., Neale, J., & Strang, J. (2020). Addiction stigma and the production of impediments to take-home naloxone uptake. *Health*, 1363459320925863. doi:10.1177/1363459320925863.

Frank, A. W. (2013). *The Wounded Storyteller: Body, Illness, and Ethics*. Chicago, IL: University of Chicago Press.

Frei, M. Y., Nielsen, S., Dobbin, M., & Tobin, C. L. (2010). Serious morbidity associated with misuse of over-the-counter codeine-ibuprofen analgesics: A series of 27 cases. *The Medical Journal of Australia*, 193(5), 294–296. http://www.ncbi.nlm.nih.gov/pubmed/20819050.

Goffman, E. (2009). *Stigma: Notes on the Management of Spoiled Identity*. New York, NY: Simon and Schuster.

Hawton, K., Bergen, H., Simkin, S., Wells, C., Kapur, N., & Gunnell, D. (2012). Six-year follow-up of impact of co-proxamol withdrawal in England and Wales on prescribing and deaths: time-series study. *PLoS Med*, 9(5), e1001213.

Independent Expert Working Group. (2017). *Drug Misuse and Dependence: UK Guidelines on Clinical Management*. London: Department of Health.

Jackson, J. E. (2005). Stigma, liminality, and chronic pain: Mind–body borderlands. *American Ethnologist*, 32(3), 332–353.

Juurlink, D. N. (2018). Critiquing the CDC Opioid Guideline: Some light from the heat. *Clinical Pharmacology & Therapeutics*, 103(6), 966–968.

Lazare, A. (1987). Shame and humiliation in the medical encounter. *Archives of Internal Medicine*, 147(9), 1653–1658.

Lewis, M. (1998). Shame and stigma. In Paul Gilbert & Bernice Andrews, (Eds.) *Shame: Interpersonal Behavior, Psychopathology, and Culture* (p. 126). New York, NY and Oxford, UK: Oxford University Press on Demand.

Marsden, J., White, M., Annand, F., Burkinshaw, P., Carville, S., Eastwood, B., Kelleher, M., Knight, J., O'Connor, R., & Tran, A. (2019). Medicines associated with dependence or withdrawal: A mixed-methods public health review and national database study in England. *The Lancet Psychiatry*, 6(11), 935–950.

Maslow, A. H. (1966). *The Psychology of Science a Reconnaissance*. New York, NY: Harper and Row.

McCrorie, C., Closs, S. J., House, A., Petty, D., Ziegler, L., Glidewell, L., West, R., & Foy, R. (2015). Understanding long-term opioid prescribing for non-cancer pain in primary care: a qualitative study. *BMC Family Practice*, 16(1), 121. doi:10.1186/s12875-015-0335-5.

McIntosh, J., & Mckeganey, N. (2000). Addicts' narratives of recovery from drug use: Constructing a non-addict identity. *Social Science & Medicine*, 50(10), 1501–1510. doi:10.1016/S0277-9536(99)00409-8.

Medicines and Healthcare products Regulatory Agency. (2009). *MHRA Public Assessment Report. Codeine and Dihydrocodeine-Containing Medicine: Minimising the Risk of Addiction*. London, UK: Department of Health and Social Care.

Newton, B. J., Southall, J. L., Raphael, J. H., Ashford, R. L., & LeMarchand, K. (2013). A narrative review of the impact of disbelief in chronic pain. *Pain Management Nursing*, 14(3), 161–171.

NHS Digital. (2019). *Statistics on Drug Misuse, England, 2019*. Leeds, UK: NHS Digital.

OECD. (2019). Addressing Problematic Opioid Use in OECD Countries. *OECD Health Policy Studies (OECD Health Policy Studies)*. OECD. doi:10.1787/a18286f0-en.

Paterson, C., Ledgerwood, K., Arnold, C., Hogg, M., Xue, C., & Zheng, Z. (2016). Resisting prescribed opioids: A qualitative study of decision making in patients taking opioids for chronic noncancer pain. *Pain Medicine, 17*(4), 717–727.

Polkinghorne, D. E. (1988). *Narrative Knowing and the Human Sciences*. Albany, NY: Suny Press.

Portenoy, R. K., & Foley, K. M. (1986). Chronic use of opioid analgesics in non-malignant pain: Report of 38 cases. *Pain, 25*(2), 171–186.

Pound, P., Britten, N., Morgan, M., Yardley, L., Pope, C., Daker-White, G., & Campbell, R. (2005). Resisting medicines: A synthesis of qualitative studies of medicine taking. *Social Science & Medicine, 61*(1), 133–155.

Public Health England. (2018). *Over the Counter and Prescription Drug Dependence Freedom of Information Request 25/8/2018*.

Ridge, D., Kokanovic, R., Broom, A., Kirkpatrick, S., Anderson, C., & Tanner, C. (2015). My dirty little habit: Patient constructions of antidepressant use and the 'crisis' of legitimacy. *Social Science & Medicine, 146*, 53–61.

Roberts, D. M., & Nielsen, S. (2018). Changes for codeine. *Australian Prescriber, 41*(1), 2.

Rosenblum, A., Marsch, L. A., Joseph, H., & Portenoy, R. K. (2008). Opioids and the treatment of chronic pain: Controversies, current status, and future directions. *Experimental and Clinical Psychopharmacology, 16*(5), 405–416. doi:10.1037/a0013628.

Scambler, G. (2009). Health-related stigma. *Sociology of Health & Illness, 31*(3), 441–455.

Stannard, C. (2019). Tramadol is not" opioid-lite". 365(l2095). https://doi.org/doi:10.1136/bmj.l2095.

Tompkins, D. A., Hobelmann, J. G., & Compton, P. (2017). Providing chronic pain management in the "Fifth Vital Sign" Era: Historical and treatment perspectives on a modern-day medical dilemma. *Drug and Alcohol Dependence, 173* (1), S11–S21. doi:10.1016/j.drugalcdep.2016.12.002.

Van Zee, A. (2009). The promotion and marketing of OxyContin: Commercial triumph public health tragedy. *The American Journal of Public Health, 99*. doi:10.2105/AJPH.2007.131714.

Vowles, K. E., McEntee, M. L., Julnes, P. S., Frohe, T., Ney, J. P., & van der Goes, D. N. (2015). Rates of opioid misuse, abuse, and addiction in chronic pain: A systematic review and data synthesis. *Pain, 156*(4). doi:10.1097/01.j.pain.0000460357.01998.f1.

Vuckovic, N., & Nichter, M. (1997). Changing patterns of pharmaceutical practice in the United States. *Social Science & Medicine, 44*(9), 1285–1302.

Werner, A., & Malterud, K. (2003). It is hard work behaving as a credible patient: Encounters between women with chronic pain and their doctors. *Social Science & Medicine, 57*(8), 1409–1419.

Whyte, S. R., van der Geest, S., & Hardon, A. (2002). *Social Lives of Medicines* (S. Whyte, S. van der Geest, & A. Hardon (eds.). Cambridge University Press. http://scholar.google.co.uk/scholar?cluster=6992584449245752940&hl=en&as_sdt=0,5#1.

Wiechelt, S. A. (2007). The specter of shame in substance misuse. *Substance Use & Misuse, 42*(2–3), 399–409.

Zheng, Z., Paterson, C., Ledgerwood, K., Hogg, M., Arnold, C. A., & Xue, C. C. L. (2013). Chaos to hope: A narrative of healing. *Pain Medicine, 14*(12), 1826–1838.

12 The drama of medicines

Narratives of living with postural tachycardia syndrome

Karen C. Lloyd, Paul Bissell, Kath Ryan and Peri J. Ballantyne

Introduction

Telling stories about living with illness and the place of medicines in managing that illness is an important form of embodied meaning making. We posit that treating these stories as dramas (Frank, 2007) enables us to understand the place and significance of medicines in people's lives. We describe how stories about medicine taking can be conceived as dramas of (1) medicines in the body, (2) signification and the self, and (3) experimentation in accounts of living with postural tachycardia syndrome, a rare dysfunction of the autonomic nervous system. We do this to demonstrate the value of studying stories and to make a case for the narrative potential of storytelling about medicines.

Understanding this deployment of medicines in stories helps to illuminate how people living with illness, one of many actors who 'work' with medicines, make sense of illness through meaning making about pharmaceutical interventions. In particular, we focus on the salience of the signifying and experimental aspects of stories about medicines, given the predominantly neoliberal language around health – and personal responsibility for health – now commonplace in many Western societies (Lupton 1995; Peacock, Bissell & Owen, 2014). Neoliberal language around responsibility for health, we argue, increasingly frames issues around illness, with medicines now acting as key signifiers that serve to possibly protect self and identity from the potential negative connotation of malingering or other undesirable markers. Thus, constructing and reconstructing meanings around medicines may become increasingly important.

Background

Telling stories about medicines

Managing illness, including its self-management through day-to-day care practices, requires the cooperation of diverse groups of individual and collective actors, shared spaces, material things and processes in the accomplishment of what can be quite heterogeneous goals. Anthropological work on pharmaceuticals has illuminated the range of actors engaged in their 'life cycle' from development, manufacture and commercial marketing, to prescribing, dispensing and consumption (van der Geest, Reynolds Whyte, & Hardon, 1996). As Pellegrino states:

> Few human experiences are so universal and have such symbolic overtones as the ordinary acts of prescribing and ingesting of medicines. Their meaning far transcends the pharmacological properties of the substances ingested. This symbolism is amongst the most ancient and deeply placed in human nature.
>
> (Pellegrino, 1976, p. 624)

Paying attention to stories about medicines might offer 'ways in' to make sense of these meanings referred to by Pellegrino and their symbolism across multiple professional and lay social worlds. While we can imagine doctors, nurses, pharmacists and even pharmaceutical marketing representatives each having their own dramas to tell about medicines in their professional lives, meaning making through stories about medicines is especially critical for understanding the experience of being ill for users of medicines (Bissell, Ryan and Morecroft, 2006).

Studying stories created by people taking medicines represents one means of unpacking how meaning about medicines is produced and re-produced. Where multiple professional practices exist for sharing stories about medicines among various professionals (case conferences, medication review, etc.) in the time-pressured nature of the clinical consultation, there may be limited opportunities for people with illness to engage in storytelling about them. Often this storytelling takes place where people use medicines in the private spaces of the home (Dew, Chamberlain, Hodgetts, Norris, Radley, & Gabe, 2014) and within communities of people living with illness, including in virtual spaces (blogs, forums, online support groups and the websites of patient organisations). Indeed, one feature of medicines that marks them out from other modalities of biomedicine, is their relative democracy. Medicines can be prescribed by various parties (Cooper et al., 2012), provide a level of relative autonomy for the user to take in prescribed and un-prescribed ways and often require little detailed specialist knowledge to consume (van der Geest & Whyte, 1989). It is their relative democracy as therapeutic modalities, and the embodied, signifying and experimental work they perform in the context of postural tachycardia syndrome that is the subject of this chapter.

Medication narratives and late modern illness experience

According to Arthur Frank, when telling stories about illness, people are engaged in an ethic of care of the self (Frank, 1998). Stories are creative, active and productive. Medicines are things that people living with illness touch, taste, consume, refuse and draw on symbolically as they seek ways to live as people who are 'successfully ill' and thus take care of the self (Frank, 2013). We focus here on what medicines as stories are *doing* with bodies, identities and the dilemmas posed by unexplained illness, and elaborate on how medicines are constructed in ways that are embodied, signifying and experimental.

We frame our analysis via Frank's (2013) work on narratives and illness experience. People who are ill need to manage their responsibilities and obligations in line with the sick role, in the classic Parsonian sense (1951), but also do so in terms of the meaning that illness has for them in their lives. This ethical work of meaning making takes place through the telling of stories about illness (Frank, 2013). Storytelling can be a highly personal, yet distinctly *social* practice, of making meaning about living with illness. Using illness narratives as a template for exploring stories about medications, Bissell, Ryan, and Morecroft (2006; see also Ryan, Bissell, & Morecroft, 2007) asserted the value of studying 'medication narratives'. Stories about medicines and illness often take the form of moral stories about social connections with others, including health professionals, family, friends and others living with illness, and focus on the (re)construction of self-identity. They may be embedded in broader stories of power and control. In our analysis, these broader stories were often ones of battles for legitimacy and recognition of the subjective experience of illness by the institutions of medicine, and doctors themselves.

Bissell et al. (2006) and Ryan et al. (2007) emphasised how studying medication narratives can enhance our understanding of the effects of illness and its treatment both for health professionals and for medication users. Qualitative research on medication taking, however, has traditionally focused on 'compliance' with treatment expectations rather than the lived experience of and meanings constructed around the use of medicines (Bissell et al. 2004, 2006; Pound et al. 2005; Britten, 2008; Nørreslet, Bissell & Traulsen, 2010).

Stories about medicines as dramas

Frank (2007) describes four kinds of illness narratives based on the thematic content, or dramas, around which they are organised and the work the storyteller wants them to do. An illness narrative that focuses on the drama of *genesis* elaborates on what caused the illness to happen when it did. Gareth Williams (1984) explored these types of narratives in terms of identity reconstruction in the face of chronic illness. What Frank describes as the drama of *emotion work* draws on Arlie Russell Hochschild's (1979) conception of emotion work as the labour that people do to modulate their emotions in the presentation of self to other. In illness narratives, emotion work can be seen in stories of individuals regulating their emotions when disclosing illness to others or seeking to appear cheerful in the face of a dire prognosis. Telling these kinds of narratives can be especially therapeutic for those who tell them. Stories about the *drama of meaning* allow people with illness to make sense of their illness and to find new meaning in a life lived through illness. Lastly, for Frank, stories about the *drama of self* involve the construction of a new kind of self, a changed self, but one made new through the experience of living with illness. It is possible to imagine how medicines could be scripted into each of these narrative types. Understanding this scholarly work on illness narratives can inform research on medication narratives.

This chapter explores how Frank's (2007) conceptualisation of illness narratives as 'dramas' can be drawn on to explore stories about medicines in everyday life with a particularly uncertain illness, postural tachycardia syndrome. We draw on this theoretical framing for our analysis for several reasons. Firstly, it allows us to convey the meaningfulness of the dramatic and the uncertainty in stories about medicines. For Frank, the term 'drama' is used to signal how stories about illness are not only *dramatic*, involving uncertainty, conflict, the building of dramatic tension, cliff hangers, and emotional peaks and troughs, but also that they have the potential to be places for *play, joy and pleasure*.

Secondly, it is through stories as 'dramas', both troubling and playful, that the private is shaped through storytelling into 'a well-wrought narrative' that becomes part of the public discourse on illness, medicines and bodies (Frank, 2007). Quoting Jerome Bruner (2002), Frank tells us that 'It is the conversion of private trouble… into public plight that makes well-wrought narrative so powerful, so comforting, so dangerous, so culturally essential' (Bruner, 2002, p. 35 as cited in Frank, 2007, p. 380). It is in this sense that stories about medicines become ethical and political projects, ones that are particularly critical in the late modern neoliberal present.

Lastly, dramas are both social products and produced as part of collective meaning making. Crafting dramas about illness, or as we argue, about medicines, is a practice of 'enacting stories to teach others how to live' (Frank, 2013, p. 381) but it is through this crafting of stories for others that we also learn how to live in our own selves, bodies and with medicines. We become who we are not only to others, but also to ourselves, when we tell stories. Drawing on the concept of dramas encourages an engagement with the performative and with storytelling as performance.

Postural tachycardia syndrome

Postural tachycardia syndrome (PoTS) describes a heterogeneous group of dysautonomic disorders involving abnormal functioning of the autonomic nervous system (Kavi, Gammage, Grubb & Karabin, 2012), triggered by standing upright, leading to orthostatic intolerance, or the experience of symptoms, such as significant increases in heart rate and blood pressure, digestion, bladder control and sweating upon standing that are alleviated by lying down (Low et al., 1995). The experience, at times in concert with one or a number of co-morbid chronic conditions, makes PoTS an especially disruptive illness that can cause anxiety and interfere with education, work, mobility and many activities of daily living (Kavi et al., 2016). Although there is only a limited social epidemiology of PoTS, the available evidence suggests that it primarily affects those in early to middle adulthood (McDonald, Koshi, Busner, Kavi & Newton, 2014) and is four times more common in women than men (Raj, 2006). Onset is usually sudden, occurring after some sort of acute event or trauma, such as viral illness, pregnancy, an operation, immunisation, or a stressful life event. The patho-physiological mechanisms underlying PoTS are poorly understood, and diagnosis is often slow, uncertain and accomplished via exclusion of other conditions, and involves the use of tilt-tables, active stand tests or electro-cardiographs.

The management of PoTS tends to involve both pharmacological and non-pharmacological approaches (Grubb, 2008; Mattias, Low, Iodice, Owens, Kirbis & Grahame, 2011; Parsaik et al., 2012). Non-pharmacological approaches include dietary management, gentle to moderate exercise, and wearing compression garments. There is presently no standard pharmacological treatment protocol and there are no medicines licensed specifically for its treatment: all medicines are prescribed 'off-label' (Conner, Sheikh & Grubb, 2012). These medicines include those designed to increase blood volume, increase vasoconstriction, reduce tachycardia, improve central cardiovascular control and treat anxiety (Grubb, 2008; Thieben et al., 2007 Kanjwal et al., 2011). McDonald et al. (2014) found that among the 91 respondents in their survey who reported medication use to manage PoTS, there were 21 unique combinations of medication regimens. Some of these medications have significant adverse effects (Benarroch, 2012).

We chose to study stories of living with and taking medicines for PoTS for two reasons. People living with this rare and sometimes contested condition and their advocates have created virtual communities of practice (Lave & Wenger, 1991) for sharing their stories and learning from each other, which provided rich data for analysis. Further, the path from onset of symptoms to diagnosis and long-term management of PoTS is often slow, uncertain and contested, and the heterogeneity of treatment modalities and inconsistency in their effectiveness means that the journey to finding medicines that 'fit' can be a long and winding one. Studying the stories of seeking out, experimenting with and resisting medicine taking among people with PoTS offered strong, illustrative examples of medication narratives in the living of pharmaceutical lives.

Methods

Stories of living with postural tachycardia syndrome

The accounts included in this paper are extant narratives written by people living with PoTS collected from the websites of three patient organisations. *PoTS UK* is a UK-based registered charity that developed in 2010 out of a Facebook support group for people with PoTS. It provides information, support and education and is managed by a board of trustees, many with medical backgrounds. Syncope Trust and Reflex Anoxia Seizures (STARS), 'The Blackouts Trust', is a UK-based information and support group for people experiencing syncope (fainting) that was founded in 1993 by the mother of a child with reflex anoxic seizures (RAS), a form of syncope. The Dysautonomia Information Network (DINET) is a US-based, volunteer-run, non-profit organisation that provides information, support and health professional resources on a number of dysautonomias, including PoTS.

Our sample consisted of 64 stories of living with PoTS that contained talk about medications drawn from a total of 99 stories posted publicly to the websites of these three organisations. Stories were accessed in January of 2017, with the approval of the organisations. Of storytellers, 92% were female, 59% were living in the United Kingdom and 41% were in the United States. Only slightly more than half (n = 34) discussed their age at the onset of symptoms or age at diagnosis. Of these, the average age at onset of symptoms was 18 years (range, 4–41 years), and the average age at diagnosis was 24 years (range, 16–43 years). Among those who discussed both their age at onset and at diagnosis, the average time to diagnosis was 7 years. Among those who did not provide a numerical age, the majority described symptom onset as occurring during secondary school or university.

Analysing medication narratives

Frank notes, 'Storytelling is *for* an other just as much as it is for oneself' (Frank, 2013, p. 17). In his view, telling stories about living with illness involves both an ethic of solidarity, of speaking with others who are living through their own experiences of being ill, as well as an ethic of inspiration, of serving as exemplars to inspire others to 'live well' through illness. This is why Frank considers storytelling an ethical practice, imbued with the responsibility not only to self but also to others (Frank, 2013). We chose to study extant narratives of using medications because we wanted to explore stories created by individuals as communicative body-selves (Frank, 2013) in dialogic interaction with others outside of the environment of the research interview. Our interest in these stories about medicines is specifically in the work they do of sharing with others in spaces, particularly virtual spaces, where storytellers and audiences engage with each other as communities of practice (Lave & Wenger, 1991).

Our analysis is informed by Riessman's (2008) thematic approach to narrative analysis and strategies for narrative coding and analysis described by Fraser (2004). While coding the stories thematically, we sought to treat them as full accounts even as we excerpted discrete sections of text. The stories were first collated from across the three sources into a single data file. They were then read in their entirety by the first author. Those that included stories about medicines embedded within narratives of living with PoTS were collated into a separate data file. This set of 'stories about medicines' was then reread as a whole by the first author to increase familiarity with their content. The stories were then coded thematically using deductive, inductive and in vivo codes, utilising NVivo 11 qualitative analysis software. Coded stories were reread and analytic memos were written for each story reflecting on codes of interest and including textual excerpts most relevant to these codes. The coded stories were reviewed and revised by the research team. These analytic memos became the basis for the analysis that follows.

We conceived of medicines as symbolic and material objects that are productive of and produced by the stories told to make sense of the experience of managing chronic illness. Our analysis focused on the dramatic within these stories told about medicines, seeking to answer the question: what narrative work is accomplished by telling stories about what medicines do and what do these stories tell us about the dramas of living with illness.

Findings

Each of the stories in our analysis was one of making sense of taking medicines and living with PoTS. Some were stories of having lived for many years with inexplicable heart palpitations, dizziness, fainting and other symptoms. Others were stories about making sense of the biographical disruption (Bury, 1982) created by a recent onset. They were stories of quests for legitimacy, to have an illness diagnosed and acknowledged as 'real', and of butting up against a health care system that could not initially explain these strange and frightening symptoms or that sought to explain them in ways that did not make sense within individuals' frameworks of being ill. As 'quest narratives' (Frank, 2013), many of these stories drew to a close with reflections on the journey from medically unexplained symptoms, through diagnosis and treatment, to making the best of a life lived with a disruptive, at times highly debilitating chronic illness. Embedded within them are narratives about making sense of medicines as one among a number of 'things' that are engaged with in the work of 'living well' with PoTS. Medicines, as symbolic and material objects, were drawn into narratives like 'props' on a stage that enabled storytellers to tell of action done on their bodies, their selves and the problem posed by illness itself. We identified three kinds of dramas in the narratives studied: (1) dramas of embodiment, (2) dramas of signification and the self, and (3) dramas of experimentation, which illuminate something novel about the narrative work of medicines in illness narratives.

Dramas of embodiment: Medicines in the body

Many narratives constructed medicines as things doing work in physical bodies, organ systems and at the molecular level, at times drawing on the language of biomedicine. That is, medicines were storied in as things consumed by users that acted on their bodies producing, or being expected to produce, specific embodied effects.

Lori, who was living with PoTS as well as sarcoidosis, an autoimmune disease, described a period of medication trialling after her dual diagnosis. She crafted her story about medicines around the actions they had on the different systems of her body and their functions, including action at the level of neurotransmitters:

> When they finally took me off the steroids, my Sarcoidosis was in remission, and I lost the rest of the water retention that I had. My medicinal [regimen] was now only for PoTS. Inderal LA to help the severe Tachycardia, Adderal XR to boost the ever-low blood pressure, and Wellbutrin SR (still not sure why I take that exactly, but Dr. Grubb explained it does something with the chemicals in my brain, and it works!)

In some of these stories, medicines worked to make bodies do things that they would not do otherwise. They acted to restore physical functioning approaching but not quite reaching pre-illness levels. This embodied work sometimes created effects on bodies that were anticipated and desired, but other times, unexpected and unwanted. Some of these undesired effects were assumed to be produced by the taking of multiple medicines together in interaction with each other. In other stories, medicines were expected to act on bodies, but in fact, were described as producing no effects at all. These stories were often ones of disappointment and uncertainty, despite much anticipation of desired embodied effects. Medicines were also narrated as acting on bodies by *producing illness*, resulting either from a genetic predisposition to illness that was then triggered by medication use, or a particular adverse medication event. One narrator believed that PoTS was triggered by an anaphylactic shock caused by her use of Protonix, a proton pump inhibitor for acid reflux. The action of medicines on bodies was also sometimes described as *productive of risk*. In these stories, what medicines did in bodies was less physiological – the slowing of a fast heart rate or the increased vasoconstriction of blood vessels – but productive *of the potential to act*, and sometimes in what were considered to be harmful ways. These dramas most often described medicines' use during pregnancy or breastfeeding.

Sophie's story illustrates the embodied dramas of medicines and how stories told about medicines can foreground what they do in and for bodies. Sophie's story opened with the sudden onset of symptoms – 'a sudden wave of nausea, shakiness and dizziness' – during an Art History study trip to Florence when she was 20. They continued undiagnosed for 16 years. During this time, she continued to experience nausea and dizziness and developed impaired vision, sweating, palpitations, muscle pains and fainting. She described these 'episodes' as the feeling that her 'whole body would go into a total "red alert"'. Thirteen years after the onset of her symptoms, Sophie experienced a significant flare-up, when she once again sought care from her GP who referred her to a neurologist. Although she did not receive a diagnosis for a further 4 years, she wrote of starting on beta blockers, medicines to control her high heart rate and blood pressure of still unknown aetiology:

> Although [the neurologist] did not know the cause of the high heart rate, he suggested I try beta blockers. Once I got used to these I stabilised a bit: beta blockers took the sharp edges off my condition. An episode would not develop into a full-blown episode anymore. A wave of dizziness would remain a wave of dizziness. Slowly I could rely on myself again. I still feel episodes and I still wake up at night with dizziness and nausea but they are a lot less severe than before.

Sophie constructed the use of medications as having had 'real' embodied effects. Their action was on the effects of PoTS on her body: taking beta blockers provided stability, a sense of equilibrium, and softened the 'sharp-edges' of her embodied experience of illness.

Embodied dramas about medicines tell of the biochemical reactions of pharmaceutical compounds in bodies ('it does something with the chemicals in my brain'.), but also of the embodied experience of being ill ('beta blockers took the sharp edges off my condition'). Such narratives echo the stories likely to be told about medications by health professionals, focusing on the physiological changes due to pharmaceutical intervention, and embedded within broader narratives of the experience of living with illness.

Dramas of signification

Medicines were also storied into dramas of signification, being invoked as part of the signifying work of being ill, specifically with a diagnosable condition. In some stories, doctors' prescribing of medicines signified that an individual was 'legitimately ill', granting permission to be ill and making it possible to take other action, such as legitimately entering the sick role, taking time off work and being absolved from other social responsibilities. Yet overwhelmingly, some medicines, specifically psychotropics, were storied in as signifying that illness was psychological in nature, that it was 'all in my head' or that 'I was losing the plot'. The narratives we studied were overwhelming 'quest narratives' (Frank, 2013), narratives of the journey to make sense of illness and the role of medicines in a life lived with illness, and for these storytellers it was difficult or impossible to make sense of what was happening to them as a sign of mental illness. They were also stories of seeking to reconstruct identities in spite of illness. When medicines signified an illness that did not fit storytellers' sense of themselves, stories about medicines were crafted as stories of resistance to the illness identities they signified. Such narratives, like Magdalene's below, make visible how medicines can be drawn into dramas about the symbolism of *who one is*, calling on narrative work to be done to make sense of or resist such identities.

Magdalene's narrative describes how, after an emergency appendectomy, she developed abdominal pain, nausea and dizziness after she ate, eventually diagnosed as gastroparesis, a condition in which the stomach fails to properly digest food, and for which she was prescribed domperidone, a drug often used to manage gastrointestinal motility disorders that is also a galactagogue, a substance that stimulates lactation. After a serious adverse reaction to domperidone, which she describes as 'all of a sudden my legs stopped working and began shaking uncontrollably. I started to have a rash all over my upper body, my vision narrowed, and I was having a hard time breathing...' Magdalene was admitted to hospital and diagnosed with anxiety. She tells of being given antianxiety medication, during what she now believes was an episode of PoTS, despite having refused consent for it previously:

> Every time I ate, I passed out. I couldn't move and could barely talk for 2 or 3 hours each time. At this time, I was on a liquid-only diet. Meanwhile, I had 8 doctors all come in one day to see me, including my primary care doctor, a neurologist, and a psychiatrist. Each one told me that this was all anxiety and that they wanted me to take a medicine for anxiety. Also, they said that I was a female and trying to do too much with school and work. I WAS SO ANGRY! After the first 3 doctors, I was so angry that by the 8th, I was enraged! NO ONE WOULD LISTEN TO ME!!!!!!!!!!!!!!!!!! I knew

that it wasn't anxiety and that there was something very wrong with me... The doctors treated me like complete crap and told me that I was a woman at the age of 23, trying to finish school, and that my body was just shutting down. They said that I was too stressed and couldn't control my emotions, so that was why I was in the position I was in!!!!!!!! At one point I passed out and was unable to talk, and the doctor ordered the nurses to give me anxiety medicine so that I would stop having the episode. I couldn't tell them that I didn't want it because I couldn't talk. They knew that I didn't want to take it because I had refused it earlier. It was unbelievable. At this point, my heart rate was at 120 beats per minute. I could barely walk. I had Parkinson-like symptoms. My breasts had filled with milk from the domperidone. Every time I threw up, I passed out, and every time I ate, I passed out.

(emphasis in original)

The imagery that Magdalene crafted in her story focused on her fight for legitimacy, recognition of her illness experience and a diagnosis that was appropriate for what she believed she knew about herself. Her story reinforced the powerful claim for the legitimacy of her own experience of being ill, and her own agency in rejecting not only medicines themselves as productive of undesired embodied effects, but also rejecting *who* these medicines symbolised she was. This construction of medicines as powerful signifiers of illness identity, in this case a particularly undesired and potentially discrediting one, draws attention to how medications themselves may come to be narratively entangled in the loss of self (Charmaz, 1983) experienced by people with chronic illness.

Medicines as signifiers also served as dramatic props for refracting how others viewed them. Magdalene's story poignantly demonstrates the heterogeneous work of various actors around medicines, things around which cooperation but also conflict is created as these actors work on the problem posed by medically unexplained symptoms. When there was conflict over the biomedical categorisation of illness as diagnosable disease, medicines became one battleground where disparate interpretations of the situation were played out. In this story, medicines were the props or 'the stuff of action' around which this conflict revolves. Medicines as signifiers in narratives is analytically meaningful because it makes starkly visible how storytelling is also moral work, or a form of ethical practice (Frank, 2013), with implications for the performance of illness identities. One of the reasons why medicines became key elements in the battleground over the diagnosis of illness, and storied into such dramas, at times invoked in producing appropriate illness identities, was because of the contemporary lack of legitimate spaces to be ill. With the rise of neoliberal discourses around personal responsibility for health and illness (Lupton, 2013; Peacock et al., 2014), seeking medical legitimacy is important otherwise individuals face the uncertain and negative fate of being cast as malingerers or, the often worse fate of being labelled as someone where the cause of illness is deemed psychological, a subject position that is often fraught with difficulty (Nettleton, 2006).

Dramas of experimentation: Solving the riddle of illness

These latter points can also be seen in what we describe as the third theme running through these narratives. Dramas of experimentation in medication and illness narratives involve stories of both health care professionals and people with illness using medicines to conduct experiments to solve the body/mind problem posed by illness, particularly where there is uncertainty around a diagnosis. This is especially salient in narratives about medically unexplained symptoms or, as is the case with PoTS, in narratives of living with a chronic illness with no standardised or widely accepted treatment protocol. Much of the experimentation in these dramas is also embodied but is distinct from what we have discussed earlier about dramas of embodiment because the cooperation and also the conflict around the acting on and with medicines within these dramas is preoccupied with 'solving the riddle' (Lillirank, 2003) of diagnosis. Medicines were narrated as props with both material and symbolic effects that could be deployed by health professionals to work on the uncertainty created by illness, both before and after diagnosis. These stories emphasise our protagonists' own narrative efforts to make sense of this experimentation. Such stories are analytically meaningful because they illustrate how medications come to be embedded in dramas of grappling with the biomedical uncertainty created by illness.

Some of these dramas involved experimentation *prior* to diagnosis of medically unexplained symptoms, with the hope of providing some resolution to the biomedical uncertainty posed by a mysterious, debilitating condition. A resolution of symptoms through pharmaceutical trial and error could then provide a 'retro-fitted' diagnosis or at least clues for further diagnostic testing. In some stories, the trialling of multiple potential diagnoses and treatments for them led to further investigations, ultimately leading to a PoTS diagnosis, even if followed by a period of continued treatment uncertainty. In other stories, such as Joanna's below, living with PoTS was punctuated by experimentation with medicines even after being diagnosed.

Joanna described how she went through a period after diagnosis, when her health deteriorated and various treatment approaches were experimented with, before she found one that enabled her to manage her symptoms:

> My PoTS symptoms were worse than before and I was unable to hold down a job. I was fed up of being unreliable, constantly having to call in sick and letting people down on a daily basis. It was at this point I went back to my GP and he upped my dose of Fludrocortisone. My body didn't react well to this and it was at this point when I became severely unwell, left my job and spent the majority of the summer of 2013 in bed. I had severe sickness, bad headaches that involved me sitting all day in darkness, severe joint pains in my arms and legs which left me screwed up in a ball on my bed trying to tense my muscles to get rid of the pain, bad chest pains, awful brain fog and I was constantly tired. I was then put on a beta-blocker to see if this improved my symptoms at all. This had the opposite effect and I ended up in hospital on more than one occasion. Finally, after trial and error and 8 months spent

in bed I was put on Midodrine. After a few months on Midodrine my symptoms were better, I was less tired and was able to function.

Stories like Joanna's emphasise how dramas of experimentation often told of more than just a 'one off' experiment leading to a long-term effective treatment regimen but how experimentation is a process of continual trial and error, punctuated by dramatic highs and lows. Such experimentation was foregrounded in many narratives of living with PoTS because of the lack of a standardised treatment protocol.

Some dramas of experimentation involved self-experimentation with natural remedies or over the counter medicines that narrators described researching, seeking out, and using without medical supervision. In her story of her 'slow steady recovery from PoTS', Janis writes of her practices of self-experimentation:

I had refused to take SSRIs (selective serotonin reuptake inhibitors) because I did not like the way they made me feel. So, I began to study natural medicine. I got my NMD [Doctor of Naturopathic Medicine] degree and had a test on my neurotransmitter levels. I found that I was low in serotonin and epinephrine, while high in norepinephrine. I started taking natural supplements to raise serotonin and gaba. I also worked to help my norepinephrine and epinephrine levels through diet and supplements. I'd greatly improved by the first neurotransmitter retest.

For some, like Janis, experimentation ultimately generated some degree of enhanced certainty and even 'recovery'. For others, the often-extended work of experimentation on the bodily dilemma posed by PoTS produced heightened uncertainty. Some stories highlighted the recurrent biographical disruption of chronic illness (Saunders, 2017) and illustrating how such experimentation may, in fact, be productive of further uncertainty. For example, experimentation sometimes had the effect of disrupting a presumed 'certain' diagnosis, generating additional uncertainty and causing doctors and people with illness to mistrust an earlier diagnosis when medicines expected to manage it had little effect or led to worsening symptoms. When experimentation led nowhere and no medicines 'fit' the body and the illness about which these stories were told, there was no solution found to the riddle and the problem posed by embodied illness and what it symbolised. In these stories, a narrative of hope for medicines of the future and anticipated experimentation with them sustained narrators' sense of optimism for eventual treatment and recovery.

While dramas of embodiment emphasise what medicines do in bodies, and dramas of signification focus on how they are invoked in legitimising illness, these dramas of experimentation construct medicines as tools for solving the problems posed by the uncertainty of illness. The telling of such stories about medicines in narratives of living with PoTS illuminates how medicines are drawn into the dramatic, and in fact, moral sense making around the uncertainty of medically unexplained symptoms and the liminality of being chronically ill.

Discussion

Our aim for this chapter was, first, to demonstrate the value of studying stories about medicines as they are embedded within broader stories of living with illness, and second, to illustrate how medicines can be conceived of as dramatic elements invoked to accomplish embodied, signifying and experimental work for storytellers. Medicines are things, both material and symbolic, around which multiple actors do the work of making sense of and managing illness. As in the case of the stories analysed here, some of this work takes place within particular communities of practice (Lave & Wenger, 1991), emergent via patient organisations.

Medicines were drawn into dramas like theatrical props on a stage and used by storytellers to craft a story about the subjective experience of living with illness and taking medicines. These tales were both individual and personal, yet also social, seeking to share and connect with others. They are, as Frank (2013) asserted, part of an *ethical practice* of engaging with others to make meaning about medicines and living with illness. At the same time, such stories about medicines are also performative. They are a medium through which storytellers can engage in impression management, navigating various definitions of the situation at hand, to present one embodied iteration of the self to others (Goffman, 1959). We can think of these dramas of medicines as akin to Goffman's 'front stage' wherein medicines come to be props, things around which action is developing and meaning is crafted, in performances of how to live with illness.

Drawing on the theoretical framework developed by Frank (2007), we have discussed three kinds of dramas of medicines in stories of living with PoTS. *Dramas of embodiment* describe stories of medicines acting on physical bodies, organ systems, physical functions and the subjective embodied experience of living with PoTS, quite often drawing on the language of clinical medicine itself. These kinds of stories most closely align with those of health professionals about the biophysiological action of medicines in bodies. Foregrounding these embodied experiences may echo what Frank (2013) calls the modernist voice of medicine in stories of taking medications, perhaps the only voice immediately and readily accessible to some people to describe what medicines are doing in their bodies. Yet talking about the subjective experience of the effects of medicines in the body means chronicling *doing something* about being ill –something that is tangible and also performative. Through the lens of contemporary interpretations of Parsons' sick role in the context of chronic illness (Varul, 2010), these dramas of embodiment emphasise how actors perform the obligation to seek out and take guidance from experts and to desire to be restored to health.

In dramas of signification and experimentation, storytellers may position themselves as complying with the expectations placed on them as ill people, while crafting their own stories, their own lay knowledge of living with PoTS. Stories of embodied effects, particularly the undesired ones that are productive of illness or risk, also highlight how such stories convey meaning making in the face of the recurrent biographical disruption of living with (sometimes unexplained) chronic illness (Saunders, 2017).

Dramas of signification invoke the symbolic potential of medicines – their capacity to signify not only what illness one has, but also *who one is*. Medicines are intricately entangled in the identity work of narratives and the performative nature of storytelling. While medicines have the potential to signify that individuals are 'legitimately ill' and experiencing an illness that reinforces their definition of the situation and their own sense of self (Goffman, 1959), they may likewise, as in Magdalene's story, signify an illness identity that does not 'fit' individuals' sense of themselves, and dramas about these medicines may be ones of resistance and contestation. Within these dramas, a mismatch, between health professionals' definitions of the situation and that of people living with illness risk the loss, or at least the public discrediting, of the self. Charmaz (1983) has described how '[d]ramatic discrediting occurs during the course of encounters when ill persons experience public mortification. The images of self mirrored to these ill persons can be so unexpected or jarring that they shake the very foundations of their self-concepts' (Charmaz, 1983, p. 181). In dramas of signification, medicines can become the mirror held up for people to see themselves, calling on them to perhaps do narrative work to make sense of the image reflected back at them.

Dramas of signification, in particular, may be stories of narrative reconstruction (Williams, 1984), often accomplished with particular moral force. For Frank (2013, p. 18), 'Telling stories… attempts to change one's own life by affecting the lives of others'. Telling stories of resisting an illness identity that does not fit with one's subjective experience of being ill is one way of asserting agency and pushing back with narrative force against the effort to discredit and delegitimise the subjective experience of being ill. Telling stories also enables the storyteller to reconstruct a sense of self amidst biomedical uncertainty, and to engage dialogically with others potentially yet to travel this path. Dramas of signification are 'quest narratives' (Frank, 2013) *par excellence*, wherein small stories of resistance to the symbolic potential of medicines and of staking a claim to embodied expertise become the 'boons' offered up to others who themselves have yet to write their own stories. Stories about resisting medicines and the undesired illness identities they might signify may create a script, potentially to be shared within existing communities of practice formed by people living with illness, for the performance of identity, imbuing these stories with a particular narrative telos.

Dramas of experimentation describe tales of medicines deployed as tools to solve the problem posed by illness. Medicines become the props that multiple actors engage with to 'solve the riddle' of medically unexplained symptoms (Lillirank, 2003). The narrative telos of these stories is to make sense of experimentation on the problem of illness and on the body itself, and to make sense of the uncertainty of living with illness that clinical medicine cannot so easily render certain. Modernity is predicated on the assumptions of traditional forms of authority and expertise, certainty, continually striving for social and scientific progress. A key characteristic of late modernity is the deterioration of traditional authority and forms of expertise, through fragmentation, contestation, insecurity and risk (Giddens, 1991; Beck, 1992, Bauman, 1991, 1997).

This is particularly salient – and deeply problematic – for those living with medically unexplained symptoms (Nettleton, 2006). We argue this may also be the case for those experiencing undiagnosed symptoms and when diagnosed with something as poorly understood and with as little standardisation in treatment protocols as PoTS. Nettleton argues that 'modernist discourses of solutions, restitution and certainty can be constraining for those who must endure uncertainty and chaos. Searching for solutions and 'closure' can, in and of itself, form a further tyranny that people find they have to negotiate' (2006, p. 1175). In these stories of living with and taking medicines for PoTS, medicines can come to be invoked in dramas of experimentation, foregrounding their tellers' efforts to grapple with uncertainty amid expectations and desires for restitution, closure and certainty through clinical intervention. In a context where there are fewer and fewer legitimate spaces for the sick to occupy under the prevailing condition of current public health discourses (Peacock et al., 2014), it seems likely that the role that medicines play in this experimental – and legitimating – work will become increasingly problematic and contested, highlighting the importance of analyses like this one.

The overlapping fields of medical humanities and narrative medicine have already made the case for how stories, art, etc., have much insight to offer to the practice of medicine and other fields of health care. Understanding medication narratives *as dramas*, instead of simply as stories, places emphasis on the performative effects of each actor's role in both the front stage and back stage and makes space for theorising about medicines in the everyday lives of people living with illness, as well as peoples' lives with medicines for prevention and enhancement.

Conclusion

Studying the construction of stories about medicines allows space to step outside the traditional adherence/non-adherence binary that guides much research on experiences of medicine taking (Bissell et al., 2004) and to focus instead on how people who tell stories have a stake in acting on and with medicines. Such a theoretical lens holds space for conceiving of the managing of illness as unfolding in a field of practice, where stories about medicines may be a means to understanding how people with illness make sense of medicines in their lives and why they act with and on them in the ways that they do. Our analysis demonstrates how medicines enter into complex, multifaceted stories – dramas that can be full of private and public troubles, of resistance and contestation, but also of play and experimentation. Through these dramas, medicines can be seen as much more than objects in a bidirectional relationship between doctors and patients and the expectation of compliant consumption of prescribed medicines. The dramas of medicines in narratives troubles these assumptions and creates possibilities for the development of a field of narrative pharmacy, in the spirit of narrative medicine (Greenhalgh & Hurwitz, 1998; Charon, 2006, 2007), focused on medicine taking that allows for more nuance and more depth than the simplistic adherence/non-adherence binary.

We have explored meaning making about taking medicines via stories told from one particular viewpoint, that of people living with illness themselves, and produced for a particular purpose and audience. This analysis, therefore, presents a necessarily partial picture. Future research should explore stories about medicines produced by heterogeneous actors engaged in managing illness and medicines' use, including doctors, nurses, pharmacists and other health professionals, as well as family members and carers, and perhaps even producers of medicines themselves. Future research ought to query what other kinds of dramas might be found in narratives of medicines in our lives. The expansiveness of the potential for further analysis warrants continued research on stories about medicines in the context of both illness and health.

References

Bauman, Z. (1991). *Modernity and Ambivalence.* Cambridge, UK: Polity Press.

Bauman, Z. (1997). *Postmodernity and Its Discontents.* New York: NYU Press.

Beck, U. (1992). *Risk Society: Towards a New Modernity.* London: SAGE Publications.

Bennaroch, E.E. (2012). Postural tachycardia syndrome: A heterogeneous and multifactorial disorder. *Mayo Clinic Proceedings, 87,* 1214–1225.

Bissell, P., Ryan, K., & Morecroft, C. (2006). Narratives about illness and medication: A neglected theme/new methodology within pharmacy practice research. Part I: Conceptual framework. *Pharm World & Science, 28,* 54–60.

Bissell, P., May, C.R., & Noyce, P.R. (2004). From compliance to concordance: Barriers to accomplishing a re-framed model of health care interactions. *Social Science & Medicne, 58*(4), 851–862.

Britten, N. (2008). *Medicines and Society Patients, Professionals and the Dominance of Pharmaceuticals.* Camden, UK: Palgrave Macmillan.

Bruner, J. (2002). *Making stories: Law, literature, life.* New York: Clarkson Potter.

Bury, M. (1982). Chronic illness as biographical disruption. *Sociology of Health & Illness, 4,* 167–182.

Charmaz, K. (1983). Loss of self: A fundamental form of suffering in the chronically ill. *Sociology of Health & Illness, 5,* 168–195.

Charon, R. (2007). What to do with stories: The sciences of narrative medicine. *Canadian Family Physician, 53,* 1265–1267.

Charon, R. (2006). *Narrative Medicine: Honoring the Stories of Illness.* Oxford: Oxford University Press.

Conner, R., Sheikh, M., & Grubb, B. (2012). Postural orthostatic tachycardia syndrome (POTS): Evaluation and management. *British Journal of Medical Practitioners, 5,* a540.

Cooper, R.J., Bissell, P., Ward, P.R., Murphy, E., Anderson, C., Avery, T., ... Ratcliffe, J. (2012). Further challenges to medical dominance? The case of nurse and pharmacist supplementary prescribing. *Health 16*(2), 115–133.

Dew, K., Chamberlain, K., Hodgetts, D., Norris, P., Radley, A., & Gabe, J. (2014). Home as a hybid centre of medication practice. *Sociology of Health and Illness, 36,* 28–43.

Frank, A.W. (2013). *The Wounded Storyteller: Body, Illness and Ethics.* Chicago: University of Chicago Press.

Frank, A.W. (2007). Five dramas of illness. *Perspectives in Biology and Medicine, 50*(3), 379–394.

Frank, A.W. (1998) Stories of illness as care of the self: A Foucauldian dialogue. *Health*, 2, 329–348.

Fraser, H. (2004). Doing narrative research: Analysing personal stories line by line. *Qualitative Social Work*, 3, 179–201.

Giddens, A. (1991). *Modernity and Self-Identity: Self and Society in the Late Modern Age*. Cambridge: Polity Press.

Goffman, E. (1959). *The Presentation of the Self in Everyday Life*. New York: Penguin.

Greenhalgh, T., & Hurwitz, B. (1998). *Narrative Based Medicine*. London: BMJ Books.

Grubb, B.P. (2008). Postural tachycardia syndrome. *Circulation*, *117*, 2814–2817.

Hochschild, A.. (1979). Emotion work, feeling rules, and social structure. *American Journal of Sociology*, *85*(3), 551–575.

Kanjwal, K., Karabin, B., Sheikh, M., Elmer, L., Kanjwal, Y., Saeed, B., & Grubb, B. (2011). Pyridostigmine in the treatment of postural orthostatic tachycardia: A single-center experience. *Pacing and Clinical Electrophysiology*, *34*, 750–755.

Kavi, L., Gammage, M.D., Grubb, B.P., & Karabin, B.L. (2012). Postural tachycardia syndrome: Multiple symptoms, but easily missed. *British Journal of General Practice*, *62*, 286–287.

Kavi, L., Nuttall, M., Low, D.A., Opie, M., Nicholson, L.M., Caldow, E., & Newton, J.L. (2016). A profile of patients with postural tachycardia syndrome and their experience of healthcare in the UK. *British Journal of Cardiology*, *23*, 33.

Lave, J., & Wenger, E. (1991). *Situated Learning: Legitimate Peripheral Participation*. Cambridge: Cambridge University Press.

Lillirank, A. (2003). Back pain and the resolution of diagnostic uncertainty in illness narratives. *Social Science & Medicine*, *57*, 1045–1054.

Low, P., Opfer-Gehrking, T., Textor, S., Benarroch, E., Shen, W., Schondorf, R., ... Kligfield, P. (1995). Postural tachycardia syndrome (POTS). *Neurology*, *45*, 519–525.

Lupton, D. (1995) *The Imperative of Health: Public Health and the Regulated Body*. London: Sage.

Mattias, C.J., Low, D.A., Iodice, V., Owens, A.P., Kirbis, M., & Grahame, R. (2011). Postural tachycardia syndrome: Current experience and concepts. *National Review of Neurology*, *8*, 22–34.

McDonald, C., Koshi, S., Busner, L., Kavi, L., & Newton, J.L. (2014). Postural tachycardia syndrome is associated with significant symptoms and functional impairment predominantly affecting young women: A UK perspective. *BMJ Open*, *4*, e004127.

Nettleton, S. (2006). 'I just want permission to be ill': Towards a sociology of medically unexplained symptoms. *Social Science & Medicine*, *62*, 1167–1178.

Nørreslet, M., Bissell, P., & Traulsen, J.M. (2010). From consumerism to active dependence. *Health*, *14*(1), 91–106.

Parsaik, A., Allison, T.G., Singer, W., Sletten, D.M., Joyner, M., Benarroch, E.E., ... Sandroni, P. (2012). Deconditioning in patients with orthostatic intolerance. *Neurology*, *79*, 1435–1439.

Parsons, T. (1951). *The Social System*. Glencoe, IL: The Free Press.

Peacock, M., Bissell, P., & Owen, J. (2014). Dependency denied: Health inequalities in the neoliberal era. *Social Science & Medicine*, *118*, 173–180.

Pellegrino, E.D. (1976). Prescribing and drug ingestion: Symbols and substances. *Annals of Pharmacotherapy*, *10*, 624–630.

Pound, P., Britten, N., Morgan, N., Yardley, L., Pope, C., Daker-White, G., & Campbell, R. (2005). Resisting medicines: A synthesis of qualitative studies of medicine taking. *Social Science & Medicine*, *61*, 133–155.

Raj, S.R. (2006). The postural tachycardia syndrome (POTS): Pathophysiology diagnosis and management. *Indian Pacing and Electrophysiology Journal, 6,* 84–99.

Riessman, C.K. (2008). *Narrative Methods in the Human Sciences.* New York: SAGE.

Ryan, K., Bissell, P., & Morecroft, C. (2007) Narratives about illness and medication: A neglected theme/new methodology within pharmacy practice research. Part II: Medication narratives in practice. *Pharmacy World & Science, 29,* 353–360.

Saunders, B. (2017). 'It seems like you're going around in circles': Recurrent biographical disruption constructed through the past, present and anticipated future in the narratives of young adults with inflammatory bowel disease. *Sociology of Health and Illness, 39,* 726–740.

Thieben, M., Sandroni, P., Sletten, D., Benrud-Larson, L., Fealey, R., Vernino, S., … Low, P. (2007). Postural orthostatic tachycardia syndrome: The Mayo Clinic experience. *Mayo Clinic Proceedings, 82,* 308–313.

van der Geest, S., Reynolds, S., & Hardon, A. (1996). The anthropology of pharmaceuticals: A biographical approach. *Annual Review of Anthropology, 25,* 153–178.

van der Geest, S., & Whyte, S.R. (1989). The charm of medicines: Metaphors and Metonyms. *Medical Anthropology Quarterly* 3(4), 345–367.

Varul, M.Z. (2010). Talcott Parsons, the sick role and chronic illness. *Body & Society, 16,* 72–94.

Williams, G. (1984). The genesis of chronic illness: Narrative re-construction. *Sociology of Health and Illness, 6,* 175–200.

13 (Developing) pharmaceutical solutions to COVID-19

Navigating global tensions around the distribution of therapeutics and vaccines

Peri J. Ballantyne, Kath Ryan and Paul Bissell

Introduction

As the collection 'Living Pharmaceutical Lives' was being organised and contributing authors were considering the place of pharmaceuticals by groups of users in differing health contexts and social and geographic settings, we were also experiencing the emergence of COVID-19. We watched as it spread across populations in our respective countries and jurisdictions. We observed, both from our professional standpoints – as academics or health professionals – and personally, as familiar patterns in the distribution of harm and death from COVID-19 were reported through local, then international media. We thought it important to include a chapter in this collection, where an overview of the ongoing COVID-19 pandemic, and the early and emerging pharmaceutical solutions being imagined, developed and tested are considered. As we are not yet able to imagine a resolution to the COVID-19 pandemic, in this chapter, we briefly outline the emergence of COVID-19; we describe the social gradient of severe illness and deaths from the virus being documented in countries around the world; and we outline the pharmaceutical solutions that emerged and are in development to reduce its harm or eliminate its threat. Given an evident shared international expectation that pharmaceuticals will ultimately save us from COVID-19, our take-away message is that there is a need for political and global health leadership around the question of how to distribute emergent therapies and vaccines for COVID-19, and to whom. What can the familiar social gradient in COVID-related illness, suffering and death tell us about how to roll out its eventual pharmaceutical solutions?

Background

The first outbreak of a new viral illness that would come to be known as 'COVID-19' occurred in Wuhan, China, December 2019. The World Health Organization (WHO) declared a Public Health Emergency of International Concern on January 30, 2020 (WHO, n.d.-a), and named the new disease – caused by severe acute respiratory syndrome coronavirus 2 (SARS CoV-2) – 'coronavirus disease' (COVID-19) on February 11, 2020 (WHO, n.d.-b). The WHO declared a pandemic on March 11, 2020 (WHO, n.d.-a). At the time of writing, approximately 10 months since the first reported outbreak, the global case and death count for COVID-19 was 43,187,134 and 1,155,653 (Johns Hopkins University, Coronavirus Resource Centre, 2000a, 2000b). While comparable global and national infection, morbidity and mortality estimates have been thwarted by the lack of widespread systematic testing (Henriques, 2020), countries reporting the highest numbers of infections at that time included the United States, India, Brazil, Russia and France (Johns Hopkins University, Coronavirus Resource Centre, 2000a).

Social inequalities in COVID-19 morbidity and mortality

The distribution of COVID-related infection and death has already been shown to follow a well-established social gradient. Referring to the reality that inequalities in population health status are related to inequalities in social status (Kosteniuk and Dickinson, 2003, p. 26) – the *social gradient* describes the inverse association between social and economic standing in society and health and mortality risks. Those with the highest social and economic standing have the lowest likelihood of experiencing poor health and lowered life expectancy, those near the top have poorer health than those at the top but better health than those in the middle; those at the bottom have the poorest health and life expectancy (Marmot et al., 1978; Marmot, 2017) a pattern observed across countries and over time (Marmot, 2017). This gradient, documented in Britain as early as the 1930s, was associated with a corresponding gradient in the distribution of medical care resources. The 'inverse care law' was so named in response to the observation that 'the availability of good medical care tends to vary inversely with the need for it in the population served… operating more completely where medical care is most exposed to market forces, and less so where such exposure is reduced' (Tudor Hart, 1971). The inverse care law is noted to have persisted, even in the context of universal coverage for health care:

> the fact that the inverse care law remains true in the British National Health Service (NHS)… where financial barriers to care have been largely removed, means that other processes are at work.
>
> (Watt, 2002, p. 252)

Evidence suggests that location on the social gradient helps to account not only for risk of individual mental and physical illness, accidents, and mortality, but also – reasonably – for co-morbidity prevalence within social groups. For example, Barnett et al. (2012) documented that the onset of multimorbidity occurred 10–15 years earlier in people living in the most deprived areas compared with the most affluent, with socioeconomic deprivation particularly associated with multimorbidity that included mental health disorders. Walker et al. (2016) found that the social patterning of mortality in people with type 2 diabetes is explained by both differing levels of comorbid disease and other dimensions of deprivation. Evidence of the social gradient in the distribution of COVID-19 emerged as early as data was compiled, providing early support for the need to develop strategies to protect vulnerable social groups from exposure to the virus. For example, early documentation by Wu and McGoogan (2020) showed that in China, older people and those with pre-existing conditions such as cancer, cardiovascular disease, diabetes, hypertension and chronic respiratory disease experienced higher risk of severe illness and death from SARS CoV-2 exposure. Based on those and similar findings across the globe, Yashadhana et al. (2020) expressed concern about the increased risk of exposure, severe illness and death from COVID-19 facing Indigenous Australians due to high chronic disease rates (i.e., co-morbidity) in this population as well as 'marginalization from health services, food insecurity, poor access to water, sanitation and adequate housing' (p. 1). Data from other countries showing that COVID-19 risks are unevenly distributed, has mounted.

In Canada, for example, higher rates of COVID-19 infections in the major cities of Montreal and Toronto have been documented in low income neighbourhoods and neighbourhoods with higher percentages of Blacks, other visible minorities, immigrants, persons with low educational levels, and low incomes and poorer conditions of work (Bowden and Cain, 2020; CBC News, 2020a; Rocha, Shingler and Montpetit, 2020; Wherry, 2020). Reporting on COVID exposure in Canada's most populous province, Public Health Ontario reported that the most ethno-culturally diverse neighbourhoods in large urban areas were experiencing disproportionately higher rates of COVID-19 and related deaths compared to neighbourhoods that are less diverse, with COVID-19 infection, hospitalisations and deaths at three, four and two times the rate in the most diverse neighbourhoods as compared to the least (Public Health Ontario, 2020). The Canadian Human Rights Commission (n.d.) recognised the amplification of inequality resulting from the COVID-19 epidemic for vulnerable groups in this country: people with disabilities, Indigenous peoples, children, people in housing need or facing food insecurity, women and children fleeing violence, single parents, the LGBTQ2I community, people needing medical attention, the elderly and people in correctional institutions.

Similar patterns are evident in the United States. The US Centres for Disease Control and Prevention reported that African-American, Latino and Indigenous persons have 4.7, 4.6 and 5.3 times greater likelihood of hospitalisation after contracting COVID-19 as compared to White, non-Hispanic persons; African-Americans have 2.1 times greater likelihood of death (US Centres for Disease Control and Prevention, n.d.-a, 2020). Finch and Hernández Finch (2020) also reported that during the early weeks of the pandemic, a larger number of confirmed COVID-19 cases were located in more disadvantaged counties in the United States, but that '...over time this trend changed so that by the beginning of April, 2020 more affluent counties had more confirmed cases of the virus' (p. 1). Attributing these results to the overall lack of adequate testing resources as the pandemic continued, particularly in more disadvantaged counties, these authors noted that rates of death due to COVID-19 were higher in poorer and more urban counties. In the United States, the greater risks of COVID-19 for particular vulnerable populations is attributed to the greater likelihood of underlying conditions that impact health – socioeconomic status, access to health care, and increased exposure to the virus in occupations like front-line, essential and critical infrastructure workers (US Centres for Disease Control, n.d.-a, 2020).

In England/Wales, social inequalities in COVID infections and mortality are evident (Bissell, Peacock and MacDonald, 2020; Sa, 2020; UK Office for National Statistics, n.d.). For example, Sa (2020) documented infections per 100,000 population to be higher in communities where there were larger households, worse levels of self-reported health and a greater reliance on public transport; and death from COVID to be higher among those who are older aged, of Black or Asian ethnic minority status, and with poorer self-rated health. Bissell, Peacock and MacDonald (2020) summarised that men, older people and those from BAME[1] backgrounds, and those with pre-existing or underlying conditions face heightened risk of death from COVID-19, pointing out the 'brutal logic' that the social gradient in the United Kingdom is a consequence of austerity measures – particularly those introduced in the aftermath of the 2008 financial crisis – in that country. Sa reasoned that to reduce COVID-19 infection and mortality rates, policymakers ought to target social determinants of health such as improved housing conditions and strategies for safe public transportation. A key European report highlighted the relevance of the socioeconomic distribution of major chronic conditions such as high blood pressure, diabetes and heart or respiratory disease documented by McNamara et al. (2017) for predicting the distribution of COVID-19 infection and mortality (EuroHealthNet, 2020). A number of factors – the inability to self-isolate due to insecure labour conditions which do not allow for teleworking or provide statutory sick or care leave, high density and overcrowded housing, unemployment and financial insecurities stemming from labour market fluctuations resulting from the pandemic – were identified to account for the increased COVID-19 related risks facing those in disadvantaged socioeconomic circumstances.

Data on the morbidity and mortality rates associated with COVID-19 for socio-economically vulnerable groups are less accessible for some global regions, but general social, economic and health vulnerabilities are indicative of its potential severity. For example, examining Asian countries' experiences with COVID-19, Kim, Hai and Rodriquez (2020) illustrated the common thread of socio-economic marginalisation and heightened exposure and risks of COVID-19 experienced by different vulnerable groups: LGBTQ+ peoples in South Korea, migrant workers in Singapore and women in Indonesia where, since COVID-19, domestic violence and sexual abuse has soared while access to reproductive health care has ground to a halt. In India, the heightened incidence and mortality from COVID-19 infection observed among the poorest segments of that country's population are attributed to the 'multi-layered vulnerability and deprivation of rural, urban and tribal toiling classes… in a context of a poorly equipped and understaffed public health system' (Lingam and Suresh Sapkal, 2020, p. 174). In Latin America and the Caribbean, and in African countries, estimates of morbidity and mortality effects of COVID-19 have been more difficult to gather due to the challenging logistics of counting infections, illness and death (Horton, 2020; Nordling, 2020; Oyesola et al., n.d.). Reports from these regions emphasise the economic crisis that has emerged and is expected to continue as a result of the COVID-19 pandemic, and that will deepen poverty and severe poverty among already-marginalised social groups (United Nations, 2020; Ndulu, 2020).

Why do we care about these notable inequalities in the distribution and effects of COVID-19? It is our view that we are at a unique historical juncture where the inequalities associated with COVID-19 could be mitigated/minimised through strategies that ensure access to anticipated COVID-19 treatments and vaccines for those most vulnerable to the virus – a reversal of the 'inverse care law' we mention above. At a socio-political level, international groups led by the WHO have already raised concern along these lines, in their anticipation of an effective vaccine, and the particular vulnerabilities to COVID-19 facing poor countries. The WHO describes the global access facility for COVID-19 vaccines:

> COVAX, the vaccines pillar of the Access to COVID-19 Tools (ACT) Accelerator, is co-led by the Coalition for Epidemic Preparedness Innovations (CEPI), Gavi, the Vaccine Alliance, and the World Health Organization (WHO) – working in partnership with developed and developing country vaccine manufacturers. It is the only global initiative that is working with governments and manufacturers to ensure COVID-19 vaccines are available worldwide to both higher-income and lower-income countries.
>
> (WHO, 2020c)

At the level of individual nations, however, plans for the fair and ethical distribution of therapeutics and vaccines are unclear, and will be challenging (British Medical Association, n.d.; Chung, 2020; Griffin, 2020). There is a need now – as vaccines and therapeutics for COVID are in development – to envision a radical approach that will prioritise treatment and immunisation for the most vulnerable groups across and within nations – in response to long-standing and unyielding social inequalities in health.

Anticipated pharmaceutical solutions

In this section, we briefly describe current efforts being made towards the development of safe and effective treatments and vaccines for COVID-19. Because it has become so evident in public discourse, we also address tensions between scientific/public health and political/economic interests in the 'race' to discover and market effective COVID-19 treatments.

Therapeutics for COVID-19

Readers might recall that the earliest claimed treatments for COVID-19 – the antiviral agent chloroquine and its less toxic derivative hydroxychloroquine – raised the spectre of political interference in claims-making about pharmaceuticals for COVID-19. Interest in using these decades-old antimalarial drugs for coronaviruses dated to the 2003 SARS CoV-1 outbreak, where preliminary findings indicated that chloroquine might inhibit the spread of SARS CoV-1 (Schmidt, 2020). While the European Medicines Agency urged caution around their promotion for COVID-19 (Miller and Burger, 2020), in the early days of the epidemic, before human trials for its use were undertaken, hydroxychloroquine was promoted by then US president Trump as a 'game changer' (Perez, 2020; Associated Press, 2020). Responding to public demand, in March 2020, the US Food and Drug Administration issued an emergency-use authorisation for chloroquine or hydroxychloroquine[2], but a safety warning quickly followed in April 2020 as heart rhythm problems were observed in treated COVID-19 patients (Food and Drug Administration, 2020a). Tensions continued as the virus spread, the research community compiled further evidence of its risks (Kunzmann, 2020; Thomson Reuters, 2020a; Yu, 2020), and Trump and Brazilian president Bolsonaro proclaimed personal use for prevention and treatment purposes (Lovelace, Jr. & Breuninger, 2020; Londoño, 2020). The US emergency use authorisation was withdrawn in June 2020 after clinical trials showed hydroxychloroquine provided no benefit while potentially increasing risks of fatal heart arrhythmia (Heidt, 2020), and clinical trials examining the use of hydroxychloroquine for COVID-19 have since been terminated (WHO, 2020d; Craven, 2020a).

By early September 2020, however, two antiviral drugs had been approved to treat COVID-19: favilavir in China, Italy and Russia, and remdesivir in the United States, Japan, Australia and Canada[3] (Cennimo & Bronze, 2020a; Craven, 2020a; Pinkerton, 2020); several other antivirals remain under investigation (Cennimo & Bronze, 2020b). Details about the mechanisms of antivirals are described in Şimşek Yavuz and Ünal (2020). Corticosteroids – dexamethasone, hydrocortisone and methylprednisolone – have also been found to improve survival rates of SARS CoV-2 infected patients with severe illness (Craven, 2020a; Thomson Reuters, 2020b; WHO Rapid Evidence Appraisal for COVID-19 Therapies (REACT) Working Group, 2020). The pros and cons of steroid use in COVID-19 patients are described in Berton et al. (2020).

Antibody therapy – a form of 'passive immunisation' – has also been under investigation as a treatment for SARS CoV-2 infection. Antibody therapy is a technique to achieve immediate short-term immunisation against infectious agents by administering pathogen-specific antibodies drawn from the serum of stimulated animals or obtained by collecting whole blood or plasma from a [human] patient who has survived a previous infection (Marano et al., 2016, p. 152). Antibody therapy for COVID-19 received an emergency use authorisation by the US Food and Drug Administration for patients hospitalised with suspected or laboratory-confirmed COVID-19 (Food and Drug Administration, 2020b; CBC News, 2020b), despite lack of evidence of benefit in large-scale randomised controlled trials (Craven, 2020a) that are only now (as of late October 2020) underway (see National Institutes of Health, 2020). As with hydroxychloroquine, the emergency use authorisation for antibody therapy was thought to have emerged under pressure from the Trump administration to show any progress over the COVID-19 epidemic, and to have oversold the benefits of an approach that remains an experimental treatment (CBC News, 2020b; CBC News, 2020c; Kupferschmidt & Cohen, 2020). Observers were quick to caution against being overly enthusiastic about the prospects of antibody treatment for COVID-19 because the anticipated production costs would make it likely to be inequitably available, especially for populations in poor countries[4] (Ledford, 2020; Cohen, 2020).

Vaccines

Around the globe, an unprecedented effort is being made to find a safe and effective vaccine that will neutralise the SARS CoV-2 virus. As of late October 2020, the Regulatory Affairs Professional Society (RAPS) COVID-19 vaccine tracker showed 7 SARS-2 vaccines in Phase 3 clinical trials, 2 at the Phase 2–3 stage, 3 at Phase 2, 10 at Phase 1–2, and many more at Phase 1 and preclinical stages (Craven, 2020b; Craven, 2020c; see also Steckelberg et al., 2020; WHO, 2020c). To date, two vaccines have been approved by the Russian Ministry of Health – the Sputnik V and the EpiVacCorona. Both were introduced to the market before the completion of Phase 3 clinical trials (Craven, 2020c). Experts have cautioned that the vaccine development process requires adequate time to assess for safety and efficacy (Craven, 2020b; Craven, 2020c, Callaway, 2020). Indeed, a tension has emerged, based on a global interest in and competition over vaccine development and distribution. On the one hand, there appears to be an unprecedented global effort to collaborate on vaccine development in the face of this pandemic, reflected in this statement from the WHO:

> Immunization currently prevents 2–3 million deaths every year from diseases like diphtheria, tetanus, pertussis, influenza and measles. There are now vaccines to prevent more than 20 life-threatening diseases, and work is ongoing at unprecedented speed to also make COVID-19 a vaccine-preventable disease. There are currently over 169 COVID-19 vaccine candidates under development, with 26 of these in the human trial phase. WHO is working in collaboration with scientists, business, and global health organizations through the ACT Accelerator to speed up the pandemic response. When a safe and effective vaccine is found, COVAX (led by WHO, GAVI and CEPI) will facilitate the equitable access and distribution of these vaccines to protect people in all countries. People most at risk will be prioritized.
>
> (WHO, n.d.-e)[5]

On the other hand, concern is emerging over 'vaccine nationalism' or a 'my nation first' approach to developing and distributing potential vaccines (Weintraub, Bitton & Rosenberg, 2020) that threatens the prospects of the democratic distribution of safe and effective vaccines or of prioritising the most at risk or vulnerable groups (Kupferschmidt, 2020; Nebehay & Lema, 2020; Taylor, 2020). For example, the United States, Europe and Australasia have placed advance orders for hundreds of millions of doses of successful vaccines, raising concern of their being little supply for those in poorer parts of the world, including health care workers and people at higher risk of severe disease (Kupferschmidt, 2020). Enhancing the sense of inequity is the expectation that a country like India – having among the highest number of cases of COVID-19 in the world as well as enhanced vaccine manufacturing capacity – will manufacture vaccines for the world but be unable to secure sufficient doses needed for the 400 million people estimated to be most at risk of exposure and severe infection from COVID-19 in that country (Vaidyanathan, 2020).

An ongoing concern is regarding the safety of fast-tracked vaccines, amidst political wrangling over the timing of (eventually) approved vaccines. The extent of this concern was evident in early September when the chief executives of nine pharmaceutical manufacturers issued a pledge that safety and efficacy protocols established through Phase 3 clinical trials would be fully undertaken before regulatory approval for an experimental COVID-19 vaccine is sought (Rowland, 2020). Later in September, Trump proclaimed to the American public that a vaccine is 'just around the corner' and that his administration would make vaccines free and available to all (Alonso-Zaldivar, 2020), putting vaccine politics front and centre of ongoing campaigns leading up to the November 3, 2020 US Federal Election.

In this context of promises of accelerated delivery of vaccines (see US Health and Human Services, 2020), evidence of the public's concern over their trustworthiness is mounting. For example, Xue and Kaplan (2020) examined vaccine perceptions in a representative sample of 1,000 US residents, and found that antivaccine sentiment was more pronounced than expected: 36% said they thought vaccines have harmful effects that are not being disclosed to the public, 10.3% said childhood vaccines are not very safe or not safe at all, and 21.1% reported refusing vaccines in the past; 21.8% said they definitely would not get a coronavirus vaccination. Noting that participants did express their trust in public health leaders when considering a potential coronavirus vaccine, these authors concluded that 'any future coronavirus vaccination campaign will require strong leaders who support good science, not leaders who manipulate or obstruct science for their own political agendas' (Xue and Kaplan, 2020, para 14).

Taking a COVID-specific perspective, in their recent publication, Romer and Jamieson (2020) reported on the findings of a panel survey involving a nationally representative sample of US residents who were interviewed at two periods since the start of the COVID-19 pandemic: March (N = 1,050) and July 2020 (N = 840). An inverse relationship was documented between three conspiracy theories about COVID[6] and (a) the perceived threat of the pandemic; (b) the taking of preventive actions such as wearing a face mask; (c) the perceived safety of vaccination and (d) the intention to be vaccinated. Romer and Jamieson argued that it is critical to confront conspiracy theories and vaccination misinformation to prevent further spread of COVID-19 in the United States.

The critical issue for global and national interests in quelling the COVID-19 pandemic is the problem individual rights advocates/anti-maskers/anti-vaxxers pose for the possibility of widespread uptake of vaccination required for herd immunity – which experts claim is the optimal strategy to stop the spread of SARS CoV-2 (D'Souza and Dowdy, 2020). As Thompson argues, herd protection is an important public good – a benefit to be shared by all individuals, but:

> it is the… kind of public good that neoliberalism has systematically obscured and undermined with its singular focus on individual responsibility for

health, its focus on the management of risks in individual patients instead of the population, and the privatisation of public goods necessary for health...

(Thompson, this volume, p. 99)

Discussion

Unless the COVID-19 crisis is to deepen already entrenched inequalities (Bissell et al., 2020), the current situation demands that action is taken to de-couple the development and production of pharmaceuticals – needed for the benefit of the public's health – from political or commercial interests, through reinforcing governments' responsibility for public health, and in this case, for getting essential drugs into bodies, and saving lives. The WHO-led vaccine initiative for COVID-19 suggests that progress is being made along these lines:

> The COVAX Facility is a Gavi-coordinated pooled procurement mechanism for new COVID-19 vaccines, through which COVAX will ensure fair and equitable access to vaccines for each participating economy, using an allocation framework currently being formulated by WHO. The COVAX Facility will do this by pooling buying power from participating economies and providing volume guarantees across a range of promising vaccine candidates, allowing those vaccine manufacturers whose expertise is essential to large scale production of the new vaccines, to make early, at-risk investments in manufacturing capacity – providing participating countries and economies with the best chance at rapid access to doses of a successful COVID-19 vaccine.
>
> (WHO, 2020c)

Clearly, the COVID-19 Vaccines Global Access (COVAX) approach challenges the principles of neoliberal capitalism and the pandemic seems to have reinvigorated appeals for a new global social and economic paradigm (Flood, MacDonnell and Venkatapuram, 2020; Schwab, 2020). Will this apparent resistance to neoliberal principles by the WHO and COVAX participating-nations (in late August 2020, 172 nations were negotiating potential participation (WHO, 2020c)) materialize in political collaboration in the earliest and ongoing distribution of therapies and vaccines? Can we sustain these early indications of global health leadership and collaboration in the face of unprecedented political upheaval coincident with the COVID-19 pandemic, including the general rise of nationalism, and the Black Lives Matter movement?

New concepts linking biopolitics, biomedical developments and citizenship rights that have been animated by contemporary global health events that have affected (or created) vulnerable populations may be applicable to our analysis of COVID-19. An example is Petryna's (2003/2013) concept of *biological citizenship* – applied in her ethnography of the Chernobyl disaster in the Ukraine in 1986, and used in reference to 'the damaged biology of a population that became the grounds for social membership and the basis for staking citizenship claims' (2003/2013: 5). For Petryna, the concept was related to 'a massive demand for, but selective access to a form of social welfare based on medical, scientific and legal criteria that both acknowledge biological injury and compensate for it' (2003/2013: 6) – a statement which characterises the current COVID-19 situation. Rose and Novas consider *biological citizenship* as part of the political history of citizenship projects and the biologisation of politics, and emphasise its individualising (referring to how individuals have come to shape their relations with themselves in terms of knowledge of their somatic individuality; part of the regime of the self) and collectivising (referring to the emergence of biosocial groupings based on a biological conception of a shared identity) features that have resulted in contemporary citizenship being manifested 'in a range of struggles over individual identities, forms of collectivization, demands for recognition, access to knowledge, and claims to expertise' (Rose and Novas, 2005, p. 442). In related research examining the politics of HIV/AIDs and access to treatment, Nguyen and colleagues (Nguyen, 2005; Nguyen et al., 2007) use the concept of *therapeutic citizenship* to refer to changes in people's identity resulting from their viral status and their rights to and responsibilities around engagement with HIV support organisations. Nguyen (2005) argues that these organisations exert power through the resources they offer and the accepted discourses about how to tackle and live with HIV (a topic taken up by Balogun-Katung et al., this volume). Nguyen et al. (2007) submit that, through interactions with HIV support organisations, particular kinds of subjects are fashioned – encouraged not only to assert their rights and make claims for treatment, but also to behave as 'responsible' HIV citizens who are adherent to antiretroviral therapy (Nguyen et al., 2007). We suggest that the spirit of these interrelated concepts – biological citizenship and therapeutic citizenship – are embedded in current statements of commitment to a human rights agenda for the management of COVID-19:

> Embracing human rights as an integral part of our public health response will not only provide ethical guidance during these difficult times but set the foundation for how the world responds to public health crises going forward.
> (WHO, 2020f)

> Now, and as we emerge from this crisis, all governments must ensure that legislation, policies, services and programs aimed at supporting Canadians and bringing our economy back to health have human rights principles baked-in. While we recognize the tremendous efforts of governments during this pandemic, we must all ensure that those people living in vulnerable circumstances are front and centre in our minds and our actions.
> (Canadian Human Rights Commission, n.d.)

The question is whether these aims will translate into action. Nguyen was perhaps prescient in her observation that 'in many Northern countries, national health insurance has meant that citizenship automatically confers access to treatment' (2005, p. 142) – of course suggestive that such privilege is unlikely available to citizens of the global South. Also prescient was another statement made in reference to the HIV/AIDS epidemic in Africa:

Therapeutic citizenship is emerging as a salient force in the local African settings that have been explored here, where widespread poverty means that neither kinship nor a hollowed-out state can offer guarantees against the vicissitudes of life. It has also emerged as a rallying point for transnational activism in a neoliberal world in which illness claims carry more weight than those based on poverty, injustice or structural violence.

(Nguyen, 2005, p. 143)

One test will be whether – as therapeutics and vaccines are being manufactured – a transnational movement will emerge to follow the principle of the WHO COVAX collaboration to challenge the market model for the distribution of pharmaceuticals so that the world's most vulnerable are prioritised for treatment. Moving forward then, will require leadership that takes a global, 'all nations' perspective. For as Flood and colleagues remark:

As nations around the world fumble through their response to COVID-19 with more or less success, the early experience reveals the desperate need for a well-resourced, central agency to spread the best scientific evidence on precautions and treatments for differently situated countries, and distribute resources to those countries that need additional support to control COVID-19... Let us be clear: a world in which a vaccine and other treatments are not made available for all will exacerbate existing health inequalities and poverty. And sooner or later these conditions will help spread the current or other novel diseases, and the next global pandemic... in our interconnected and interdependent world, protecting ourselves requires raising the quality of life and health resilience of everyone.

(Flood, MacDonnell & Venkatapuram, 2020, para 10, 12, 13)

Along a similar line, Bissell, Peacock and MacDonald assert that:

what the world is going to be like when we emerge from the COVID-19 pandemic is not an inevitability. Our newfound solidarity and awareness of mutual dependency can shape a different world, where the poorest and most disadvantaged do not face worse health outcomes as a result of broader political choices. It is down to the sort of world we demand and that is one in which the health damages of the past are recognised and not repeated.

(Bissell et al., 2020, para 7)

Conclusion

While highly anticipated, it is not yet possible for those at risk of or infected with SARS CoV-2 to 'live [through] pharmaceutical lives'. In this chapter, we outline the emergence of coronavirus-19 disease, associated with severe acute respiratory syndrome coronavirus 2 (SARS CoV-2); we describe the social gradient in the distribution of illness and deaths attributed to COVID-19; and we illustrate the current (as of late October 2020) state of development of therapeutic medicines and vaccines for COVID-19. Our aim in this chapter is to emphasise the need to reconcile public health interests in protecting vulnerable individuals and groups from COVID-19 through pharmaceutical technologies, and the political and commercial interests in winning the 'race' to approve and distribute medicines, including vaccines, for profit when they are available. Drawing on the concepts of biological citizenship – the shared biological identity of persons at risk of COVID-19 – and therapeutic citizenship – relating to claims over the right to biomedical resources including to the services of health care and to pharmaceuticals – we suggest that we are at an historic juncture where global political leadership is called on to prioritise the needs of citizens – especially the most vulnerable citizens – over political interests and commercial opportunities emanating from the COVID-19 pandemic. While we promote treatment access from a human rights perspective, we recognise that some individuals and collectives have claimed the right to resist social restrictions related to controlling the spread of the virus and vaccination programs that would enhance the likelihood of achieving global herd immunity from SARS CoV-2.

Notes

1 In the UK, the acronym 'BAME' refers to Black Asian, minority ethnic status.
2 https://www.fda.gov/media/136534/download
3 Health Canada granted authorization with conditions. https://www.canada.ca/en/health-canada/services/drugs-health-products/covid19-industry/drugs-vaccines-treatments/about.html
4 Reflective of this concern, after contracting the virus on October 2, 2020, observers were quick to note that US President Trump received the experimental antibody treatment on 'compassionate' grounds (Thomas & Kolata, 2020; Lanese, 2020).
5 The United States recently declared that it would not participate in the WHO's COVID-19 Vaccines Global Access (COVAX) facility (Taylor, 2020).
6 The conspiracy theories posed included: 'the pharmaceutical industry created the coronavirus to increase sales of its drugs and vaccines', 'the coronavirus was created by the Chinese government as a biological weapon', and 'some in the US Centres for Disease Control and Prevention, also known as CDC, are exaggerating the danger posed by the coronavirus to damage the Trump presidency' (Romer and Jamieson, 2020, p. 4).

References

Alonso-Zaldivar, R. (2020, September 16). U.S. releases plan to provide free coronavirus vaccine. *Associated Press*. Accessed on September 21, 2020 from https://globalnews.ca/news/7338230/u-s-free-coronavirus-vaccine-rollout/.

Associated Press. (2020, July 29). Hydroxychloroquine again in U.S. spotlight as video is widely shared by Trump, conservative groups. *CBC News*. Retrieved September 14, 2020 from https://www.cbc.ca/news/world/hydroxychloroquine-video-trump-1.5666923.

Barnett, K., Mercer, S.W., Norbury, M., Watt, G., Wyke, S., & Guthrie, B. (2012). Epidemiology of multimorbidity and implications for health care, research, and medical education: A cross-sectional study. *Lancet, 380*, 37–43.

Berton, A.M., Prencipe, N., Giordano, R., Ghigo, E., & Grottoli, S. (2020). Systemic steroids in patients with COVID-19: Pros and contras, an endocrinological point of view. *J Endocrinol Invest*, 1–3. doi:10.1007/s40618-020-01325-2.

Bissell, P., Peacock, M., & MacDonald, S. (2020). Health inequalities and COVID-19: Why the poor and disadvantaged are more likely to die. *Cost of Living*. Retrieved August 4, 2020 from https://www.cost-ofliving.net/health-inequalities-and-covid-19/.

Bowden, O., & Cain, P. (2020, June 2). Black neighbourhoods in Toronto are hit hardest by COVID-19 – and it's 'anchored in racism': experts. *Global News*. Retrieved August 31, 2020 from https://globalnews.ca/news/7015522/black-neighbourhoods-toronto-coronavirus-racism/.

British Medical Association. (n.d.). COVID-19 ethical issues. A guidance note. Retrieved September 11, 2020 from https://www.bma.org.uk/media/2360/bma-covid-19-ethics-guidance-april-2020.pdf.

Callaway, E. (2020, August 11). Russia's fast-track coronavirus draws outrage over safety. *Nature*. Retrieved September 10, 2020 from https://www.nature.com/articles/d41586-020-02386-2.

Cataldo, F. (2008). New forms of citizenship and sociopolitical inclusion: Accessing antiretroviral therapy in Rio de Janeiro favela. *The Sociology of Health and Illness*, 30(6), 900–912.

CBC News. (2020a, May 12). Lower income people, new immigrants at higher COVID-19 risk in Toronto, data suggests. Retrieved August 31, 2020 from https://www.cbc.ca/news/canada/toronto/low-income-immigrants-covid-19-infection-1.5566384.

CBC News. (2020b, August 23). Trump announces plasma treatment authorized for COVID-19. Retrieved September 8, 2020 from https://www.cbc.ca/news/health/trump-plasma-treatment-covid-19-1.5697206.

CBC News. (2020c, August 25). Blood plasma from recovered COVID-19 patients is still an experimental treatment. Here's why. Retrieved September 8, 2020 from https://www.cbc.ca/news/health/plasma-covid19-1.5698395.

Canadian Human Rights Commission. (n.d.). Statement – Inequality amplified by COVID-19 crisis. Retrieved August 31, 2020 from https://www.chrc-ccdp.gc.ca/eng/content/statement-inequality-amplified-covid-19-crisis

Cennimo, D.J., & Bronze, M.S. (2020a, September 4). What is the role of the antiviral drug remdesivir in the treatment of coronavirus disease 2019 (COVID-19)? *MedScape*. Retrieved September 10, 2020 from https://www.medscape.com/answers/2500114-197451/what-is-the-role-of-the-antiviral-drug-remdesivir-in-the-treatment-of-coronavirus-disease-2019-covid-19.

Cennimo, D.J., & Bronze, M.S. (2020b, September 4). What other antiviral agents are being investigated for the treatment of coronavirus disease 2019 (COVID-19)? Retrieved September 10, 2020 from https://www.medscape.com/answers/2500114-197454/what-other-antiviral-agents-are-being-investigated-for-the-treatment-of-coronavirus-disease-2019-covid-19.

Chung, E. (2020, August 1). When a COVID-19 vaccine arrives, which Canadian will get it first? *CBC News*. Retrieved September 10, 2020 from https://www.cbc.ca/news/technology/covid-vaccine-priority-canada-1.5669216.

Cohen, J. (2020, August 4). Designer antibodies could battle COVID-19 before vaccines arrive. *Science Magazine*. Retrieved September 14, 2020 https://www.sciencemag.org/news/2020/08/designer-antibodies-could-battle-covid-19-vaccines-arrive#.

Craven, J. (2020a, September 4). COVID-19 Therapeutics tracker. *Regulatory Affairs Professional Society (RAPS)*. Retrieved August 31, 2020 from https://www.raps.org/news-and-articles/news-articles/2020/3/covid-19-therapeutics-tracker.

Craven, J. (2020b, September 3) Vaccine tracker. *Regulatory Affairs Professional Society (RAPS)*. Retrieved August 31, 2020 from https://www.raps.org/news-and-articles/newsarticles/2020/3/covid-19-vaccine tracker#:~:text=To%20date%2C%20just%20one%20coronavirus,Russian%20Federation%20on%2011%20August.

Craven, J. (2020c, October 15). COVID-19 Vaccine tracker. *Regulatory Affairs Professional Society (RAPS)*. Retrieved October 22, 2020 from www.raps.org/news-and-articles/news-articles/2020/3/covid-19-vaccine-tracker.

D'Souza, G., & Dowdy, D. (2020, April 10). What is herd immunity and how can we achieve it with COVID-19? *Johns Hopkins Bloomberg School of Public Health*. Retrieved September 29, 2020 from https://www.jhsph.edu/covid-19/articiles/achieving-herd-immunity-with-covid19.html.

EuroHealthNet (2020) What COVID-19 is teaching us about inequality and the sustainability of our health systems. Retrieved September 21, 2020 from https://eurohealthnet.eu/COVID-19.

Flood, C., MacDonnell, V., & Venkatapuram, S. (2020, August 24). A response to COVID-19 requires global Action. *Policy Options Politiques*. Retrieved from https://policyoptions.irpp.org/magazines/august-2020/a-response-to-covid-19-requires-global-action/.

Food and Drug Administration. (2020a, April 24). FDA drug safety communication. Retrieved September 8, 2020 from https://www.fda.gov/media/137250/download.

Food and Drug Administration. (2020b, August 23). FDA issues emergency use authorization for convalescent plasma as potential promising COVID-19 treatment, another achievement in administration's fight against pandemic. Retrieved September 13, 2020 from https://www.fda.gov/news-events/press-announcements/fda-issues-emergency-use-authorization-convalescent-plasma-potential-promising-covid-19-treatment.

Finch, W.H., & Hernández Finch, M.E. (2020). Poverty and Covid-19: Rates of incidence and deaths in the United States during the first 10 weeks of the pandemic. *Frontiers in Sociology*, 5(17), 1–10.

Griffin, P. (2020, June 26). Worth a shot? The economics of the race for a vaccine. *Two Cents' Worth*. Retrieved September 8, 2020 from https://www.rnz.co.nz/programmes/two-cents-worth/story/2018752315/worth-a-shot-the-economics-of-the-race-for-a-vaccine.

Heidt, A. (2020, June 16). FDA pulls emergency use authorization for antimalarial drugs. *The Scientist*. Retrieved September 8, 2020 from https://www.the-scientist.com/news-opinion/fda-pulls-emergency-use-authorization-for-antimalarial-drugs-67638.

Henriques, M. (2020, April 1). Coronavirus: Why death and mortality rates differ. *BBC Future*. Retrieved September 1, 2020 from https://www.bbc.com/future/article/20200401-coronavirus-why-death-and-mortality-rates-differ.

Horton, J. (2020). Coronavirus: What are the numbers out of Latin America. *BBC World News*. Retrieved September 8, 2020 from https://www.bbc.com/news/world-latin-america-52711458.

Johns Hopkins University, Coronavirus Resource Centre (2000a). *COVID-19 Dashboard by the Centre for Systems Science and Engineering*. Retrieved October 22, 2020 from https://coronavirus.jhu.edu/map.html.

Johns Hopkins University, Coronavirus Resource Centre (2000b). Mortality analyses. Retrieved October 22, 2020 from https://coronavirus.jhu.edu/data/mortality.

Kim, D., Hai, T.T., & Rodriquez, D. (2020, June 14). Pushed to the margin: Vulnerable groups in the Asia pacific during COVID-19. *Asia Pacific Foundation of Canada*. Retrieved September 14, 2020 from https://www.asiapacific.ca/publication/pushed-margin-vulnerable-groups-asia-pacific-during-covid-19.

Kosteniuk, J.G., & Dickinson, H.D. (2003). Tracing the social gradient in the health of Canadians: Primary and secondary determinants. *Social Science & Medical, 57*(2), 263–276.

Kunzmann, K. (2020, May 25). WHO suspends hydroxychloroquine treatment in COVID-19 solidarity trial. Trials Suspended by WHO. Retrieved September 14, 2020 from https://www.contagionlive.com/news/who-hydroxychloroquine-treatment-covid-19-solidarity-trial.

Kupferschmidt, K. (2020, July 28). Vaccine nationalism threatens global plan to distribute COVID-19 shots fairly. *Science.* Retrieved September 14, 2020 from https://www.sciencemag.org/news/2020/07/vaccine-nationalism-threatens-global-plan-distribute-covid-19-shots-fairly.

Kupferschmidt, K., & Cohen, J. (2020, August 24). FDA's green light for treating COVID-19 with plasma, critics see thin evidence – and politics. *Science.* Retrieved September 9, 2020 from https://www.sciencemag.org/news/2020/08/fda-s-green-light-treating-covid-19-plasma-critics-see-thin-evidence-and-politics.

Lanese, N. (2020, October 6). Trump is 1 of 10 people to get antibody drug outside of clinical trial. *LiveScience.* Retrieved October 16, 2020 from https://www.livescience.com/antibody-cocktail-president-trump-coronavirus.html.

Ledford, H. (2020, August 11). Antibody therapies may be a bridge to a Coronavirus vaccine – but will the world benefit? *Nature.* Retrieved September 9, 2020 from https://www.nature.com/articles/d41586-020-02360-y.

Lingam, L., & Suresh Sapkal, R. (2020). COVID-19, physical distancing and social inequalities: Are we all really in this together? *International Journal of Community and Social Development, 2*(2), 173–190. Doi:10.1177%2F2516602620937932.

Lovelace, J.B., & Breuninger, K. (2020, May 18). Trump says he takes hydroxychloroquine to prevent coronavirus infection even though it's an unproven treatment. Retrieved September 9, 2020 from https://www.cnbc.com/2020/05/18/trump-says-he-takes-hydroxychloroquine-to-prevent-coronavirus-infection.html.

Londoño, E. (2020, July 9). Bolsonaro hails anti-malaria pill even as he fights Coronavirus. *New York Times.* Retrieved September 9, 2020 from https://www.nytimes.com/2020/07/08/world/americas/brazil-bolsonaro-covid-coronavirus.html.

Marano, G., Vaglio, S., Pupella, S., Facco, G., Catalano, L., Liumbruno, G.M., & Grazzini, G. (2016). Convalescent plasma: New evidence for an old therapeutic tool? *Blood Trans,* 14, 152–157. doi: 10.2450/2015.0131-15.

Marmot, M. (2017). The health gap: Doctors and the social determinants of health. *Scandinavian Journal of Public Health,* 45, 686–693.

Marmot, M., Rose, G., Shipley, M., & Hamilton, P.J.S. (1978). Employment grade and coronary heart disease in British civil servants. *Journal of Epidemiology and Community Health,* 32, 244–249.

McNamara, C.L., Balaj, M., Thomson, K.H., Eikemo, T.A., Solheim, E.F., & Bambra C. (2017). The socioeconomic distribution of non-communicable diseases in Europe: Findings from the European Social Survey (2014) special module on the social determinants of health. *Europ J Publ Health,* 27(1), 22–26. doi:10.1093/eurpub/ckw222.

Miller, J., & Burger, L. (2020, April 1). EMA urges caution on malaria drugs' use for COVID-19 in absence of evidence. Reuters. Retrieved September 8, 2020. https://www.reuters.com/article/us-health-coronavirus-ema/ema-urges-caution-on-malaria-drugs-use-for-covid-19-in-absence-of-evidence-idUSKBN21J5XN.

National Institutes of Health (NIH). (2020, August 4). NIH launches clinical trial to test antibody treatment in hospitalized COVID-19 patients. Retrieved September 10, 2020 from https://www.nih.gov/news-events/news-releases/nih-launches-clinical-trial-test-antibody-treatment-hospitalized-covid-19-patients.

Ndulu, B. (2020, August 6). The COVID-19 pandemic and its impact on sub-Saharan African economies. *Centre for International Governance Innovation.* Retrieved September 14, 2020 from https://www.cigionline.org/articles/covid-19-pandemic-and-its-impact-sub-saharan-african-economies.

Nebehay, S., & Lema, K. (2020, August 21). *'Vaccine nationalism' will make the coronavirus pandemic worse,* WHO says. Reuters. Retrieved September 4, 2020 https://globalnews.ca/news/7283673/who-vaccine-nationalism-coronavirus/.

Nguyen, V.K. (2005). Antiretroviral globalism, biopolitics and therapeutic citizenship. In Ong A., Collier S. J. (Eds.), *Global Assemblages: Technology, Politics and Ethics as Anthropological Problems* (pp. 124–144). Oxford, UK: Blackwell.

Nguyen, V.K., Ako, C. Y., Niamba, P., Sylla, A., & Tiendrébégo, I. (2007). Adherence as therapeutic citizenship: Impact of the history of access to antiretroviral drugs on adherence to treatment. *AIDS, 21*(5), S31–S35.

Nordling, L. (2020, August 11). The pandemic appears to have spared Africa so far: Scientists are struggling to explain why. *Science.* Retrieved September 17, 2020 https://www.sciencemag.org/news/2020/08/pandemic-appears-have-spared-africa-so-far-scientists-are-struggling-explain-why.

Oyesola, O., Happi, C., Adekola, A.A., Agwu, A.C., Heeney, J., & Adewale-Fasoro, O. (n.d.). Getting to grips with the COVID-19 outbreak in Nigeria. *The Conversation.* Retrieved September 8, 2020 from https://theconversation.com/getting-to-grips-with-the-covid-19-outbreak-in-nigeria-143943.

Perez, M. (2020, September 3). Prescriptions skyrocket for hydroxychloroquine: A dubious Coronavirus treatment endorsed by Trump. *Forbes.* Retrieved September 14, 2020 https://www.forbes.com/sites/mattperez/2020/09/03/prescriptions-skyrocket-for-hydroxychloroquine-a-dubious-coronavirus-treatment-endorsed-by-trump/#2f-75d2e43bb7

Petryna, A. (2003/2013). *Life Exposed: Biological Citizens after Chernobyl.* Princeton, NJ: Princeton University Press.

Pinkerton, C. (2020, July 28). Health Canada makes Gilead's remidisivir drug first approved COVID-19 treatment. *I-Politics.* Retrieved September 8, 2020 from https://ipolitics.ca/2020/07/28/health-canada-makes-gileads-remidisivir-drug-first-approved-covid-19-treatment/.

Public Health Ontario. (2020, May 12). Enhanced epidemiological summary COVID-19 in Ontario – A focus on diversity. Retrieved August 31, 2020 from https://www.publichealthontario.ca/-/media/documents/ncov/epi/2020/06/covid-19-epi-diversity.pdf?la=en.

Reuters, T. (2020a, June 5) Hydroxychloroquine 'useless' on COVID-19 patients, researcher says. *CBC News.* Retrieved September 10, 2020 from https://www.cbc.ca/news/health/hydroxychloroquine-covid-recovery-trial-1.5600821.

Reuters, T. (2020b, September 2). Steroids cut death rates among critically ill COVID-19 patients, studies suggest. *CBC News.* Retrieved September 9, 2020 from https://www.cbc.ca/news/health/steroids-covid-19-1.5709073.

Rocha, R., Shingler, B., & Montpetit, J. (2020, June 11). Montreal's poorest and most racially diverse neighbourhoods hit hardest by COVID-19, data analysis shows. *CBC News.* Retrieved August 31, 2020 from https://www.cbc.ca/news/canada/montreal/race-covid-19-montreal-data-census-1.5607123.

Romer, D., & Jamieson, K.H. (2020). Conspiracy theories as barriers to controlling the spread of COVID-19 in the U.S. *Social Science & Medicine.* doi:10.1016/j.socscimed.2020.113356.

Rowland, C. (2020, September 8). Vaccine CEOs issue safety pledge amid Trump's quest for pre election approval. *Washington Post.* https://www.washingtonpost.com/business/2020/09/08/vaccine-safety-pledge-ceos/.

Rose, N., & Novas, C. (2005). Biological citizenship. In Ong, A. & Collier, S.J., (eds). *Global Assemblages: Technology, Politics, and Ethics as Anthropological Problems* (pp. 439–463). Oxford, UK: Blackwell.

Sa, F. (2020). Socioeconomic determinants of COVID-19 infections and mortality: Evidence from England and Wales. IZA Policy Papers 159, Institute of Labor Economics (IZA). Retrieved August 31, 2020 from https://ideas.repec.org/p/iza/izapps/pp159.html

Schmidt, M. (2020, June 5). What is hydroxychloroquine and does it treat COVID-19?. *Discover Magazine.* Retrieved September 8, 2020 from https://www.discovermagazine.com/health/what-is-hydroxychloroquine-and-does-it-treat-covid-19.

Schwab, K. (2020). Post COVID capitalism. *Gavi The Vaccine Alliance.* Retrieved October 22, 2020 from https://www.gavi.org/vaccineswork/post-covid-capitalism.

Şimşek Yavuz, S., & Ünal, S. (2020). Antiviral treatment of COVID-19. *Turkish J Medical Science, 50*(3), 611–619. doi:10.3906/sag-2004-145.

Steckelberg, A., Johnson, C.Y., Florit, G., & Alcantara, C. (2020, September 8). These are the top Coronavirus vaccines to watch. *Washington Post.* Retrieved September 9, 2020 from https://www.washingtonpost.com/graphics/2020/health/covid-vaccine-update-coronavirus/?itid=ap_carolyny.%20johnson&itid=lk_interstitial_manual_6.

Taylor, A. (2020, September 3). Why vaccine nationalism is winning. *Washington Post.* Retrieved September 10, 2020 from https://www.washingtonpost.com/world/2020/09/03/why-coronavirus-vaccine-nationalism-is-winning/.

Thomas, K., & Kolata, G. (2020, October 3). President Trump received Regeneron experimental antibody treatment. *New York Times.* Retrieved October 15, 2020 from https://www.nytimes.com/2020/10/02/health/trump-antibody-treatment.html.

Tudor Hart, J. (1971). The inverse care law. *Lancet, 297,* 405–412. doi:10.1016/SO140 6736(71)92410-X.

UK Office for National Statistics (n.d.). Coronavirus (COVID-19) related deaths by ethnic group, England and Wales: 2 March 2020 to 10 April 2020. Retrieved August 31, 2020 from https://www.ons.gov.uk/peoplepopulationandcommunity/birthsdeathsandmarriages/deaths/articles/coronavirusrelateddeathsbyethnicgroupenglandandwales/2march2020to10april2020.

United Nations. (2020, July). Policy brief: The impact of COVID-19 on latin America and the Caribbean. Retrieved September 16, 2020 from https://www.un.org/sites/un2.un.org/files/sg_policy_brief_covid_lac.pdf.

US Centres for Disease Control and Prevention. (n.d.). People at increased risk and other people who need to take extra precautions. Retrieved August 31, 2020 from https://www.cdc.gov/coronavirus/2019-ncov/need-extra-precautions/index.html.

US Centres for Disease Control and Prevention (n.d.-b, updated Aug 18, 2020). COVID-19 hospitalization and death by race/ethnicity. Retrieved August 31, 2020 from https://www.cdc.gov/coronavirus/2019-ncov/covid-data/investigations-discovery/hospitalization-death-by-race-ethnicity.html.

US Health and Human Services. (2020, June 16). Fact sheet: Explaining operation warp speed. *HHS Press Office.* Retrieved September 22, 2020 from https://www.hhs.gov/about/news/2020/06/16/fact-sheet-explaining-operation-warp-speed.html.

Vaidyanathan, G. (2020, September 3). India will supply coronavirus vaccines to the world – will its people benefit? *Nature.* Retrieved September 10, 2020 from https://www.nature.com/articles/d41586-020-02507-x.

Walker, J., Halbesma, N., Lone, N., McAllister, D., Weir, C.J., Wild, S.H., on behalf of the Scottish Diabetes Research Network Epidemiology Group. (2016). Socioeconomic status, comorbidity and mortality in patients with type 2 diabetes mellitus in Scotland 2004–2011: A cohort study. *Joournal of Epidemiology and Community Health, 70,* 596–601.

Watt, G. (2002). The inverse care law today. *Lancet, 360,* 252–254.

Weintraub, R., Bitton, A., & Rosenberg, M.L. (2020, May 22). The danger of vaccine nationalism. *Harvard Business Review* Retrieved September 15, 2020 from https://hbr.org/2020/05/the-danger-of-vaccine-nationalism.

Wherry, A. (2020, June 13). One country, two pandemics: what COVID-19 reveals about inequality in Canada. *CBC News.* Retrieved September 8, 2020 from https://www.cbc.ca/news/politics/pandemic-covid-coronavirus-cerb-unemployment-1.5610404.

World Health Organization (WHO). (n.d.-a). Timeline: WHO's COVID-19 response. Retrieved August 31, 2020 from https://www.who.int/emergencies/diseases/novel-coronavirus-2019/interactive-timeline?gclid=Cj0KCQjwv7L6BRDxARIsAGj 34ogsS4V08k-TOAWNIl8X_WqzFXD7ipXC0jEXT3hwyEGsJ6bjloBoLY4aArmSEALw_wcB#!.

World Health Organization (WHO). (n.d.-b). Naming the Coronavirus disease (COVID-19) and the virus that causes it. Retrieved September 8, 2020 from https://www.who.int/emergencies/diseases/novel-coronavirus-2019/technical-guidance/naming-the-coronavirus-disease-(covid-2019)-and-the-virus-that-causes-it.

World Health Organization (WHO). (2020c). 172 countries and multiple candidate vaccines engaged in COVID-19 vaccine Global Access Facility. Retrieved September 22, 2020 from https://www.who.int/news-room/detail/24-08-2020-172-countries-and-multiple-candidate-vaccines-engaged-in-covid-19-vaccine-global-access-facility.

World Health Organization (WHO). (2020d, July 4). WHO discontinues hydroxychloroquine and lopinavir/ritonavir treatment arms for COVID-19. Retrieved September 14, 2020 from https://www.who.int/news-room/detail/04-07-2020-who-discontinues-hydroxychloroquine-and-lopinavir-ritonavir-treatment-arms-for-covid-19.

World Health Organization (WHO). (n.d.-e). The push for a COVID-19 vaccine. Retrieved from https://www.who.int/emergencies/diseases/novel-coronavirus-2019/covid-19-vaccines?gclid=Cj0KCQjwwOz6BRCgARIsAKEG4FVBWngefxlcnc5-w32mpr360x-JoslQl8TWlv4etLigzFAb6rdMOG_QaArgTEALw_wcB Accessed Sept. 11, 2020.

World Health Organization (WHO). (2020f, April 21) Addressing human rights as key to the COVID-19 response. Retrieved September 21, 2020 from https://www.who.int/publications/i/item/addressing-human-rights-as-key-to-the-covid-19-response.

World Health Organization Rapid Evidence Appraisal for COVID-19 Therapies (REACT) Working Group. (2020). Association between administration of systemic corticosteroids and mortality among critically ill patients with COVID-19. A meta analysis. *JAMA.* doi:10.1001/jama.2020.17023.

Wu, Z., & McGoogan, J.M. (2020). Characteristics of and important lessons from the coronavirus disease 2019 (COVID-19) outbreak in China: Summary of a report of 72,314 cases from the Chinese Centre for Disease Control and Prevention. *JAMA, 323*(13), 1239–1242. doi:10.1001/jama.2020.2648.

Xue, J., & Kaplan, R.M. (2020, September 21). Op-Ed: A Covid-19 vaccine is one thing. Getting Americans to take it is another. *L.A. Times* Retrieved September 21, 2020 from https://ca.movies.yahoo.com/op-ed-covid-19-vaccine-100053843.html.

Yashhadhana, A., Pollard-Wharton, N., Zwi, A.B., & Biles, B. (2020). Indigenous Australians at increased risk of COVID-19 due to existing health and socioeconomic inequities. *The Lancet Regional Health – Western Pacific.* doi: 10/1016/j.lanwpc.2020.

Yu, G. (2020, April 11). Trump suggests hydroxychloroquine may protect against COVID-19. Researchers say there's no evidence of that. *CNN.com.* Retrieved from https://www.cnn.com/2020/04/05/health/trump-lupus-hydroxychloroquine-coronavirus-protection/index.html.

14 Conclusion

What of pharmaceutical lives?

Peri J. Ballantyne and Kath Ryan

Introduction

We introduced the collection by reference to the reality that pharmaceuticals have become increasingly promoted as solutions to human health problems, health risks and the challenges of everyday life. Yet, as demonstrated in the contents of this collection, using pharmaceuticals rarely reflects a straightforward choice and rational decision – but rather is a negotiated process undertaken by users in the context of their lives. In this final chapter, we identify and discuss three central but overlapping themes embedded in the preceding chapters: (a) users' observation and navigation of medicines' varied impacts – positive, mixed or uncertain and negative; (b) the negotiation of medicines by users as 'work'; and (c) the social and political contexts of medicine access and use. Together, these themes capture the complexity of 'living pharmaceutical lives'. As illustrated in the chapters here, complexity refers to the benefits as well as the challenges of using medicines on an everyday basis, as these relate to the expectations associated with their use, the uncertainty about a condition or about the duration of a medicine regimen for it; the need to negotiate the stigma associated with a condition or the medicine used to treat it; the challenges of accessing and paying for medicines and scheduling them into daily routines; and the need to manage medicines' effects and side effects in the context of the demands of everyday life.

Medicines' varied effects

Several contributions in this collection highlight the expected or experienced positive outcomes of using different types of medicines. For example, McIntosh asserts that 'HPV vaccinations offer virtually complete protection against select serotypes and thus are an effective primary preventive strategy' and Thompson refers to 'the success of public health in the near eradication of many formally endemic diseases'. Balogun-Katung et al. observe that:

> the general consensus amongst participants was that consistent use of ART offered an abundance of health benefits. All MSM reported that they experienced an overall improvement in their health and wellbeing, and improved CD4 counts and viral loads within a few months of starting their treatment.
> (Balogun-Katung et al., this volume, p. 144)

Participants in Rathbone's study referred to cancer medications as 'life giving'; and participants in the Eassey et al. study conveyed that their very lives depend on the ongoing and appropriate adherence to medications prescribed for severe asthma. However, for all medicine types described by these authors, their positive bodily effects were complicated and, often, undermined by other impacts associated with their use – these complicating features are central in the chapters herein.

Some medicines examined in this collection are used in conditions of uncertainty, and as producing mixed or uncertain effects. Most clearly, for example, Rosenlund Lau et al. describe taking statins as a 'practice of anticipation' that is 'a way to manage uncertain health futures and actively reorient possible future lives towards imagined safe and healthy trajectories'. Describing statins as one of the most sold classes of pharmaceuticals in western countries, used as a preventive medicine for heart-healthy individuals and as a secondary prophylaxis among people with cardiovascular disease, these authors point out that in the medical community 'widespread use of statins is both a matter of course and a matter of concern'. For most of their participants, a diagnosis of elevated cholesterol was unexpected and not linked to experiential signs of illness. Yet, the diagnosis – and the recommendation of its treatment with statins – was consequential: many participants were appreciative and generally positively evaluated the opportunity for cholesterol screening, while others were left with a sense of dread about their risks of future serious illness, or interpreted having high cholesterol as a serious disease itself. Some experienced physical side effects of statin use, others experienced psychological side effects associated with the heightened sense of risk and vulnerability when statins were declined, or their use terminated.

Uncertainty is also a theme in the Lloyd et al. chapter examining medicine use in the face of postural tachycardia syndrome, a medically unexplained and misunderstood condition with no standard pharmacological treatment protocol and no medicines licensed specifically for its treatment; and in the Ghouri et al. chapter where women expressed conflict in not wanting to take medicines while pregnant but also not wanting to jeopardise their pregnancy with an untreated urinary tract infection. In 'Drugs at Work: Implicated in the Making of the Neoliberal Worker', Ballantyne emphasises the uncertainty of effects of several types of drugs commonly used by workers at work. Particularly concerning are those used over long periods of time in the absence of clinical evidence to guide their safe long-term use (i.e., amphetamines used by long-haul truck drivers), or used for short periods, but having long term embodied consequences (i.e., mefloquine, for military enlistees deployed to tropical settings). In this chapter, the poor pharmaceutical management of medical conditions (i.e., diabetes, chronic pain) in the restrictive environments and schedules of the workplace (i.e., prolonged work shifts) are also associated with the theme of uncertainty. For example, consider the reality that some workplaces and work schedules impede optimal management of diabetes, including the optimal use of pharmaceutical therapies; or that work causes pain, which motivates pharmaceutical treatment, which produces iatrogenic outcomes associated with the long-term use of analgesics. Finally, Ballantyne et al. also emphasise uncertainty about but anticipation of the benefits of eventual therapies and vaccines for a new viral infection – SARS CoV-2 – affecting populations around the globe. As these authors elaborate, in the context of COVID-19, uncertainty is related not only to the effectiveness of treatments and preventives over the short- and long term, but also to the allocation of these in a context of limited supplies and high demand, and even higher need.

Consideration of the explicit negative effects of some types of pharmaceuticals must be central to any discussion of 'living pharmaceutical lives'. For example, irrespective of the effectiveness of opioid analgesics for pain management, their negative effects are the particular focus in Cooper's discussion of stigma, shame and identity-disrupting effects of using them. Similarly, Balogun-Katung and colleagues emphasised the negative physical effects of antiviral therapies that are prominent during the initial weeks and months of commencing treatment: skin rashes, scars, drunken feeling, dizziness, unusual or bad dreams, hot flushes and fever, fat redistribution; and the negative 'side effect' of being observed to use antiretroviral therapies in a context where doing so is highly stigmatised, criminalised or otherwise punished. Lloyd and colleagues described the negative effects of health professionals' interpretation of symptoms (of postural tachy-cardia syndrome) as indicative of stress or poor mental health rather than 'real' illness.

Thus, whether in a context of perceived or experienced benefits of using med-icines for the prevention of future potential illness, or for the treatment of med-ical conditions like HIV/AIDS, cancer, severe asthma, urinary tract infection or for the harms of work – fatigue, pain and sleep disruption – medicine-taking is also characterised by uncertainty and sometimes associated with explicitly neg-ative outcomes. This means that a decision to use or not to use medicines, the 'negotiation' of medicines, involves 'work' on the part of users, as we discuss below.

Pharmaceutical healthwork

In her chapter, examining the management of diabetes for people living in mar-ginal social and economic circumstances, Epstein draws on the concept of med-icine-taking as *healthwork*. Borrowing the term from Myhalovskiy and colleagues – the 'everyday/everynight activities through which people look after health' (Mykhalovskiy et al., 2004, p. 323), Epstein argues that as healthwork, medi-cation use is much more complex than cognitive remembering or simple acts of swallowing or injecting medical products. Instead, it involves an often-pro-longed effort to create and sustain effective and meaningful medication practices and routines. Epstein emphasises that this *healthwork* occurs in temporal and spatial context, asserting that:

> As a mass-produced technology, pharmaceuticals are designed (ideally) to deliver uniform and mechanically predictable effects with every dose taken. In turn, the bodies they work on become (again ideally) equally uniform and predictable, inseparable from routinised medication schedules and greater

regimentation of the user's daily life. In contrast, I show how successful diabetes control comes from creating social space that is local, unique and rooted in embodied experience. Focusing on the spatial and temporal forms provides a unique insight into the ways alienation between body and self is both produced and resisted through pharmaceutical use. It moves the focus away from individual psychology or labels of 'non-adherence' and studies how people creatively construct (or struggle to construct) medication self-care practices within the macro forces of modern capitalism.

(Epstein, this volume, p. 28)

Employing life history methodology, and defining 'control' as 'the ability to examine one's past behaviours and to put learned experience into practice', Epstein organises her participants' explanations of *healthwork* involving pharmaceuticals into three categories that reflect time needed and the stops and starts of learning to negotiate a life with diabetes and its treatment. She remarks:

In the Just Beginning group… narratives revealed how clinicians presented routinisation and quantification as useful tools for orderliness often at odds with the marginal social control many people actually experienced. Instead of being a useful tool, routinisation and quantification were resisted as another added burden. In the Cycling group, people cycled between Just Beginning and Care of the Self. Rational decision-making and medical facts could be incorporated into self-care practices but this did not motivate sustained transformation. Control was therefore not defined in terms of medication compliance, technical skills or creating routines, but rather in terms of the meanings underlying practices of self-care.

(Epstein, this volume, p. 32)

Epstein emphasises control (of diabetes and its treatment) through meaning-creation, a central aspect of healthwork that only developed over time.

We suggest that the *healthwork* undertaken to establish meaning and control of diabetes described in Epstein's research, and her emphasis on the time and space needed to approach and negotiate one's bodily and treatment experiences, are also evident in several other of the empirical studies outlined in the collection. For example, in their research examining experiences of postural tachycardia syndrome, Lloyd et al. illustrate how participants' health and medication narratives relayed their negotiations of the meaning of symptoms, and of pharmaceutical treatments that functioned in three ways: to produce embodied effects that were then evaluated as being positive, negative and uncertain; to signify their illness status – to legitimise or fail to legitimise their illness and the story-teller's entrance into the sick role; and to experiment with treatments in a context of clinical uncertainty about their condition. Participants emphasised the important and often extended role of medicines in the experimental work undertaken to make sense of their medically unexplained illness. These authors conclude that:

Studying the construction of stories about medicines allows space to step outside the traditional adherence/non-adherence binary that guides much research on experiences of medicine taking and to focus instead on how people who tell stories have a stake in acting on and with medicines. Such a theoretical lens holds space for conceiving of the managing of illness as *unfolding in a field of practice*, where stories about medicines may be a means to understanding how people with illness make sense of medicines in their lives and why they act with and on them in the ways that they do.

(Lloyd et al., this volume, p. 183)

Their comment reflects the spatiotemporal perspective on meaning-making that is central in Epstein's writing.

Similarly, in their work examining the experience of severe asthma, Eassey et al. also show the work of managing medicines, even in the context of 'adherent' practices, where 'control' is not necessarily achieved, and seeking it is an ongoing practice requiring work by the person with asthma and others (including health professionals) whose support may or may not be forthcoming. Ghouri et al. also illustrate the work of negotiating competing health priorities for pregnant women with urinary tract infections – of protecting the health of their unborn babies, and of minimising the use of antibiotics understood to be a societal and public health concern. In this study, women's decisions reflect what they viewed as the best interest of their babies; the risks of antimicrobial resistance are eclipsed by mothers' prenatal attachment and the perceived risks of a urinary tract infection in pregnancy.

Also illustrating *healthwork* in the context of their responsibility for babies and children, Thompson examines the moral work of middle-class mothers who negotiate childhood vaccinations for their children. Thompson locates this work in the context of mothers' duty for the health of themselves and their family members – part of the neoliberal mandate for individuals' personal responsibility for health:

> The current phenomenon of parents choosing to not vaccinate their children, on non-religious grounds, is in part attributable to the fact that the diseases against which childhood vaccines are given are now rare, thanks to the success of immunisation programs. Or so the thinking goes. This leads parents to believe that the risks of vaccination are now greater than the risks associated with getting the disease… I posit that the decline in parental uptake of childhood vaccines – within the segment of society that is well educated and middle-class – is indeed because of the success of public health. It is, however, not only because of the success of public health in the near eradication of many formally endemic diseases that risk perception among this group of parents has shifted. Neoliberal public health regimes have rendered this group of parents, and mothers in particular, hypervigilant risk managers who place self-and-infant-care above care for the other.

(Thompson, this volume, p. 88)

Thompson effectively argues that public health in the context of neoliberalism has created the very maternal subjectivities that made the emergence of this form of resistance inevitable.

In another example, asking *what* it means to live with preventive pharmaceuticals rather than *whether or not* one should live with them, Rosenlund Lau and her colleagues show the work of negotiating statins – whose use is recommended as a way of anticipating futures without cardiovascular disease. These authors assert that:

> ... testing for high cholesterol and taking statins becomes a way of optimising life through the effort to secure one's future and preparing the body by changing biomechanisms that might or might not cause future disease. Yet, the work associated with optimisation and preparedness is not always simple. Pharmaceutical prevention may affect the way we see ourselves and the way we live our lives. In some instances, statin use becomes a moral failure because it is indicative of a dysfunctional body and unmanageable health. In other cases, optimisation and preparedness result in actions imposed on or by others. We have thus shown that the preventive work is never just about taking a pill. It also includes daily moral contestation over food and medicine and about living life the 'right' way.
>
> (Rosenlund Lau et al., this volume, pp. 112–113)

Rathbone – examining decisions about medicine use for cancer and the trajectory from diagnosis to early and later experience as a cancer survivor – also showed that acceptance of cancer treatment wasn't a simple yes or no, but a process that was undertaken over time, dependent on experiences with the disease, ongoing objective tests of its status, etc. His research shows that the *healthwork* undertaken by older persons with cancer is further complicated because, in the setting of Rathbone's study, participants frequently reported co-morbid conditions, many of which were also treated with pharmaceuticals.

We suggest that the above examples depict *healthwork* – and *pharmaceutical healthwork* – and reflect the medicine user's central role in negotiating medicines use in a context of complex lives, illness conditions or risks and medicine outcomes.

Medicine access and medicine use in social and political contexts

Several chapters explicitly problematise the broad social and political contexts that shape individuals' access to, and negotiation of medicines. Most explicitly and alarmingly, Balogun-Katung et al. show how a social-political context that supports and institutionalises homophobia and criminalises same-sex relationships resulted in impeded access to, sub-optimal use or avoidance of antiretroviral therapy by HIV positive men, even while those men accepted it's benefits for their health and life expectancy. Several other chapters focus on how key principles of neoliberalism, including *healthism*, have reinforced the emergence and expansion of pharmaceuticals in peoples' lives and complicated their orientations to them. As Ballantyne describes, neoliberal capitalism organises the social world and individuals' roles within it in particular ways. Emphasising capitalist economic growth and consumerism, neoliberalism supports the individual as rational agent – whose value is demonstrated through participation in the labour market and consumption of its goods – both of which, she argues, support the expansion of the pharmaceutical economy. Neoliberalism demands individual responsibility for health and supports the proliferation of pharmaceuticals as consumer goods for the treatment of illness, the management of risk, and enhancement of 'health'.

Rosenlund Lau and colleagues examine the structural shaping of heart disease as a risk category and the moral obligation of citizens to act to minimise the risk of future cardiovascular disease. Borrowing from Jenkins' (2010) research focused on psychological medicines, Rosenlund Lau et al. distinguish between the *pharmaceutical imaginary* and the *pharmaceutical self*:

> Jenkins depicts the pharmaceutical self as the aspect of the self that is oriented by and towards pharmaceuticals… and the pharmaceutical imaginary as the global shaping of consumption. With the dual concept of self/imaginary, Jenkins' point is that subjective experiences of pharmaceuticals are tightly linked to the social and cultural conundrums of pharmaceuticals' local and global lives.
>
> (Rosenlund Lau et al., this volume, pp. 104–105.)

While Rosenlund Lau et al., examine the promotion of statins for cardiovascular health, another social and cultural 'conundrum' is elaborated in Thompson's examination of (middle-class mothers') vaccine hesitancy and resistance. Thompson argues that individual health behaviour can be understood in relation to the neoliberal emphasis on individual responsibility for health, and that the logical conclusion to the imperative of individual responsibility for health is resistance to collective action in favour of a singular focus on individual behaviours. This is, she asserts, an orientation that is in keeping with the moral discourse of public health, which prioritises lifestyle factors over social and political determinants of health. As addressed by Thompson, and briefly by Ballantyne, Ryan and Bissell in their discussion of the COVID pandemic, successful collective immunisation programs rely at least in part on citizens having a duty to each other to contribute to herd immunity. However, as asserted by Thompson 'it is precisely this kind of public good that neoliberalism has systematically obscured and undermined with its singular focus on individual responsibility for health, its focus on the management of risks in individual patients instead of the population' (Thompson, this volume, p. 99).

The social and political organisation of medicines access and use is evident too in McIntosh's chapter examining the serious but unintended consequences of the HPV vaccination programme rolled out in Ontario, Canada in 2007; and in Epstein's chapter examining the management of Type 2 diabetes mellitus in a socio-political context that normalises health insurance as a commodity not a right of citizenship.

In McIntosh's study, while the example of a federal government decision to fund a (sexually transmitted infection prevention) vaccination program for presexually active girls might be laudable, the failure to follow other national and international covenants, most notably, the right to informed consent, means that when put into practice, the program did not follow expected practice ethics. McIntosh also examines how the HPV vaccination program was coupled with other changes in health services available to girls and young women (i.e., changes in pap testing, STI testing, etc.), with additional negative, but preventable health consequences.

Epstein examined how, for people with diabetes, a social context of low-paying work, working multiple jobs, or unemployment, of family health issues, the lack of health insurance, and overwhelming stress contributed to both an over-dependence on medications for diabetes, and underuse of them – and to participants' difficulties in reaching an understanding of their condition and establishing routines for its effective everyday management.

Two other chapters emphasise the vulnerable lay medicine user – and reinforce the importance of social or political responses. For example, Cooper's focus is on persons afflicted with chronic pain, whose vulnerability is heightened when they are required to navigate the stigma attached to seeking and using opioid analgesic medicines. Cooper emphasises the legitimacy of a person's seeking relief from chronic pain (and Cooper and Ballantyne describe evidence suggesting the ubiquity of pain-filled lives), the legitimating role of opioid analgesics, that is, in validating pain and the right to pain medicines; and identifies the potential settings of stigma, shame and identity disruption: pharmacy counters, prescribers' offices and clinics, or online support groups. Cooper's insights reinforce that, for individuals, accessing opioid analgesics is fraught with peril and possibilities, and that social- and political-level action in response to chronic pain-related suffering is required.

Addressing another vulnerable sub-group of medicine users, Ghouri and colleagues sought to understand women's views of antibiotic use during pregnancy, and their views of antimicrobial resistance. The latter issue was understood by participants to be a serious societal issue, but the authors reported that most were unclear about how resistant bacteria transfer among people and spread across society to cause a rise in treatment resistant infections – leaving participants to depict antibiotic resistance as a hypothetical rather than a real and imminent problem. Ultimately, in their study, participants held prescribers responsible for the overuse of antibiotics. Given the context of the current COVID-19 pandemic and heightened sensitivity to global risk of treatment resistant infections, their findings that antibiotic users view antimicrobial resistance as a matter not for individual users but for health professionals and perhaps for health care systems is notable. Indeed, similar to Thompson's findings illustrating mothers' concern to minimise their children's health risks, Ghouri and colleagues report that women gave priority to the short-term health and safety of their unborn babies over broader societal concerns that (hypothetically) could affect their own or others' health in the future.

In sum, the chapters in this collection illustrate the varying political and social contexts that influence access to and the distribution of medicines; and that produce varying outcomes, including those that may not be optimal for individual medicine users and/or for the public.

Conclusion

The three overlapping themes above – medicines' varied effects, medicines negotiation as [health]work, and the social and political contexts of pharmaceuticals
and pharmaceutical lives – overlap with each other, and depict pharmaceutical
use as a sociological phenomenon, that is at once a 'private trouble' negotiated
by individuals (or their mothers), and a public issue – having relevance for any/
everyone who may be impacted by the potential benefits and harms of medicines
sought out (or not), accessed (or not), and used (or not). We draw here on the
distinction made by sociologist C. Wright Mills (Mills, 1959) who suggested
that many problems ordinarily considered private troubles are best understood
as public issues – emerging from and reflecting the structural context of peoples'
lives. The works in this collection illustrate that the negotiation of access to and
use of medicines is of public relevance – a topic to be addressed in the public
realm. A return to our introductory chapter will remind readers of the growing
and central place of pharmaceuticals in health care, and for health care budgets,
and the included chapters show a broad range of contexts where *pharmaceutical
healthwork* is undertaken – by users, but also by those who control users' access to
medicines. We suggest that the details gathered for this collection illustrate the
complexity of pharmaceuticals and users' ambivalence about 'living pharmaceutical lives' – emerging from contradictory ideas, expectations and experiences of
pharmaceuticals in the diverse and specific contexts of their use.

References

Jenkins, J. H. (2010). *Pharmaceutical Self – The global shaping of experience in an age of psychopharmacology*. Sante Fe: School for Advanced Research Press.
Mills, C. W. (1959). *The Sociological Imagination*, Oxford, UK, Oxford University Press.
Mykhalovskiy, E., McCoy, L., Breslier, M. (2004). Compliance/Adherence, HIV, and the
critique of medical power *Social Theory and Health 2*, 315–340.

Index

Page numbers in italics indicate *figures*, page numbers in bold indicate **tables** and page numbers followed by 'n' indicate notes.

Printed in the United States
by Baker & Taylor Publisher Services